Ethics in Health Services and Policy

A Global Approach

DEAN M. HARRIS

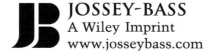

JOSSEY-BASS
A Wiley Imprint
www.josseybass.com

Published by Jossey-Bass
A Wiley Imprint
989 Market Street, San Francisco, CA 94103-1741—www.josseybass.com

Jossey-Bass books and products are available through most bookstores. To contact Jossey-Bass directly call our Customer Care Department within the U.S. at 800-956-7739, outside the U.S. at 317-572-3986, or fax 317-572-4002.

Jossey-Bass also publishes its books in a variety of electronic formats. Some content that appears in print may not be available in electronic books.

Library of Congress Cataloging-in-Publication Data
Harris, Dean M., 1951-
   Ethics in health services and policy : a global approach / Dean M. Harris.
      p. cm.—(J-B public health/health services text ; 43)
   Includes bibliographical references and index.
   ISBN 978-0-470-53106-8 (pbk.); 978-0-470-94064-8 (ebk.); 978-0-470-94066-2 (ebk.); 978-0-470-94067-9 (ebk.)
   1. Medical ethics. 2. Medical care. I. Title.
   R724.H238 2011
   174.2—dc22
                                                                        2010047563

Printed in the United States of America
FIRST EDITION
PB Printing   10 9 8 7 6 5 4 3 2 1

CONTENTS

To Deborah McLaughlin Harris

INTRODUCTION

This book analyzes the ethical issues of health policy and health services in global perspective. The global perspective is both comparative and transnational. Applying a comparative, or multicultural, approach, the book compares and contrasts different perspectives on ethical issues in various countries and cultures, such as different views about informed consent, withholding or withdrawing treatment, physician-assisted suicide, reproductive health issues, research with human subjects, the right to health care, rationing of limited resources, and health system reform. Applying a transnational, or cross-border, approach, the book analyzes ethical issues that arise from the movement of patients and health professionals across national borders, considering such matters as medical tourism and transplant tourism, ethical obligations to provide care for undocumented aliens, and the *brain drain* of health professionals from developing countries.

As explained in this book, people in different cultures have their own perspectives on the ethical issues of health services and policy. However, some ethical values are universal in the sense that they apply to all human societies and transcend the values of a particular culture. The theme of universal values will be revisited throughout this book, especially in the chapters on issues such as autonomy and informed consent, reproductive concerns, female genital mutilation, rationing, health reform, and corruption in health systems.

Another major theme of this book is evaluating ways to encourage people and organizations in the health system to *do the right thing* and determining the best ways to accomplish that goal in different circumstances. In addition to analyzing ethical theories, this book takes a practical approach to resolving ethical dilemmas in health services and policy. Each chapter of the book concludes with an activity that provides an opportunity to evaluate potential solutions to practical problems in global health. This book is useful for students of public health, medicine, nursing and allied health professions, public policy, and ethics. It will help students in all these areas to develop important competencies in their chosen fields.

Chapter One provides the analytical background on ethical theories and bioethics in a global perspective. This chapter should be read first. However, the remaining chapters can be read in any order. Chapter Two evaluates the ethical obligation to obtain a patient's informed consent and analyzes the theoretical and practical problems of obtaining informed consent in developed and developing countries. Chapter Three applies the principles of informed consent and autonomy in the context of physician-assisted suicide and withholding or withdrawing life-sustaining treatment. Chapter Four analyzes ethical issues in reproductive health, including abortion and emergency contraception, and Chapter Five analyzes the ethical issues surrounding female genital mutilation. Chapter Six explains the ethical issues in conducting research with human subjects and evaluates the particular ethical problems that arise in conducting research with human subjects in developing countries.

Chapter Seven examines the ethical right to health care and evaluates the ethical obligations of both health care professionals and the private companies that provide health care goods and services. Chapter Eight analyzes the ethical issues in the rationing and allocation of limited health care resources. Chapter Nine describes the fundamental values on which the health systems of various countries are based and analyzes the ethical issues in designing a fair system of health insurance and reforming a health system.

Chapter Ten evaluates the ethical problems in the movement of patients across national borders, as in medical tourism and transplant tourism, as well as the ethical obligations to provide care for undocumented aliens and people who have limited proficiency in the language of the health care provider. In contrast, Chapter Eleven evaluates the ethical problems arising from the movement of health care professionals across national borders, including the brain drain of health professionals from resource-poor to resource-rich countries and the fair treatment of health care workers from other countries. Finally, Chapter Twelve explains the problem of corruption and informal payments in health systems and analyzes the relationship between corruption and the health of a population.

ACKNOWLEDGMENTS

I appreciate the support and encouragement that I have received from Dr. Peggy Leatt, chair of the Department of Health Policy and Management, UNC Gillings School of Global Public Health, and from my colleague, Dr. Bruce J. Fried.

My research assistant on this project, Corrie Piontak, did an excellent job. In addition, it was a real pleasure to work with the staff at Jossey-Bass.

My mother, Felice Harris, provided useful ideas and perspectives for this book. Finally, I appreciate the constant help and support of Deborah, David, and Devon Harris.

THE AUTHOR

Dean M. Harris is clinical associate professor in the Department of Health Policy and Management, UNC Gillings School of Global Public Health, University of North Carolina at Chapel Hill, where he teaches courses on comparative health systems, health law, and global perspectives on ethical issues.

In addition, he has been appointed adjunct professor in the Health Economics and Management Institute at Peking University. He frequently provides lectures and seminars at universities in Asia and Eastern Europe. He has also helped to conduct training programs for a unit of China's Ministry of Health and a medical university in Beijing.

He received his B.A. degree in Asian Studies from Cornell University in 1973 and his J.D. degree with high honors from the UNC School of Law in 1981.

CHAPTER ONE

ETHICAL THEORIES AND BIOETHICS IN A GLOBAL PERSPECTIVE

LEARNING OBJECTIVES

- Acquire proficiency in analyzing the major theories of ethics, such as utilitarianism, and be able to apply those theories to health (bioethics).

- Understand and be able to explain the recent trend in bioethics of moving beyond clinical issues of the doctor-patient relationship to broader issues of social justice and population health.

- Learn how to evaluate whether traditional theories of ethics are truly global and whether there are any universal values that transcend culture.

- Learn how to evaluate whether theories of ethics are useful in helping individuals and organizations in the health system to do the right thing. Begin to debate the best ways of encouraging desirable conduct.

THICS has been defined in many different ways. According to Tom Beauchamp and James Childress (1994), ethics refers to "various ways of understanding and examining the moral life" (p. 4). Ethics is sometimes referred to as "moral philosophy," and can also be defined as a system for distinguishing right conduct from wrong (Blocker, 1986, p. 7). "Ethics, in other words, is a theoretical discipline within the broader study of philosophy which attempts to discover *why* any action is right or wrong; that is, what *makes* an action right or wrong" (Blocker, p. 8). As a practical matter, what difference does it make if we know *why* a particular action is right or wrong? The answer is that we want to be able to extrapolate or generalize from the particular situation, in order to develop ways to determine what is right or wrong in other situations.

Bioethics is the application of ethical principles and processes to health, including, but not limited to, health services, systems, policies, and technologies. In the latter half of the twentieth century, bioethics in the United States focused on clinical issues of the doctor-patient relationship, rather than issues of social justice or population health (Marshall and Koenig, 2004, p. 254). During that period the role of the physician became less paternalistic than it had been, and bioethics emphasized the principle of patient autonomy, as expressed in concepts such as informed consent and the right to refuse treatment (Brock, 2000, pp. 21–22). In contrast, the recent trend in bioethics in the United States and many other countries is to move beyond the individual patient and the medical relationship and to address the broader issues of health disparities, public health, allocation of limited resources, and social determinants of health (Marshall and Koenig, 2004; Brock, 2000; Illingworth and Parmet, 2009). This recent trend reflects a concern for social justice both within individual societies and from a *global* (or worldwide) perspective. The ethical issues addressed in this book are part of this broader focus and include problems of fairness and population health from the global perspective as well as problems that arise in caring for individual patients in different cultures.

This chapter begins by analyzing theories of ethics, focusing primarily on utilitarianism, Kantian ethics, and the doctrine of prima facie moral duties, which is also known as principlism. These theories of ethics can provide a framework for discussion of specific issues, but they raise two potential problems. First, are these theories of ethics really global—in the sense that they apply to all societies and cultures throughout the world—or is each theory limited to the society and culture in which it was developed? This chapter addresses that question by evaluating whether there are any universal values that transcend culture. Are all systems of ethics cultural? The possible existence of universal values that supersede culture is one of the major themes of this book. This theme is introduced in this chapter and then considered in greater specificity in the chapters on autonomy and informed consent, withdrawal of care, reproductive issues, female genital mutilation, health care rationing, health care reform, and corruption in health systems.

The second potential problem with applying theories of ethics to health care is the question of whether those theories are useful in helping individuals and organizations in the health system to *do the right thing*. If not, how can we encourage people and organizations to do the right thing? This is another major theme of this book, which will also be considered in the chapters that follow. Finally, the activity at the end of this chapter provides an opportunity to evaluate the usefulness of ethical theories in a specific context, establishing a new hospital in a developing country.

THEORIES OF ETHICS

For thousands of years of human experience, people have looked for ways to differentiate right conduct from wrong. Systems have been developed for the purpose of helping individuals to try to make ethical decisions and determine the right thing to do in particular situations. Many people have sought simple rules of decision making that could be used in every situation, such as the Golden Rule of treating others as one would like to be treated, but those simple rules often fail to provide specific guidance in complex circumstances (Shaw and Barry, 1992, pp. 9–10). Therefore the search for methods of identifying the right conduct has led to the development of more complex theories of ethics. Even these more complex theories, however, may be based on attempts to distill a single rule that could be used in every situation. As Bonnie Steinbock and others (2003) have explained, "Traditionally, ethical theories tend to be reductionist; that is, they offer one idea as the key to morality, and attempt to reduce everything to that one idea" (p. 9).

In developing ethical theories, some people have relied on the concept of a social contract as the ultimate source of ethics. Under that approach, morality is based on some type of voluntary agreement. Others have concluded that ethics is based on religion or on the concept of natural law. In his 1963 "Letter from Birmingham Jail," Martin Luther King Jr. reasoned that ethical conduct is based on natural law, which can supersede unjust human law:

> One may well ask, "How can you advocate breaking some laws and obeying others?" The answer is found in the fact that there are two types of laws: there are just laws, and there are unjust laws. [. . .] I would agree with St. Augustine that "An unjust law is no law at all."

Now, what is the difference between the two? How does one determine when a law is just or unjust? A just law is a man-made code that squares with the moral law, or the law of God. An unjust law is a code that is out of harmony with the moral law. To put it in the terms of St. Thomas Aquinas, an unjust law is a human law that is not rooted in eternal and natural law. Any law that uplifts human personality is just. Any law that degrades human personality is unjust. All segregation statutes are unjust because segregation distorts the soul and damages the personality . . . [King, 1963].

Under this approach an action is ethical if it is consistent with natural law. The way we know the action is consistent with natural law is that it has the effect of uplifting human personality.

However, all of these possible sources of ethics pose problems for the practical matter of applying ethics. If the source of ethics is religion or divine will, that would seem to imply that believers in different religions could have very different standards of ethical conduct. Moreover, how could we expect those who believe in a minority religion, or no religion at all, to follow ethical standards derived from the religion followed by the majority in their society?

If the source of ethics is natural law and natural law can supersede unjust human law, every individual could decide not to obey those human laws that he or she considers to be unfair. That approach would seem to give people the option to make individual decisions about which laws to obey and which laws to violate. Of course we can sympathize with and support civil disobedience against laws that enforce racism and segregation. But what would we conclude about a modern-day Robin Hood who steals from the rich and gives to the poor and who defends the theft by arguing that natural law takes precedence over the unfair human laws of private property?

If the source of ethics is a social contract, what are the terms of that contract? Who agreed to that contract on our behalf? Moreover, contracts involve mutual obligations among all parties to the contract. If an individual has failed to meet his or her obligations to society under the social contract, would that mean the contract has been breached and society no longer has any obligation to that individual?

Serious problems exist with applying values derived from each of the possible sources of ethics; moreover it is probably impossible for us to reach complete agreement about the underlying source of ethical standards. Nevertheless we can analyze and categorize various ethical theories without having reached agreement on their ultimate source.

A useful method of categorizing ethical theories is to distinguish between consequentialist and nonconsequentialist theories (Shaw and Barry, 1992, p. 57).

Consequentialism is the idea that only results determine whether an action is right or wrong, whereas **nonconsequentialism** is the idea that consequences are not the only thing that matters.

One consequentialist theory is **utilitarianism**. In focusing solely on the results of an action, utilitarianism holds that an action is right if it results in the greatest good for the greatest number of people (Steinbock and others, 2003, pp. 9–10). It is important to identify both the people who would be helped by a proposed course of action and the people who would be harmed by it. This process of identification is similar to performing a stakeholder analysis. That is only the starting point, however. Merely counting the numbers of people who would be helped or harmed would be an oversimplification of utilitarianism. In determining the greatest good for the greatest number of people, utilitarians also consider the degree of benefit or harm to each person, and not merely the absolute numbers of people who are benefited or harmed. Utilitarianism can be contrasted with **egoism**, which is another consequentialist theory but which holds that an action is right if it results in the greatest good for the only person who really matters—that one individual! (Shaw and Barry, 1992, pp. 57–58).

As stated earlier, nonconsequentialists argue that ethics do not depend solely on results. Nonconsequentialist theories of ethics are also referred to as **deontological** theories (Beauchamp and Childress, 1994, p. 56). One of the most important theories in this category is **Kantian ethics**, named for Immanuel Kant, a German philosopher and professor who lived from 1724 to 1804. As a nonconsequentialist, Kant believed that an action might be wrong even if it results in good consequences, and therefore that "the ends do not justify the means" (Steinbock and others, 2003, p. 14). Kant argued that a proposed action would be ethical if it is an action that we would want everyone to perform in a similar situation. In other words, could we "consistently will" that under a particular set of circumstances everyone else should act in that manner? (Steinbock and others, pp. 9, 15). This concept of Kant's is called the **categorical imperative**. In addition, Kant believed that individuals should be treated as ends, and not as a means to an end, or at least not only as a means to an end (Beauchamp and Childress, 1994, p. 58).

Another approach to ethics is **principlism**, so called because it is based on a set of ethical principles, including autonomy, justice, and beneficence (Beauchamp and others, 2008, p. 22). Sometimes the principle of beneficence is broken down into separate principles of beneficence, or helping other people, and nonmaleficence, or not harming people. In contrast to **monistic** theories, such as utilitarianism or Kantian ethics, which try to reduce ethical conduct to a single idea, principlism is **pluralistic,** in the sense that more than one ethical principle may apply in a particular situation (Beauchamp and Childress, 1994,

p. 100; Steinbock and others, 2003, pp. 9, 36–37). The moral duties represented by those principles are not absolute but rather apply **prima facie**, or at first glance (Beauchamp and Childress, pp. 100, 104; Steinbock and others, p. 37). In other words, one moral duty might outweigh another in the circumstances of a particular case. "A prima facie duty, then, is always right and binding, all other things being equal; it is conditional on not being overridden or outweighed by competing moral demands" (Beauchamp and others, 2008, p. 27). According to the proponents of principlism, prima facie moral duties are based on "common-morality theory" and "shared moral beliefs" (Beauchamp and Childress, 1994, p. 100). "A common-morality theory takes its basic premises directly from the morality shared in common by the members of a society—that is, unphilosophical common sense and tradition" (Beauchamp and Childress, p. 100). (The next section of this chapter addresses the question of whether ethical principles that are derived from the shared beliefs of society can be truly global and universal.)

Which of these ethical approaches, if any, is the best one? Steinbock and others (2003) argue against selecting one theory or approach as the exclusive answer to all ethical questions: "In a typical introduction to ethical theory class, each theory is presented and subjected to devastating criticism. The unfortunate result is that students frequently conclude that all of the theories are wrong—or worse, are pretentious nonsense.... We conclude that it is a mistake to view the various theoretical alternatives as mutually exclusive claims to moral truth. Instead, we should view them as important but partial contributions to a comprehensive, although necessarily fragmented, moral vision" (p. 9). Steinbock and colleagues are correct that no single theory has conclusively demonstrated its correctness and applicability in all situations. However, that seems to leave us with a "buffet approach" to ethical theory. Individuals are left to say to themselves, "I will look over the menu of ethical theories, and then choose some of each. Perhaps, I will take an order of utilitarianism, with a side order of principlism." In addition to causing uncertainty, this buffet approach would allow individuals simply to make their own decisions and then to justify whatever they have already chosen to do. How, if at all, would this individualized buffet approach help people to make difficult ethical decisions in the real world of health policy and services?

Throughout this book we will consider the various ethical theories described in this chapter. In particular we will consider two fundamental questions: (1) are these ethical theories really global, in the sense of being applicable to all societies and cultures; and (2) are these ethical theories really useful in helping individuals and organizations to make the hard decisions in the real world of health policy, health services, and global health? Then, if these ethical theories are not really useful, how can we encourage individuals and organizations in the health system to do the right thing?

ARE THEORIES OF ETHICS GLOBAL?

It is beyond dispute that people of different cultures will perceive the same things in different ways and make very different decisions when faced with the same circumstances. For example, as discussed in Chapter Eight (about allocation of resources), the Akamba people of Kenya have preferences for rationing limited health care resources on the basis of age that are very different from the preferences of most people in the United States (Kilner, 1984, p. 19). It is also clear that different cultures have different values, or at least that they place very different priorities on particular values. Although Western societies generally place a high priority on individual autonomy and equality, some other societies place their high priorities on values such as solidarity of the community, fulfillment of duty, or obedience to a hierarchical order. As Blackhall and others (2001) have written, "Beliefs commonly held in the European-American culture about individuality, self-determination, and the importance of maintaining control too often have been treated as if they were universal ethical principles" (p. 70).

Does this mean that there is no common morality of ethical principles, one that is shared by all human beings, regardless of the society in which they live? Does it mean that there are no universal ethical values that transcend the values of any particular culture? Those two questions are not necessarily the same. As discussed previously, Beauchamp and Childress, who are well-known proponents of principlism, have argued that the prima facie moral duties are based on "common-morality theory" and "shared moral beliefs" (1994, p. 100). It is difficult to conclude, however, that the moral duties of justice and autonomy are really shared by those societies that do not believe in self-determination for women, equal rights for racial and ethnic minorities, or freedom of speech and religion. Patricia Marshall and Barbara Koenig (2004) have described the distinction that Beauchamp has tried to make between those values of common morality that are shared universally and those "particular moralities" that are not shared by all human societies. As Marshall and Koenig also note, however, Beauchamp's distinction is not helpful as a practical matter in addressing difficult questions of bioethics (p. 256). (An excerpt from Marshall and Koenig's article appears later in this chapter.)

In fact, different societies can and do reach very different conclusions about important ethical issues. Whether we characterize those differences as a lack of universality or as "particular moralities" about specific issues, such disagreement among societies requires us to address the second question set forth earlier and to ask whether any universal ethical values exist that transcend the values of a particular culture. When societies disagree about ethics, can we ever conclude that the values or practices of one society are unethical and therefore should give way to overriding universal values? Proponents of ethical relativism argue that ethics is dependent on culture and that actions are ethical if they are considered to be ethical by the culture in which they take place (Steinbock and others, 2003, pp. 6–8). For example, an ethical relativist might even argue that slavery is ethical within the context of a culture that considers slavery to be ethical. Of course many people would strongly disagree with that proposition. Many people would insist that there are indeed universal values of ethics and that these universal values transcend the values of that particular society and make slavery, wherever it occurs, horribly unethical. The issue of ethical relativism is addressed in more detail in Chapter Five of this book, with regard to the problem of female genital mutilation, which is accepted in some cultures and vehemently rejected in others.

The following excerpt from an article by Marshall and Koenig offers further insights into the question of whether a common morality exists. It also traces the evolution of Western bioethics from its former focus on clinical issues to its current concerns with issues of social justice and population health.

EXCERPT FROM "ACCOUNTING FOR CULTURE IN A GLOBALIZED BIOETHICS"

BY PATRICIA MARSHALL AND BARBARA KOENIG

As we look to the future in a world with porous borders and boundaries transgressed by technologies, an inevitable question is: Can there be a single, "global" bioethics? Intimately intertwined with this question is a second one: How might a global bioethics account for profound—and constantly transforming—sources of cultural difference? Can a uniform, global bioethics be relevant cross-culturally? . . .

Although there appears to be agreement about bioethics as a field of study, there is much less consensus about the relevance and applicability of bioethics as a set of guidelines and practices that can be implemented in diverse cultural settings . . . . Currently, the exportation of a Western approach to bioethics in clinical and research settings worldwide mirrors the globalization of biomedicine itself. However, unlike the acceptability of biomedical techniques across the world—from efficacious low-tech interventions like antibiotics to complex surgical procedures like heart transplantation and intensive care units—the adoption of bioethics' concepts and practices has been more contentious, in part because the moral meanings of illness, health, and healing systems are culturally and religiously grounded. Thus, bioethics practices such as advance care planning, full disclosure of a terminal diagnosis, or informed consent in clinical research may be in fundamental conflict with local traditions and beliefs. As anthropologists engaged in a pragmatic vision of bioethics, we have to ask: do such practices actually improve the care of the ill, enhance the well being of populations, or protect subjects in biomedical research?

In this paper, we reflect on the tensions produced as various visions of bioethics circulate in a rapidly globalizing world. Commentators concerned with global health equality and human rights have been vocal critics of an American bioethics focused on the "quandary ethics" of affluence. The physician and anthropologist Paul Farmer contrasts his experiences treating patients in rural Haiti with his work as an attending physician at Harvard. As an infectious disease specialist he uses the same tools in both places; but in Haiti obtaining the drugs that are the tools of his trade is the greatest challenge. Discussions during clinical ethics rounds at a Boston teaching hospital of withholding antibiotics (considered to be futile) stand in stark contrast to the imperative to save lives lost prematurely to treatable infections in Port au Prince . . . It seems unlikely that a bioethics developed in American hospitals will prove up to the challenges of rural poverty without significant refinements. We are deeply concerned with the implications of exporting American bioethics practices throughout the world. The problem is not simply one of national wealth or access to resources, although these are critical considerations. Given the diversity of human values, we ask if bioethics can only flourish in the context of a liberal democratic state, one that is—at least theoretically—based upon respect for individual rights and recognition of diverse cultural and religious values? . . .

. . . In configuring a global bioethics, how do we resolve fundamental cultural and religious differences about the foundations of medical morality? How do we accommodate human rights while maintaining a posture of respect for cultural difference, particularly when there is evidence of abuse or injustice towards individuals or groups? How do we avoid the promulgation of a Westernized bioethics that fosters only an illusion of global consensus about the morality of medical practices? In "real" worlds, morally complex challenges abound . . . .

Bioethics' Reluctant Engagement with Social Context and Cultural Difference

The past is a necessary prologue in looking toward the future. Moral pluralism and cultural difference have not been central topics of concern in the first decades of American academic bioethics....

Possibly linked to this disregard of "difference" is the field's failure to engage with questions of global health equity or population health. In the post World War II period, bioethics' focus on the doctor/patient dyad mirrored the concerns of American biomedicine, which disregarded population health issues and ignored the growing disparities in health care across the U.S. population related to social inequality. In an era of boundless hope and belief in the power of biomedicine, belief in the research enterprise and its applicability to individual health was unquestioned.

Much critical ink has been spilled rehearsing the deficiencies of an individualistic, de-contextualized, American bioethics focused on a limited number of abstract principles: the Georgetown mantra....

The topics engaged by bioethicists reveal the "Americanness" of bioethics. The early focus was invariably on quandary ethics in the context of "high tech" biomedicine, with analyses targeted to "high drama" cases like heart transplantation or refusal of blood products by Jehovah's Witness patients. This orientation calls attention to specific cases, to the individual, to the "local"—not the global—it is case specific, diminishing the potential for broader social critique.

Cultural Analysis: Adding a Reflexive Critique of Bioethics

We opened this essay by making a distinction between bioethics as an academic field and bioethics as a set of observable cultural practices that circulate independently of their theoretical foundations.... Often the bioethics practices utilized in the clinic or as part of a research protocol take on a life of their own, emphasized as procedures only, disconnected from the foundational theory on which they were once based. Indeed, since practices have rarely been studied empirically, we often have little evidence of their usefulness. In the case of some innovations, for example the widespread adoption of advance directives to guide end-of-life care, we actually have evidence that bioethics practices have generally failed, and that they are differentially valued by ethnically diverse U.S. populations....

...A full cultural critique will continually evaluate how bioethics itself is tied into global power structures, perhaps inadvertently serving to maintain the status quo in biomedicine or in the rapidly changing clinical trials industry. Who funds the bioethics enterprise? What interests are served by its existence? One might argue that the rote purpose of informed consent in research—empowering human subjects—has been transformed by socio-political-economic structures into a legalistic informed consent document that now functions more to protect the interests of institutions (both academic health science centers and pharmaceutical companies) than of subjects. And bioethicists are employed by those same institutions . . . .

Is There a Common Morality?

We acknowledge that our claims about the relevance of cultural context run counter to standard accounts within bioethics. The suggestion that it is impossible to understand (and thus to critique) a moral system without attention to historical contingencies and social traditions is very problematic for many philosophers and philosophically-trained bioethicists. From the vantage point of philosophy, the primacy of the moral sphere—and the objectivity of ethical inquiry—may be threatened by social science claims about the relevance of empirical descriptions of cultural variation to the sphere of ethics . . . .

. . . The notion of "common morality" is gaining currency in the field of bioethics . . . . In defending his views about the legitimacy of the concept and how it might be empirically examined, Beauchamp is careful to differentiate between universally shared values and principles which are "located in the common morality" and moral norms ("particular moralities") that are not universally shared by individuals or populations. This parsing of universality and particularity may help explain the diversity and malleability of behavioral norms for morality across cultures (or religions, or institutions) but it is less helpful in relation to the application of bioethics practices in particular international or culturally "different" settings . . . .

In general, we accept a more nuanced view, arguing that the application of general principles is impossible to accomplish without detailed local knowledge. However, there is one universal principle or claim that requires special attention in our analysis: the claim of universal human rights, and the accompanying claim of a right to health care as central to the implementation of global justice. Increasingly, bioethics' attention to human rights follows from critical self-examination of the cultural sources of past errors, specifically, the field's reification of individual choice and quandary ethics paired with a neglect of global equity. Although others may disagree, in our view these blind spots stem from bioethics' American roots and its strong link with powerful interests, such as high-technology biomedicine. From the perspective of the clinic, it was hard to develop a vision that crossed borders.

Scholars in bioethics have begun to consider carefully broader structural issues contributing to global population health, including social, economic, and political factors influencing the disproportionate burden of disease throughout the world. Theorists directly link health with basic human rights. Considerations of social justice and health disparities—both within and between nations—are key dimensions of the new critique . . . .

Looking Ahead in Bioethics

Bioethics must widen its focus beyond its Western view to incorporate and acknowledge moral pluralism and cultural variation or it will lose its relevance and applicability for most of the worlds' [sic] population. Perhaps the key question for reconfiguring bioethics in a way that recognizes and accounts for cultural difference is simply this: Can bioethics lose the stamp of its American cultural origins? At stake here is the saliency and credibility of the profession—and the practices it upholds—in the global arena. At stake is the ability of bioethicists and others associated with the field to actively engage in thoughtful debate about the implications of cultural difference and its consequences for the production of science and its applications worldwide. At stake is our capacity to achieve praxis in the way we promulgate and "do" bioethics in diverse cultural terrains.

How does bioethics need to change to be more relevant cross-culturally? If it sheds its American focus on individualism will it become "something" else? Bioethics will necessarily change as it continues to incorporate the arguments and sensibilities of cultural difference into its fundamental underlying ideology. As contextual approaches to ethics have shown in recent years, the Georgetown mantra loses its principled rigidity as soon as social context and its inherent moral ambiguity become a part of its interpretive structure.

There are two particular areas in which it is imperative for bioethics to revise its basic orientation in order to become culturally relevant and globally "aware." First, as we suggest above, it is vitally important that bioethics attend to social justice and focus attention on the broad goals of population health . . . . Second, bioethics must consider social context, especially the impact of political economy on the moral dimensions of science and healthcare . . . .

Attention to Social Justice and Human Rights

In the arena of human rights and population health, bioethics must address the systematic and powerful ways in which structural forces influence morbidity and mortality in diverse populations . . . .

Attention to Social Context

The second broad area that bioethics must systematically address is social context, particularly political and economic factors that influence profoundly the quality of life and the experience of suffering or health for individuals and populations worldwide . . . .

The African American experience of health disparities in the U.S. provides a good example of why it is imperative for bioethics to consider the primacy of social context in thinking about ethics, science, and biomedicine at all levels, including research, clinical care, and access to health services. Studies indicate that African Americans are reluctant to limit or forego medically futile treatment at the end of life. A lack of "trust" is frequently implicated to explain choices for aggressive medical care. However, African American concerns about the potential for mistreatment or neglect in clinical settings is historically well justified. Consider the legacy of Jim Crow segregation in hospitals, or the abuses of the Tuskegee Syphilis Study . . . . Ignoring the political economy of social context, including the long term consequences of entrenched racism, severely limits our capacity to analyze critically the underlying ethical dimensions of biomedical practice or research . . . .

Conclusion

Predicting the future is inevitably a risky business. In this essay we have tried to show how a bioethics informed by attention to social context, and sensitive to cultural difference, might look in future decades. Detailed analysis of and attention to the social, political, and economic context will not necessarily solve every ethical dilemma, but it will certainly avoid mistakes based on the naive assumption that applying solutions derived from the U.S. to resource-poor, developing world problems is adequate. Exporting the American institutional review board system to sub-Saharan Africa may allow compliance with federal regulations, but without attention to the local cultural context does little to protect research subjects . . . .

For those working in the field of bioethics, our greatest challenge is maintaining the reflexive stance characteristic of the best social science. We have argued that a culturally-informed bioethics will remain critical of its own goals, re-examining them when challenged. The emerging emphasis on issues of population health and global justice is heartening. Our global environment precludes "business as usual"; the field of bioethics can no longer focus its energy and attention on the ethical dilemmas experienced by individual patients privileged by social status with too much medical care....

Source: Excerpted from "Accounting for Culture in a Globalized Bioethics," by P. Marshall and B. Koenig, 2004. *Journal of Law, Medicine & Ethics, 32*(2), 252–266 (citations, references, and some text omitted). Copyright 2004 by American Society of Law & Medicine, Inc. Reprinted by permission.

In their article, Marshall and Koenig (2004) took what they described as "a more nuanced view" (p. 257) on the issue of the existence of a common morality. They recognized the need for local knowledge in applying general principles. However, they also recognized the existence of some universal principles and called particular attention to the universal principles of human rights and the right to health care as matters of global justice. The right to health care is discussed in detail in Chapter Seven of this book, together with an analysis of ethical obligations to provide health care goods and services.

CAN THEORIES OF ETHICS ENCOURAGE PEOPLE TO DO THE RIGHT THING?

Throughout human history, societies have searched for the best ways to encourage desirable conduct and discourage undesirable conduct. For example, in ancient China, the Legalists argued that society could not be controlled by means of morality or virtue but only by means of strict laws and severe punishments (Chen, 1999, p. 10). The Confucianists strongly disagreed with the Legalists. According to the Confucianists, regulations and punishments are ineffective, and the only way to maintain social order is to educate people by means of morality and lead people by means of virtue (Chen, p. 7). Other countries and cultures have had similar debates about the best ways to promote the good of individuals and societies.

Several chapters of this book consider the usefulness of ethical theories in handling practical problems of health policy and services. For example, Chapter Four, which addresses reproductive health issues, evaluates whether ethical theories are helpful in resolving the morality of abortion, concluding that they are not particularly helpful. If we were to use utilitarianism to address that issue, we would still need to consider whether to address the interests of fetuses when considering the greatest good for the greatest number. If we were to use Kantian ethics, we would first need to decide whether fetuses are people and thus entitled to be treated as ends. Under each of the theories of ethics, a threshold issue would essentially beg the question and that would be likely to determine the outcome of ethical analysis. If we were to try to use principlism to address the ethical issue of abortion, the analysis might be so flexible that it would fail to give us any real guidance. Because no moral duty is absolute, each person could decide for himself or herself which duty outweighs the others in the particular circumstances. Rather than helping us to determine the most ethical course of conduct, the open-ended analysis of principlism would probably lead to any desired result. Then the chosen result could be justified by declaring that one moral duty outweighs all of the others in this particular situation. Additional examples of this phenomenon can be found in the activities at the end of each chapter of this book. These activities provide opportunities to consider whether theories of ethics are really helpful in solving practical problems in health services and systems. In addition these practical activities can help individuals to develop the ability to identify ethical problems in health policy and services and to consider the effect of potential solutions on each stakeholder.

If ethical theories are not particularly helpful, how can we encourage individuals and organizations in the health system to do the right thing? There are many possibilities. Each would have advantages and disadvantages, and some would be more effective than others. Theoretically, we could require everyone who works in health policy or services to take a college-level course in ethics as a job requirement before being hired or to participate in on-the-job training on ethics. It is not at all clear, however, that this type of education or training would actually encourage ethical conduct on the job. Employers in the health system could try to use preemployment testing to evaluate the ethical standards of all potential employees, but answers on preemployment tests would not necessarily indicate a greater likelihood of ethical conduct. Health care organizations could monitor and supervise the conduct of all employees by means of inspections and internal auditing and by making confidential hotlines available so that individuals could inform the management anonymously about unethical conduct in the organization. In the United States, health care organizations have been encouraged by the government to adopt compliance programs that include these types of activities. However, compliance programs usually devote more time and resources to avoiding legal or financial problems for the organization than they give to helping the organization and its personnel to make difficult ethical decisions, such as determining the most ethical way to allocate the organization's limited health care resources. Perhaps the most effective method of encouraging ethical conduct would be for managers and board members of organizations in the health system to lead by example, and to encourage an ethical culture at all levels of the organization. In particular, leaders should make it clear that in considering proposed courses of action for the organization it is completely appropriate for all personnel in the organization to raise potential ethical concerns and to discuss each of the alternatives from an ethical perspective.

SUMMARY

Since the latter half of the twentieth century, bioethics in the United States and a number of other countries has made an important transition, from an emphasis on individual autonomy in the doctor-patient relationship to a serious concern about broader issues of social justice and public health (Marshall and Koenig, 2004; Brock, 2000; Illingworth and Parmet, 2009). This recent trend reflects a new and global perspective, as well as a commitment to fairness on the national level. This chapter began by analyzing various ethical theories, including utilitarianism, Kantian ethics, and principlism. Some theories of ethics may be limited to the societies and cultures in which they were developed. Nevertheless there are some overriding ethical values, even if they have not been adopted by a particular culture. Those overriding ethical values are universal in the sense that they apply to all human societies and they transcend the values of a particular culture. Contrary to the arguments of ethical relativists, there are some circumstances, such as slavery, in which we can and should conclude that the values of a particular society are unethical and therefore should give way to overriding universal values. This chapter also evaluated the usefulness of ethical theories as methods of making ethical decisions, and considered other potential methods of encouraging people and organizations to do the right thing. Finally, the activity at the end of this chapter, along with the activities in the other chapters, can help people develop the ability to identify ethical problems and consider potential solutions.

KEY TERMS

bioethics	ethics	prima facie
categorical imperative	Kantian ethics	principlism
consequentialism	monistic	utilitarianism
deontological	nonconsequentialism	
egoism	pluralistic	

DISCUSSION QUESTIONS

1. Which ethical theory, if any, is the best one?
2. Are ethics dependent on culture, such that all actions considered to be ethical by a particular culture are ethical when they occur in that culture?
3. In the latter half of the twentieth century, why was bioethics in the United States focused on the doctor-patient relationship rather than on broader issues of public health?
4. What are the most effective ways of helping individuals and organizations in the health system to make ethical decisions and act in an ethical manner?

ACTIVITY: BUILDING AND OPERATING A NEW HOSPITAL IN A DEVELOPING COUNTRY

A developing country in sub-Saharan Africa, which we will call the Republic of Tuvunu, has a population of about forty million people. In Tuvunu, millions of people are suffering from diseases such as HIV/AIDS, TB, and malaria. Every year, tens of thousands of children and adults die unnecessarily as a result of diseases that could be managed by means of appropriate medical treatment and drugs.

An academic medical center in a wealthy, industrialized country, which we will call the University Health System (UHS), operates several hospitals and other health care facilities in its local area and draws patients from a wide region. However, UHS has not developed or operated health facilities in any other country.

Tuvunu's Ministry of Health (MOH) has requested UHS to build and operate a new hospital in an isolated area of Tuvunu that currently has no health care facility. Specifically, MOH has asked UHS to provide $100 million for construction of the hospital and $10 million per year for ten years as annual operating costs. Under this proposal, UHS would own and operate the hospital, which would be known as UHS-Tuvunu. The administrator, physicians, nurses, and all other workers at UHS-Tuvunu would be salaried employees of UHS. In addition, some physicians and managers from the home campus of UHS would travel to Tuvunu on a periodic basis, for one month at a time, in order to assist in providing care to patients and operating the hospital.

UHS is seriously considering this proposal. UHS already has sufficient funds in its accumulated reserves to build the hospital and operate it for ten years. Although the project is expensive, it is estimated that the new hospital will save more than one thousand lives per year and will significantly improve the lives of thousands more.

At this point in the negotiations the only serious concern is the list of conditions that MOH recently presented to UHS. According to MOH, UHS will be required to respect Tuvunu's cultural practices and religious beliefs in operating the hospital. For its part UHS is committed to multiculturalism and does not want to impose its views on the government or people of Tuvunu. The conditions presented by MOH are as follows:

1. No abortion may be performed at UHS-Tuvunu, unless it is absolutely necessary to save the life of the mother.
2. UHS-Tuvunu will respect Tuvunu's longstanding cultural practice of female circumcision (FC) and will perform FC when requested by the patient or, if the patient is a child, when requested by the parent.
3. In accordance with Tuvunu's culture, informed consent to the performance of medical or surgical treatment will be granted or denied by the eldest male in the patient's extended family.
4. In sending physicians and managers from the home campus of UHS to UHS-Tuvunu, UHS may not send any Jews or homosexuals to Tuvunu.
5. The top floor of UHS-Tuvunu will be designed and advertised as the VIP Floor. It will be used by patients who are capable of paying higher charges, including wealthy residents of Tuvunu and foreign medical tourists.
6. As a condition of receiving a license to operate UHS-Tuvunu, UHS will sign a consulting agreement with a local company to be designated by MOH, and UHS will pay $1 million to that company.

Your task is to evaluate the ethical issues raised by these conditions. In evaluating these ethical issues, please apply the ethical theories or approaches of utilitarianism, Kantian ethics, and principlism (prima facie moral duties). In other words, how would a follower of each ethical theory or approach resolve these ethical issues? In addition, please feel free to consider any other ethical theories or approaches that you think may be relevant, including your own ethical views. In evaluating the ethical issues, please consider two alternative scenarios, as follows:

In the first scenario, please assume that the complete list of conditions presented by MOH is nonnegotiable. MOH will not change its position on any of those issues. Therefore the proposal is all or nothing, and UHS must either take it or leave it. Under this scenario, no other institution is considering building or operating a hospital in Tuvunu. Even if another institution could be identified to build or operate a hospital in Tuvunu, that institution would be subject to the same set of nonnegotiable conditions. Under these circumstances, is it ethical for UHS to build and operate the proposed hospital in Tuvunu? Is it ethical for UHS to refuse to build and operate the proposed hospital in Tuvunu?

In the second scenario, please assume that the conditions are negotiable to some extent. Under this scenario, UHS has the flexibility to eliminate some of the conditions but cannot eliminate all of the conditions. As an ethical matter, which of the conditions are the most important to eliminate? Which of the conditions, if any, could be tolerated as a compromise, in order to make it possible for UHS to build and operate a new hospital in a severely underserved area of Tuvunu?

CHAPTER TWO

AUTONOMY AND INFORMED CONSENT IN GLOBAL PERSPECTIVE

LEARNING OBJECTIVES

- Acquire proficiency in analyzing the ethical duty of health care providers to obtain a patient's informed consent to treatment.

- Understand and be able to explain the practical problems of obtaining truly informed consent in both developed and developing countries.

- Be able to evaluate whether informed consent really matters to patients.

- Be prepared to debate whether informed consent is a value of a particular culture or a universal principle of ethics.

THE Hippocratic Oath does not mention any ethical duty on the part of a physician to obtain the consent of a patient, or even any obligation to provide information to a patient. Jay Katz (1994) has pointed out that as recently as 1847, the American Medical Association's Code of Ethics instructed patients to simply obey orders, despite their own "crude opinions" (p. 73). Nevertheless, the concept of informed consent has become so much a part of modern practice that people in many countries tend to take it for granted.

This chapter begins by analyzing the ethical principles and practical issues of informed consent, including the problems of obtaining informed consent in developing countries, looking at these principles and issues specifically in the context of clinical practice. (Chapter Six analyzes the ethical issues of informed consent in the context of research with human subjects.) Developing country issues are exemplified through an excerpt from an article by scholars from Pakistan about the practice of informed consent at two hospitals in Lahore. Then two additional questions are evaluated. First, does informed consent really matter to patients? Second, is informed consent a universal principle or a value only of a particular culture? An activity at the end of this chapter addresses the ethical aspects of informed consent procedures at a rural health facility in a developing country in light of the opportunity cost of spending limited time and resources on informed consent.

ETHICAL PRINCIPLES AND PRACTICAL ISSUES OF INFORMED CONSENT

The patient's right to choose is based on the ethical principle of **autonomy**, or self-determination. Pursuant to that ethical principle, **informed consent** refers to the right of a patient to make his or her own decisions regarding diagnosis and treatment and to do so after receiving all of the necessary information from the health care provider. Thus, informed consent includes both a decisional component and an informational component.

In the United States, the American Medical Association (AMA) has adopted standards for both of these components of informed consent, as expressed in Opinion 10.01 of the AMA Code of Medical Ethics, which is titled "Fundamental Elements of the Patient-Physician Relationship" (American Medical Association, 1992). With regard to the decisional component, Opinion 10.01(2) provides that the "patient has the right to make decisions regarding the health care that is recommended by his or her physician. Accordingly, patients may accept or refuse any recommended medical treatment." In regard to the informational component, Opinion 10.01(1) states that the "patient has the right to receive information from physicians and to discuss the benefits, risks, and costs of appropriate treatment alternatives." These ethical principles have been accepted as standard practice in many countries around the world. In fact, the International Code of Medical Ethics of the World Medical Association (WMA) explicitly provides that "a physician shall respect a competent patient's right to accept or refuse treatment" (World Medical Association, 2006). As discussed in Chapter Six, in many countries research projects that use human subjects must comply with the requirements of informed consent. Moreover, some people have argued that the ethical duty of disclosure includes an obligation for health care providers to inform patients even about medical errors the providers have made (Wu and others, 1997).

The ethical principle of informed consent has also been adopted as a legal requirement in many countries. In one frequently quoted decision, a U.S. state court explained that "[e]very human being of adult years and sound mind has a right to determine what shall be done with his own body; and a surgeon who performs an operation without his patient's consent, commits an assault, for which he is liable in damages" (*Schloendorff* v. *Society of New York Hospital*, 1914, p. 93). The Law of the People's Republic of China on Medical Practitioners contains this provision: "Doctors should truthfully explain the patients' conditions to the patients and their family members provided that attention is paid to avoid an adverse effect on the patients" (People's Republic of China, 1999, art. 26). The point here is not to focus on the laws in particular countries but rather to recognize that in many countries informed consent has become so well accepted as a matter of ethical theory and medical practice that it has become enshrined as a legal requirement, with potentially severe consequences for a health care provider's failure to comply.

However, practical problems exist in providing understandable information to patients and obtaining truly informed consent, even in industrialized countries with relatively well educated patients. Immigration and the movement of people across national borders mean that large numbers of patients are not fluent in the dominant language of the country in which they need to receive health care and thus face additional communication barriers that can inhibit their access to care, as discussed in Chapter Ten. For example, millions of people in the United States have limited English proficiency, and immigration is resulting in similar language barriers in other developed and developing countries as well. It is axiomatic that a patient cannot give informed consent unless that patient can obtain information and provide consent in a language that he or she understands.

In developing countries, resource limitations and educational levels pose additional problems in obtaining truly informed consent. As Yousuf and others (2007) have pointed out, overworked doctors in a developing country may lack the time and the patience to comply with all of the procedures of informed consent (p. 562). Sastry and others (2004) have noted the difficulty of implementing informed consent procedures in those parts of India where resources and staff time are limited and where educational levels are very low. These authors described the practice of informed consent for pregnant women in India as follows:

> Typically, informed consent for pregnant women in most Indian hospitals and clinics is for operative procedures such as cesarean section or laparotomy. It is usual for the doctor or resident on duty to put down in his or her own handwriting the text of the consent on a patient's case papers . . . . This is signed (or a thumbprint given) by the patient, her husband or an accompanying relative, and is generally considered to serve as legal consent; therefore, it is not interpreted as voluntary. Most often, due to time constraints, very little is explained to the patient about the procedure, risks, and benefits, or what her signature actually means. As found in other regions in India, there is a general perception by clinicians and other healthcare workers that women are "unable" to understand any of the procedures even if explained, because they are illiterate or have no medical background [Sastry and others, 2004, citations omitted].

Ayesha Humayun and others (2008) have noted similar problems in Pakistan with informed consent, privacy, and confidentiality. Pakistan is a Muslim country. The practice of medicine is subject to the Code of Ethics issued in 2002 by the Pakistan Medical and Dental Council (PMDC), which is a government regulatory authority. Farhat Moazam and Aamir Jafarey (2005) have identified an inherent tension in the PMDC's Code of Ethics, which contains aspects of both the moral values of Islam and the contemporary principles of bioethics, such as autonomy, beneficence, and justice (p. 252). As stated in the PMDC's Code of Ethics, "If secular Western bioethics can be described as rights-based, with a strong emphasis on individual rights, Islamic bioethics is based on duties and obligations (e.g., to preserve life, seek treatment), although rights (of Allah, the community, and the individual) do feature in bioethics, as does a call to virtue (Ihsan)" (Pakistan Medical and Dental Council, 2001, sec. 7.0).

The following excerpt from the article by Humayun and colleagues mentioned previously describes some of the practical limitations of obtaining informed consent in Pakistan, as well as differences between practices at public and private hospitals. Significantly, the article authors have treated informed consent as an ethical requirement for all health care professionals, even in developing countries, and they have not questioned the importance of informed consent or the applicability of that principle to every country and culture.

EXCERPT FROM "PATIENTS' PERCEPTION AND ACTUAL PRACTICE OF INFORMED CONSENT, PRIVACY AND CONFIDENTIALITY IN GENERAL MEDICAL OUTPATIENT DEPARTMENTS OF TWO TERTIARY CARE HOSPITALS OF LAHORE"

BY AYESHA HUMAYUN AND OTHERS

Introduction

...The concepts of privacy and confidentiality are closely related. Privacy is a broader term including physical privacy, informational privacy, protection of personal identity and the ability to make choices without interference. Confidentiality is a narrower term referring to informational privacy and the duty not to disclose any patient information without prior approval from the patient. Privacy and confidentiality are not only basic rights of the patients but also serve to further a trustful, frank and open relationship with the doctor, thus improving patient care. It has also been noted that patients often over- or underestimate their ethical rights in medicine.

While most western countries have enshrined these concepts of informed consent, privacy and confidentiality in federal or state laws and codes of ethics, such law-making is almost non-existent in Pakistan although there have been some recent efforts to create ethical guidelines for research and medical practice. Significantly, Pakistan Medical and Dental Council (PMDC), the regulatory body of medical practitioners[,] has formulated a code of ethics for all doctors, although no concrete steps have been taken to ensure their application. However, most other work on this subject focuses on research ethics and is currently limited to individual institutions or some non-governmental organizations. At the same time, cultural values in Pakistan offer a challenge to the practice of medical ethics in Pakistan. This is because crucial decision making is often done by family members or is left entirely up to the physician, and there seems to be a general acceptance of this shifting of focus from the individual to other people. Public (patient) awareness of their rights to informed consent and privacy is often low. Previous qualitative research has shown that a significant number of physicians do not think it is necessary to obtain a proper consent after providing the patients with thorough information. Furthermore, general observation points to wide differences between the quality of medical care offered at private and public hospitals. In view of these observations, this study was conducted to explore the degree to which the ethical practices of informed consent, privacy and confidentiality are observed in medical out-patient departments of public and private hospitals in Lahore, Pakistan. We follow it up with an assessment of patients' perceptions of these practices in comparison to the assessment performed by our data collectors.

Materials and Methods

A cross-sectional study was conducted at general medical out-patient departments (OPDs) of two tertiary care hospitals of Lahore during the period March–June 2005. One hospital was from the public sector while the other was from the private sector. The sample was selected using multistage random sampling....

Prior consent had been obtained from all doctors so as to be allowed to observe and evaluate any doctor-patient interaction during the study period. However, in order to minimize bias, at no point were the doctors informed of the individual patient selection. Hence they remained unaware of which patient interaction was being graded for ethical practices. This had been made clear to them while obtaining consent for their participation. In Pakistan, the nursing departments are often understaffed so that the role of nurses in the out-patient departments is limited and it is almost always the doctors who obtain informed consent from the patients regarding their examination/treatment. Therefore, nurses were not included in the study.

Ethical approval for the study was obtained from the review committee of the Center for Health Research, Lahore. The study was conducted in compliance with the "Ethical Principles for Medical Research involving Human Subjects" of [the] Helsinki Declaration. Patient names were not recorded to assure confidentiality. Verbal consent was obtained from all subjects and documented in the presence of a witness....

Results

We enrolled and followed 93 patients in each of the two hospitals....

...Observance of ethical practices was inadequate or improper in most instances. The practice of informed consent in the private hospital was much better compared to the public hospital (p: < 0.0001). No informed consent was taken at all in 90.3% cases in the public hospital compared to 53.3% of the patients in the private hospital. Similarly, confidentiality was adequately practised more often in the private hospital than in the public hospital (p: < 0.0001). On the other hand, the differences in the provision of privacy were not statistically significant....

...Compared to the public hospital, more patients in the private hospital believed that the ethical principles had been well observed by the doctors interacting with them (p: < 0.0003)....

Discussion

The present study was designed with a purpose to assess the actual practice of informed consent, privacy and confidentiality by the doctors through direct observation of the entire process of patient care provided in outpatient departments (OPDs) of public and private hospitals, and correlate these ethical practices with patient perception of doctors' ethical practices. Our results show that the doctors took proper informed consent from very few patients coming to these hospitals. One of reasons behind such practice is that the cultural trends in Pakistan still tend to accept the paternalistic model of medical care. This is in line with the Asian culture as a whole, where the decision-making is often left purely to the doctors or other family members. Studies from Kashmir and Japan reflect similar practices wherein patients are willing to accept what doctors choose for them, while doctors are satisfied with their role of a decision-maker. For example in a study by...[Yousuf] RM et al, 65% [of] physicians in Kashmir and 35% [of] physicians in Malaysia said they would listen to the family's request to withhold information from the patient. A study from Hong Kong also shows the patients and physicians to be more willing to accept the role of families in crucial decisions regarding medical care. Even in countries like Lithuania and South Africa, the practices of doctors often do not meet the moral and legal requirements for medical ethics, although the observance of ethics is better than what our study has found in Pakistan.

While the situation in US was not much different till the 1960s, the current medical practice in US lays significant focus on the concepts of informed consent and shared decision-making. This differs substantially from the trends in Asia and experts have gone to the extent of calling it a "cultural artifact" in that reliance on this concept is not universal. Even in US, there is often a clash between these ethical standards and the moral intuitions of many physicians.

Improper consent of some form was taken from a large number of patients at the private hospital but just a few from public hospital. No informed consent was taken from an alarming proportion of patients (90%) at the public hospital. Even in the private hospital more than half the patients were denied their right to informed consent. On the whole, the practice of informed consent was better at the private hospital but still far from the ideal. Several reasons may account for the differences. Firstly, doctors at private hospitals are better paid than their colleagues in the public sector, something that may translate into better performance at work and greater care for the patients. Secondly, doctors in the private sector are often employed on contracts that need regular renewal. Doctors' work is regularly monitored and assessed, and this renewal is often linked to patient satisfaction with care. Hence doctors in the private sector are more likely to respect the patients' fundamental rights related to their medical management. On the other hand, jobs in the public sector are secure and more or less permanent in nature. At the same time, there is little or no accountability of the doctors since there is usually no effort to elicit patients' opinion about the care provided to them. The results of our study are in line with those from a study conducted in a public sector hospital in Karachi that concluded that the current practice of informed consent was below the internationally acceptable standards. Even though that study commented only on preoperative informed consent, it is pertinent to note that the trend of both our studies is similar. Another study from a private hospital in Karachi also reported that the number of patients complaining of lack of privacy was greater than in the west.

Similarly, the principle of confidentiality (informational privacy) was also inadequately practised in our study. This is not surprising since even a study in a country like Canada, has shown that quite a few of the family physicians do not fully understand their obligations towards patient confidentiality. Furthermore, the practice of confidentiality was more inadequate/unsatisfactory in the public sector hospital than the private one. While the reasons cited above may also contribute to this difference as well, there are others factors that must also be explored. Significant patient burden at general OPDs of public hospitals often makes it impossible for the doctors to follow the full protocol of informed consent and confidentiality. Usually the OPDs are in the form of big rooms in which on one side the patients are waiting (a part of their total waiting time in and outside the OPD room) while on the other, there are some examination tables (with or without a screen). In the center of the room, many doctors are interviewing and examining multiple patients and/or writing medical prescriptions. 2 to 4 patients are dealt with simultaneously. Seldom if ever are the attendants requested to leave the room while the patient is being interviewed or examined. Hence the patient and his/her problems are discussed in front of all present in the room. Such practice may prevent the patients in revealing their complete history and list of symptoms.

Provision of privacy during physical examinations was also inadequate in both hospitals. However, privacy-related practices were still somewhat better than the practices of informed consent and informational privacy. The private hospital again showed better ethical practices than the public hospital although in this case the difference was not statistically significant. This may be because in both settings, doctors have no choice but to carry out these examinations behind a screen, especially examinations requiring significant exposure . . . .

Our study shows that compared to the public hospital, more patients in the private hospital believed that ethical practices were well observed by doctors interacting with them. This is fairly in line with the assessment of our data collectors where principles of informed consent, informational privacy and physical privacy were more often applied in the private hospitals as discussed earlier. We compared whether the patients' perception of these ethical practices matched correctly with the assessment of our data collectors. In 38/93 instances in the public hospital and 24/93 in the private hospital, patients' perception differed with the assessment of our trained data collector. This is a significant number, and again shows that many patients are unaware of, or misunderstand[,] their ethical rights. Once again, the discordance is higher in the public hospital and this may be directly related to the lower socioeconomic status of these patients compared to those in the private hospital.

It is noteworthy, that there are also some other reasons for inadequate ethical practices in Pakistan. For example, although innovative ethical curricula have been shown to improve the confidence and practice of doctors with regards to medical ethics, PMDC does not include education in bioethics as a major component of the medical curriculum. It follows, that very few medical colleges in Pakistan impart formal training in bioethics. Such education is also largely omitted from postgraduate training programs. Lack of applied ethical training is also perceived in other countries like Germany and even US, which has always championed the cause of bioethics. This lack of Pakistani education in ethics means that trainees can only learn from the practices of their consultants, most of whom belong to the era when a paternalistic approach towards the patients was in vogue. This leads to a vicious cycle where every subsequent generation of doctors believes in paternalism. Even doctors who favor practices like informed consent, often abandon these practices since they believe that most of their patients are uneducated and would not be able to decide what is best for them. It is true though, that often the patients do not want to take any decision and want the doctor to decide each and every thing for them. Furthermore, the lack of accountability and legal recourse means that doctors who do not respect patient ethics are never taken to task in this country.

However, regardless of the excuses provided for the lack of medical ethics, it should be kept in mind that the principles of informed consent, confidentiality and physical privacy must always be applied in medical practice.

Conclusion

Adherence to principles of ethics in medical practice is inadequate in Pakistan. Formal training in bioethics should be incorporated in undergraduate and postgraduate medical training so that the healthcare providers understand the concept, process and application of medical ethics. Local languages should be utilized in written and verbal consent. Forms for written consent should be easy to understand for even the less educated patients. Every patient should be interviewed and examined in a separate room to ensure informational and physical privacy and the number of medical staff should complement the patient load at any hospital. Sincere attempts need to be made at legalizing the value and processes of medical ethics and public health programs should aim at making the patients aware of their legal rights to informed consent, confidentiality and privacy.

Source: Excerpted from "Patients' Perception and Actual Practice of Informed Consent, Privacy and Confidentiality in General Medical Outpatient Departments of Two Tertiary Care Hospitals of Lahore," by A. Humayun and others, 2008. BMC Medical Ethics, 9(14), doi: 10.1186/1472-6939-9-14 (citations, references, tables, and some text omitted). Copyright 2008 by Humayun et al.; licensee BioMed Central Ltd. This is an Open Access article distributed under the terms of the Creative Commons Attribution License (http://creativecommons.org/licenses/by/2.0), which permits unrestricted use, distribution, and reproduction in any medium, provided the original work is properly cited.

In the foregoing reading, Humayun and others (2008) argued that health care professionals have an ethical obligation to obtain the informed consent of their patients, "regardless of the excuses provided for the lack of medical ethics." However, they did not consider the opportunity cost of spending time and resources on informed consent, a cost likely to be particularly high in a developing country with severe limitations in health resources. In other words, if the limited staff could treat more patients per day by dispensing with some of the time-consuming procedures for informed consent, would that increased efficiency justify a failure to comply with ethical principles of autonomy and informed consent? The activity at the end of this chapter provides an opportunity to evaluate that question in the context of a rural health facility in a developing country.

DOES INFORMED CONSENT REALLY MATTER TO PATIENTS?

We should consider the possibility that, in the real world, patients may not really care very much about informed consent. Philosophers and ethicists care very deeply about informed consent, and tell the rest of the world that they should care about it. Many academics have built their careers by writing scholarly articles and books about informed consent and related subjects. They attend conferences, participate in panel discussions, and serve on advisory committees about informed consent and other bioethical issues. There is an entire informed consent industry of highly educated, caring, and articulate experts.

Malpractice lawyers also care about informed consent. The doctrine provides a legal basis on which patients may sue their health care providers in the event of an adverse outcome, without needing to prove that the treatment was performed in a negligent manner. If a lawyer prevails on behalf of a patient, that lawyer will probably receive a contingency fee that takes a significant share of the patient's monetary damages.

It is possible, however, that many patients might not care very much about informed consent. Or if they do care, it might be because someone has told them they should care. Moreover, by insisting that doctors comply with specific procedures for informed consent, we have encouraged an attitude of distrust between patients and their doctors. We even insist that doctors provide information about potential risks when the reality is that the patient does not have much of a choice. For example, we insist that pediatricians give detailed disclosures to parents about the risks of immunizing their children, including gruesome statistics about the numbers of children who will die or become paralyzed as a result of receiving particular immunizations. As a practical matter, many parents have little choice but to agree to immunization for their children if they want their children to be allowed to attend school. Nevertheless, we require doctors and parents to go through the ritual of disclosing the frightening risks and then obtaining a signature in order to prove that there was voluntary informed consent.

Another problem is that the current practice of informed consent does not include disclosure of those risks that may be most significant to the patient. We require doctors to disclose the risks and benefits of various treatments, but we do not require doctors to disclose information about themselves, which might pose the most significant risks to the patient. For example, we generally do not require doctors to tell patients about their level of experience, mortality rate compared to that of other doctors, disciplinary board actions, malpractice cases, infectious diseases, history of alcoholism or substance abuse, or any disabilities that might affect their performance of medicine or surgery. Generally, we do not require hospitals or other health care facilities that need to obtain informed consent to inform patients about the facility's quality ratings by governmental or nongovernmental agencies. Those types of provider-specific risks might be much more important to the patient than the abstract statistical risk of an adverse outcome for each type of treatment in the nation as a whole. The failure to require disclosure of the most important risks is one more reason why the current practice of informed consent does not meet the real needs and concerns of patients.

If patients really do care about informed consent, it still might be fairly low on their hierarchy of priorities. Imagine the tragic scene in which a physician needs to tell a patient that she has cancer. Obviously, the patient will be shocked, upset, and terribly frightened. She wants to know if she is going to die. She wants the doctor to save her life, not guarantee that she will have final decision-making authority over the choice of treatment modality. Later, when she is told about various treatment options and asked to make a choice, the doctor can subtly—but effectively—influence her choice of treatment. The doctor can present and explain the alternatives in a way that makes it more likely that the patient will choose the alternative that the doctor thinks is best for that patient, after which the patient might be firmly convinced that she made her own, independent decision.

Every day, we put ourselves, our lives, and our families in the hands of other people who know how to do things that we don't know how to do, and we trust them. We don't require them to disclose all of the risks or give us the power to make decisions about how they will do their jobs. For example, imagine what passengers might hear from their pilot if we handled the risks of airplane travel in the same manner as we handle informed consent to medical care:

> Good morning, ladies and gentlemen. Welcome to Modern Airlines flight number 372. This is your captain speaking to you from the flight deck. Before takeoff, I need to tell you about some of the risks you will face on today's flight. There is a risk that we will slide off the runway during takeoff, and there is a risk that we will crash during our approach for landing. There is a risk that we will crash into a mountain. There is a risk that we will crash into the ocean.
>
> Before we take off, I will continue to explain the risks of today's flight. Meanwhile, our flight attendants will pass through the cabin handing out consent forms for you to sign. You must sign a consent form if you want to remain on this flight.
>
> In addition, there are some important decisions which need to be made about the best and safest way to reach the airport at our destination. If there is only one passenger on today's flight, that one passenger will make the decision. If there is more than one passenger on today's flight, the decision will be made by majority vote of the passengers, with our copilot voting in the event of a tie. The choice is between making a gradual descent to the airport at our destination and making a faster descent. As a matter of safety, each alternative has some advantages and some element of statistical risk. Now, I have been a professional airline pilot

for over twenty-five years, but the choice is up to you. So, please let the flight attendants know what you want me to do.

Of course that would be utterly ridiculous, but that is precisely what we require from our doctors under the current practice of informed consent. A doctor may have practiced medicine or surgery for over twenty-five years. Nevertheless, in choosing between alternatives, we require the doctor to give a tutorial to the patient in medical science, and then we let the patient tell the doctor what to do.

In addition to being impractical, informed consent demonstrates a real lack of trust in our doctors. Philosophers and ethicists have told us that patients should have the opportunity to choose, and perhaps they should. Perhaps patients should have the opportunity to choose a doctor whom they trust. If a patient does not trust his or her doctor, the patient should find a different doctor. If patients are limited in their choice of doctor by the restrictions of their insurance plans or government programs, perhaps that is where we should reform the health care system, rather than perpetuating the current ritual of informed consent.

Obviously, there are significant counterarguments that support the need for informed consent. At a fundamental level, informed consent is a crucial bulwark against the worst abuses of human rights in the health care system, such as research on human subjects without their consent and sterilization of indigent women without their consent or even without their knowledge. Chapter Six describes some of the most infamous examples of such abuses of human rights, such as the Tuskegee experiment in the United States and the medical experiments by Nazi doctors, abuses that help to explain the modern emphasis on the concept of informed consent. The ethical principle of autonomy protects human dignity by recognizing and assuring the right of the individual to decide what will—and will not—be done to his or her body. Moreover, medical treatment is distinguishable from airline travel on several grounds. Medical treatment is more invasive and more personal than taking a trip on an airplane. Airline pilots share the risks of injury or death with their passengers, whereas physicians and surgeons do not share the risks of injury or death with their patients. It is also important for health care providers to respect patients' values and preferences with regard to issues such as quality versus quantity of life, tolerance for risk, and attitudes toward particular types of treatment such as drugs, blood transfusions, or surgery. The goal of public policy on informed consent is to find a good compromise so that the process used protects the autonomy and dignity of patients but does not require excessive disclosure of potential risks and does not place undue demands on resources that could be used for other aspects of patient care and for treatment of other patients.

IS INFORMED CONSENT A UNIVERSAL PRINCIPLE OR A CULTURAL VALUE?

Many people conclude or assume that autonomy and informed consent are universal principles of human life. In its *World Health Report 2000*, the World Health Organization (WHO) used the criterion of **responsiveness** as a universal value to compare the health systems of different countries. Responsiveness includes both client orientation and respect for persons. **Respect for persons**, in turn, includes autonomy and "helping choose what treatment to receive or not to receive" (World Health Organization, 2000, pp. 31–32). Thus, WHO considered autonomy and the ability to participate in choosing one's treatment as universal values of human life against which every health system in the world should be judged.

We should consider, however, whether autonomy is really a universal value of human existence or a more limited value, applying to a particular culture or group of cultures at a particular point in time. Many observers have recognized that some modern Western cultures are preoccupied with the personal desires of the individual. In some Western countries, people tend to focus on individual rights and individual choice. Western philosophies are based to a large extent on the concept of individual free will. Many Western political systems place a high value on self-determination, as expressed through free elections with one person—one vote. In modern Western societies, bookstores are stocked with volumes offering self-help, and the criteria for mental health are deemed to include self-knowledge, self-esteem, and self-actualization.

Compared to other cultures and other times, many modern Western cultures could be described as preoccupied—or even obsessed—with personal wants and needs, as opposed to the needs of communities. Many Westerners attempt to justify their preoccupation with the individual by insisting that autonomy and self-determination are fundamental components of human dignity. But perhaps these are just culturally based values. Many people in other cultures find human dignity in meeting their responsibilities and fulfilling their roles in their extended family, community, or nation.

As discussed earlier, Katz (1994) has demonstrated that the current concern with informed consent is not a longstanding tradition of medical ethics, even in Western cultures: "Viewed from the perspective of medical history, the doctrine of informed consent, if taken seriously, constitutes a revolutionary break with customary practice" (p. 72). This does not necessarily mean that there is anything wrong with the current doctrine of informed consent. However, it does mean that informed consent is not a universal value for all periods of time and all cultures.

In some cultures, many health care providers do not follow Western practices of informed consent. In fact many people in those cultures would consider Western consent practices to be grossly inappropriate, rude, or even cruel. Akira Akabayashi and colleagues have described cultural practices in Japan, where directly disclosing a diagnosis of terminal disease to a patient may be considered cruel (Akabayashi and Slingsby, 2006; Akabayashi and others, 1999). As these authors explained, patients in Japan may prefer "a family-facilitated approach . . . in which a patient's family communicates with the attending physician and medical staff and often makes treatment-related decisions" (Akabayashi and Slingsby, p. 11). In the city of Doha in the Persian Gulf, a patient may distrust a physician who gives the patient too much information (Rodriguez del Pozo and Fins, 2008, p. 276). Describing the situation in Kashmir, Yousuf and others (2007) explained that "most patients avoid the responsibility of decision-making and defer this role to the family or the doctor. Women, in particular, do not give consent unless they get approval from their husband or the head of the family" (p. 562).

Even within the United States, some groups of immigrants have attitudes about informed consent and disclosure of medical information that are very different from typical U.S. medical practice. In one study, Leslie Blackhall and others (2001) found that most Korean Americans believe cancer patients should not be told their diagnosis and should not be told about a terminal prognosis. These researchers also found that 65 percent of Mexican Americans believe that patients should be told the truth about a diagnosis of cancer, but only 48 percent of this group believe that a person should be told he or she has a terminal condition (p. 61). In traditional Navajo culture, speaking words about a potential adverse result is believed to make it more likely that this result will occur (Marshall and Koenig, 2004, p. 260).

Nevertheless, even when physicians do not disclose complete information to their patients directly, patients in some cultures might be receiving additional information by means that are more subtle and more indirect. Blackhall and others (2001) describe a type of nonverbal communication among some Korean Americans and Mexican Americans that allows them to infer the complete truth from ambiguous statements and from context but that also maintains sensitivity and preserves hope (pp. 67–70). In Doha also, patients obtain information not only from explicit disclosures but also from context and from what is not explicitly stated (Rodriguez del Pozo and Fins, 2008, p. 276). The cultures in which this can occur are characterized as *high-context*, meaning that a large amount of information is provided by and derived from the social environment, reducing the need for the types of explicit disclosures that are necessary in *low-context* cultures, such as those found in Germany and among the majority U.S. society (Blackhall and others, pp. 69–70; Rodriguez del Pozo and Fins, pp. 274–276).

In addition, Akabayashi and others (1999) have described subtle methods of communication in Japanese culture that are ambiguous but also informative to people who understand those particular methods of communication (p. 298). Akabayashi and Slingsby (2006), characterized the Japanese style of informed consent (*informudo consento*) as being consistent with an interdependent view of the self, in which individuals see themselves as part of a set of relationships with family and other groups. "Thus it is considered that patients who hold an interdependent view will feel more comfortable participating in collaborative decision making with their family, friends or medical providers. We further believe that within this collaborative mode, an individual who holds an interdependent construal will tend to entrust decision making to his or her family or medical provider. In effect, patients who entrust their decisions to their family and/or medical provider often do not participate directly in decision making" (p. 12).

Does this mean that the ethical principle of autonomy is not relevant to patients in those cultures? Yousuf and others (2007) concluded that "in certain parts of the world, preserving community norms and family relationships are more important than individual autonomy" (p. 564). Other scholars have disagreed with that conclusion, however. Akabayashi and colleagues reasoned that honoring a patient's preference for a family-facilitated approach to informed consent might be consistent with that patient's self-determination and autonomy. However, this analysis appears to be somewhat circular, and these researchers conceded that the argument requires additional thought (Akabayashi and Slingsby, 2006, p. 13; Akabayashi and others, 1999, p. 300).

In their analysis of informed consent in Doha, Pablo Rodriguez del Pozo and Joseph Fins (2008) reasoned that Middle Eastern patients have their own form of self-determination, although self-determination is different in that type of high-context society in which individuals view themselves as part of their groups, and patients receive information through their family and their context (p. 277). It is unclear from that analysis, however, whether the Middle Eastern patient would make his or her own decision with the information provided by the family or, alternatively, whether that form of self-determination is another circular example of a supposedly autonomous choice to forgo individual autonomy.

Viewed more broadly, this type of research demonstrates the danger of viewing other cultures through the eyes of one's own culture. We may think that we are being open-minded by considering and respecting the ways in which other people appear to do things and think about things. However, we need to be vigilant to avoid analyzing the practices and views of other cultures, including their processes for informed consent, through the lens of our own cultural experience. Finally, Blackhall and others (2001) wisely caution against stereotyping, because the values and attitudes of a cultural group are not necessarily those of any particular individual in the group (p. 70).

SUMMARY

Informed consent is based on the ethical principle of autonomy, or self-determination. Pursuant to that ethical principle, patients have the right to make their own decisions regarding treatment, after receiving all of the necessary information.

However, practical problems arise in attempting to explain medical information and treatment alternatives, even in industrialized countries with relatively well educated populations. In our globalized world, widespread immigration has resulted in additional communication barriers that complicate the process of obtaining informed consent and also create problems in accessing care. Resource limitations pose further problems, especially in developing countries, and raise the question of whether limited staff time should be spent on attempting to comply with international standards for informed consent. This chapter also addressed the question of whether informed consent really matters to patients and evaluated arguments pro and con on that issue. Finally, this chapter analyzed different perspectives on communication and decision making in various cultures and demonstrated the need for more understanding about diverse approaches to autonomy and informed consent.

KEY TERMS

autonomy	respect for persons	responsiveness
informed consent		

DISCUSSION QUESTIONS

1. What are the practical problems of obtaining informed consent in developed countries? How do these problems differ from the practical problems of obtaining informed consent in developing countries?
2. As an ethical matter, should health care providers in a developing country, with severe limitations on resources, spend time attempting to fully comply with international standards on procedures for informed consent?
3. How can health care professionals meet their ethical obligation to provide the information that patients really need and at the same time avoid excessive disclosure of potential risks?

4. How can health care providers meet their ethical obligation to obtain informed consent from patients when those patients see themselves as functioning within a set of relationships rather than acting as autonomous individuals?

ACTIVITY: INFORMED CONSENT AT A RURAL HEALTH FACILITY IN A DEVELOPING COUNTRY

Please assume that you are the director of a government health care facility in a rural area of a developing country. Your facility provides a broad range of outpatient services and is staffed by two physicians, three nurses, and one maintenance worker. The facility is funded by the national government through tax revenues. The facility provides services free of charge to residents of the area, all of whom are extremely poor.

People travel long distances to seek care at the facility. The facility is open 7 days a week, 365 days a year, from 8:00 A.M. to 8:00 P.M.. People regularly arrive each day as early as 6:00 A.M. to join the queue for treatment and are treated on the basis of first-come, first-served. Only 100 people can be seen each day, and every day some potential patients are sent home without being seen.

With the current level of staff, it is not possible to increase the number of patients seen each day or the hours of service. It is not possible for the staff to work any harder or faster than they already are working. Nor is it possible to increase the level of staffing, because the government will not provide any additional funding. Therefore, 100 patients per day is the maximum number that can be seen.

A few months ago one of the physicians at your facility attended a medical conference in the nation's capital, where she heard a presentation about informed consent. She quickly concluded that your facility was not following proper procedures for informed consent, because the vast majority of patients were not advised of the risks, benefits, and alternatives of treatment and were not given an opportunity to make a truly informed choice about their treatment. She raised the issue at a recent staff meeting, where there was a heated discussion about the ethical and practical considerations of attempting to follow international standards on procedures for informed consent. The Code of Ethics of the country's national medical association provides that physicians should obtain the informed consent of their patients, but the Code of Ethics is not enforced and is routinely ignored throughout the country.

The staff members recognize that procedures for informed consent are time consuming and will reduce the amount of time available for other aspects of patient care. Last month your facility conducted some time-and-motion studies to determine the precise impact of adopting various levels of consent procedures. On the basis of those time-and-motion studies, the facility has identified three alternative courses of action, as follows:

1. The first alternative is to fully comply with international standards on procedures for informed consent, including advising each patient of the risks and benefits of the recommended treatment and also the risks and benefits of any potential alternative treatment, allowing time for the patient to ask questions and for the provider to answer those questions, giving the patient the opportunity to make his or her own decision, and documenting all of the foregoing in the patient's record. The time required to perform those tasks would reduce the number of patients treated each day from 100 patients to 80 patients.
2. The second alternative is to adopt an abbreviated consent procedure that would provide some elements of informed consent even though it would not meet international standards on procedures for informed consent. Specifically, physicians at the facility would inform each patient of the purpose of the recommended medical procedure, give the patient an opportunity to accept or reject the procedure, and document those facts in the patient's record. However, the physician would not attempt to explain the risks of the recommended procedure or the risks and benefits of any potential alternative procedure, and the physician would not encourage the patient to ask questions. The time required to perform those tasks would reduce the number of patients treated each day from 100 patients to 95 patients.
3. The third alternative is to continue to follow current practice at the facility and routinely fail to comply with procedures for informed consent. This alternative would allow the facility to continue to serve 100 patients per day.

Remembering that it is not possible to increase the level of staffing, hours of service, or funding of the facility, please evaluate the three alternatives, decide which of them is the most ethical, and explain your reasoning.

CHAPTER THREE

WITHHOLDING OR WITHDRAWING TREATMENT AND PHYSICIAN-ASSISTED SUICIDE

LEARNING OBJECTIVES

- Acquire proficiency in analyzing the ethical issues in making decisions to withhold or withdraw various types of life-sustaining treatment.

- Be able to evaluate the ethical problems that arise when health care professionals help their patients to die, including the problems that arise in developing countries with limited health care resources.

- Understand and be able to explain the value of applying a comparative, multicultural approach to understanding the different views of people in different cultures about terminating care and causing a quicker death.

- Learn how to use and apply a transnational, or cross-border, approach to understanding the phenomenon of *suicide tourism*.

IN an article provocatively titled "You Promised Me I Wouldn't Die Like This," Timothy Quill and Robert Brody (1995) wrote that one of the goals of health care professionals who treat dying patients is to help those patients have a "good death" and avoid a "bad death" (p. 1250). Other experts on medical ethics have agreed with this expansive view of the goals of health care and medicine. In 1996, under the direction of Daniel Callahan of the Hastings Center, experts from fourteen countries considered the fundamental goals of medicine. They concluded that the goals of medicine are not limited to curing disease, relieving pain, and avoiding untimely death but also include helping patients to have a peaceful death (Callahan, 1996, p. S13). In many cases patients who are terminally ill might decide to forgo medical interventions that could prolong their lives because they prefer to die in ways that they hope will be more comfortable, peaceful, and natural (Battin, 1983). According to the experts from fourteen countries, "Medical treatment should be provided in ways that enhance, rather than threaten, the possibility of a peaceful death" (Callahan, 1996, p. S13).

This chapter analyzes the ethical issues that arise at the end of life in making decisions to withhold or withdraw particular types of treatment. It also evaluates the ethical implications when health care professionals take actions that cause patients to die sooner than they would otherwise have died. In some ways the issues in this chapter are related to those in Chapter Two, which analyzed the ethical doctrine of informed consent. As explained in Chapter Two, informed consent is not limited to the patient's right to receive information but also includes the patient's right to accept or decline any particular type of treatment. Chapter Three applies the same principles in the context of life-sustaining treatment or extraordinary means of life support, such as ventilation equipment or artificial nutrition and hydration. In this context the ethical issues can become even more complex, because many patients at the end of life are unable to make their own decisions or effectively communicate their desires.

Under these circumstances, health care professionals encounter serious ethical issues in treating terminally ill patients. As Tom Beauchamp and others (2008) have explained, physicians have become more willing to respect the autonomy of patients when it comes to patients' making their own decisions about treatment at the end of life, but health care professionals are very concerned about the ethical boundaries and the lack of consensus about appropriate professional conduct. These professionals may worry about the ethical implications of withdrawing life support or allowing their patients to decline treatment that would keep them alive (p. 397). Prescribing and administering lethal drugs to dying patients raises even more complex ethical issues. All these issues are analyzed at length in this chapter.

In viewing these issues from a global perspective, this chapter applies a comparative, multicultural approach, as well as a transnational, or cross-border, approach. The comparative, multicultural approach is based on the recognition that attitudes about life and death are influenced strongly by culture and that people in different cultures can have very different views about terminating care or hastening death. Religious beliefs can also affect the views of patients and health care professionals, and thereby lead to different conclusions about the value of life and the significance of suffering.

In fact, people in different cultures can have very different views about when a person is really dead. The traditional criteria for determining death were lack of breathing and lack of circulation, so that patients were considered to be dead when their hearts stopped beating and they were no longer breathing (Truog, 2007). Since the late 1960s, medical science has developed neurological criteria for determining death, as an optional alternative to the traditional cardiorespiratory criteria. This new alternative is referred to as **brain death** and is defined as the permanent loss of all brain functions (Truog, p. 273). Defining death as brain death makes it possible to withdraw ventilation equipment from a hopelessly brain-damaged patient, because the patient is already deemed to be dead before the ventilation equipment is removed. Moreover, diagnosing a patient as brain dead makes it possible to remove donated organs from the dead patient, even though the patient's heart is still beating and the patient is still on ventilation equipment (Truog, pp. 273, 276–277). Religious and cultural groups differ, however, in their willingness to accept the concept of brain death. On the basis of a 1986 Islamic decision, or *fatwa*, Saudi Arabia uses the concept of brain death to permit cadaver organ transplants (Albar, 2007, pp. 634–635). In contrast, some orthodox Jews refuse to accept brain death (Truog, 2007, p. 277). In Japan, "there is no public consensus on whether brain death should be accepted as actual death" ("Recognition of Brain Death," 2009). Japan passed a law to recognize brain death in 2009, but a survey indicated that the Japanese people were divided almost equally on the issue of whether brain death is really death (Brasor, 2009).

Culture and nationality also affect the views of health care professionals on when it is appropriate to terminate medical care. For example, Marisa Rebagliato and others (2000) conducted a cross-cultural analysis in ten European countries about physicians' attitudes and practices in deciding to terminate treatment for seriously ill newborns. They found a lack of consensus on when to stop providing neonatal intensive care, and addressed the personal, cultural, and religious values that underlie the different positions on this issue. As they explained,

> no consensus exists on which patients might be candidates for palliative care rather than for intensive care or on the criteria on which such choices might be based. At one extreme, vitalists support the idea of an absolute intrinsic value of human life (the so-called *sanctity-of-life* position) and reject any form of discontinuation of life-sustaining treatment except for cases of imminent death. In contrast, others believe that the value of life is related to certain

present or future capacities (such as, at a minimum having self-consciousness, the ability to establish a relationship with other human beings, and the capacity to derive some pleasure from existence), which define its *quality*, and hence a physician's duty to sustain it. A number of intermediate positions that may be identified between these 2 extremes have been the source of ongoing discussions [Rebagliato and others, 2000, pp. 2451–2452, footnotes omitted].

After conducting their empirical analysis of physician attitudes and self-reported practices, Rebagliato and others (2000) found that the most important variable for predicting the attitudes and practices of physicians was their country (pp. 2451, 2458).

Such differences among countries in attitudes and practices create an incentive for patients to travel across national borders in order to obtain services more consistent with their individual values. Therefore this chapter also applies a transnational approach to the ethical problems of withdrawal of care and assistance in dying. As discussed in Chapter Ten, some people travel to other countries to obtain treatments not available in their countries of residence, such as a choice of reproductive health services (Cortez, 2008, pp. 77–78). Some patients who are terminally ill want assistance in ending their lives, but their countries of residence might prohibit health care professionals from assisting patients in that manner. Under these circumstances, terminally ill patients might travel to a country that is more flexible about allowing people to assist patients in committing suicide (Ball and Mengewein, 2010). Thus the ethical issues in terminating treatment and assisting dying patients can be analyzed from a global perspective, with both comparative and transnational approaches.

This chapter begins by analyzing the ethical aspects of withholding or withdrawing treatment from patients at the end of life, including both adult patients and seriously ill newborns. Then it evaluates the ethical issues that arise when health care professionals prescribe or administer lethal drugs in an effort to help their patients to die. Finally, the activity at the end of this chapter provides readers with an opportunity to practice developing, for a medical society, an ethics policy about withholding or withdrawing treatment and helping patients to die.

WITHHOLDING OR WITHDRAWING TREATMENT AT THE END OF LIFE

Withholding treatment refers to not beginning a particular treatment, whereas **withdrawing treatment** refers to stopping a treatment that has been started: "Something temporal, by definition, distinguishes withholding from withdrawing: the historical fact of the initiation of therapy" (Sulmasy and Sugarman, 1994, p. 218). In the United States the American Medical Association (AMA) (1996) takes the position that there is "no ethical distinction between withdrawing and withholding life-sustaining treatment." Howard Brody (1995) agrees that there is no useful distinction between withholding and withdrawing, and argues that the purported distinction can distract attention from the ethically relevant issues of the patient's wishes and the effect of the treatment (p. 716).

As an ethical matter, a patient's right to accept or decline particular treatments at the end of life is based on the principle of autonomy (Beauchamp and others, p. 397). In some cases, however, the principle of beneficence might outweigh the patient's interest in autonomy, especially if the proposed treatment would reduce pain or increase functioning without adverse consequences or if the patient were unable to make a rational decision about accepting or declining treatment. Utilitarians would also support efforts that would result in limiting expensive medical treatments for dying patients, on the ground that society would benefit more by allocating money and resources to individuals who could continue to serve the needs of society. Utilitarians might also give less weight to the autonomous choices of individual patients and might support rules of resource allocation that limit medical treatments for all dying patients.

The right of patients to make their own decisions at the end of life is also supported by the professional ethics of health care providers. According to the World Medical Association (2005), "the right to decline medical treatment is a basic right of the patient and the physician does not act unethically even if respecting such a wish results in the death of the patient." In the United States the American Medical Association (1996) agrees that the "principle of patient autonomy requires that physicians respect the decision to forego life-sustaining treatment of a patient who possesses decision-making capacity."

Physicians also have an ethical obligation to provide **palliative care**, care focused on relieving symptoms and reducing pain rather than on continuing any attempt to cure the patient's underlying disease (Stevens and others, 2006). Palliative care presents an ethical conundrum, because the administration of drugs to control pain can also cause some patients to die more quickly than they would otherwise have died. Does this mean that the physician who attempted to relieve the pain has killed the patient? Medical ethics handles this conundrum by distinguishing between intent and foreseeability. One opinion expressed in the AMA's Code of Medical Ethics recognizes that physicians have an ethical duty to relieve the suffering of their patients, and that in some cases such duty includes even "palliative sedation to unconsciousness" (American Medical Association, 2008). In the same opinion the AMA gives this warning to physicians: "Palliative sedation must never be used to intentionally cause a patient's death." However, another opinion in the AMA's Code of Medical Ethics clarifies that physicians' ethical duty to relieve suffering and advance the interests of their dying patients "includes providing effective palliative treatment even though it may foreseeably hasten death" (American Medical Association, 1996). Thus, under the principles of medical ethics in the United States, physicians may prescribe or administer drugs that can reasonably be expected to make their patients die more quickly, so long as the physicians intend only to relieve suffering and do not intend to cause death.

The American Medical Association (1996) includes artificial nutrition and hydration in the category of life-sustaining treatments that patients may decide to forgo, treating artificial nutrition and hydration as a type of medical treatment, in the same category as ventilation equipment or chemotherapy. In contrast, Catholic authorities have taken the position that nutrition and hydration is not a type of medical treatment that can be withdrawn at will but rather is part of basic care, like cleaning a patient and avoiding pressure sores (Graham, 2010). In addition to explaining religious doctrine to Catholics, such official Church positions are binding on health care facilities operated by the Catholic Church, and apply to all patients who are treated in those facilities, regardless of those patients' own religious beliefs (United States Conference of Catholic Bishops, 2009, pp. 4, 11–12). In 2009, the United States Conference of Catholic Bishops issued a new edition of the *Ethical and Religious Directives for Catholic Health Care Services*. Directive 58 of that edition provides as follows:

> In principle, there is an obligation to provide patients with food and water, including medically assisted nutrition and hydration for those who cannot take food orally. This obligation extends to patients in chronic and presumably irreversible conditions (e.g., the "persistent vegetative state") who can reasonably be expected to live indefinitely if given such care. Medically assisted nutrition and hydration become morally optional when they cannot reasonably be expected to prolong life or when they would be "excessively burdensome for the patient or [would] cause significant physical discomfort, for example resulting from complications in the use of the means employed." For instance, as a patient draws close to inevitable death from an underlying progressive and fatal condition, certain measures to provide nutrition and hydration may become excessively burdensome and therefore not obligatory in light of their very limited ability to prolong life or provide comfort [United States Conference of Catholic Bishops, 2009, p. 31, footnotes omitted].

The directives also make it clear that Catholic health care facilities will not comply with patients' requests about life-sustaining procedures when those requests are contrary to positions of the Church. Under these circumstances the ability of patients to decline the use of nutrition and hydration might depend on the ownership of the health care facilities in which they are treated. It is also interesting to note the way in which discussion of these ethical issues can be influenced by the use of particular language or terminology (Tucker and Steele, 2007). The AMA, for example, describes this type of nutrition and hydration as "artificial," whereas the Catholic authorities describe it as "medically assisted" (American Medical Association, 1996; United States Conference of Catholic Bishops, 2009, p. 31).

If health care providers are willing to follow the wishes of a patient, how do they know what the patient wants? Put another way, how do health care providers know which specific life-sustaining measures a patient does want and which ones he or she does not want? Adult patients who are mentally competent and able to communicate can simply speak for themselves about their specific desires. In some cases, patients who are no longer competent or able to communicate will have expressed their desires previously in a written **advance directive**. An advance directive is a "tool for persons to state preferences and name a surrogate decision maker in case they become mentally incapacitated later in life" (Teno, 2004, p. 159). One type of advance directive is the **living will**, in which individuals can list the treatments that they would want and those they would not want in the event they are ever in a particular medical condition. Another type of advance directive is the **health care power of attorney**, sometimes referred to as the **durable power of attorney**, in which individuals can designate someone to make medical decisions on their behalf under specified conditions.

The evidence from empirical research, however, raises serious doubts that advance directives actually have an effect on the care patients receive (Fagerlin and Schneider, 2004, pp. 36–37). Among other practical problems, individuals often do not know what types of medical interventions they would really want if they were to become seriously ill at some time in the future and were no longer competent to make life-or-death decisions (Fagerlin and Schneider, 2004, pp. 33–34). Although many ethicists support the use of advance directives, many patients who are poor or uninsured are concerned about getting enough medical care, rather than avoiding too much care (Blackhall and others, 2001, p. 60). Moreover, attitudes in the United States about the use of advance directives differ among racial, ethnic, and cultural groups, with African Americans, Hispanics, and Asians being less likely than others to use advance directives. It is likely that the lower use of advance directives among African Americans results in large part from cultural values and a distrust of the health care system that is the continuing legacy of systematic discrimination (Searight and Gafford, 2005).

If a patient is incompetent and has made no advance directive, the patient's interests might be represented by a surrogate decision maker, such as the patient's spouse, another family member, or a guardian. The surrogate might try to make the decision that the surrogate believes the patient would have been most likely to make, or alternatively, a decision that the surrogate believes to be in the best interest of the patient. Of course, both of those standards are extremely subjective.

In some circumstances physicians should not comply with the decisions of the surrogate for an incompetent patient. Principles of medical ethics in the United States provide that a physician should ordinarily comply with a decision of a surrogate but not if the physician believes that decision to be inconsistent with the patient's preferences or not in the best interest of the patient (American Medical Association, 1996). In particular, physicians might disagree with a surrogate or family member about whether treatment of a patient has become futile or whether to continue intensive treatment of a seriously ill newborn. In those situations the AMA recommends the use of ethics committees or other institutional procedures to try to resolve disputes between physicians and surrogates or family members (American Medical Association, 1994b, 1997).

According to M. Albar (2007), a scholar in Saudi Arabia, a fatwa has been issued in that country that authorizes physicians to stop resuscitation on the basis of medical criteria, regardless of the wishes of family members. That fatwa provides as follows:

> Q.6. If the treating physicians decided that resuscitation will be useless in a certain patient, is it permissible not to resuscitate even though the patient or his relatives asked for resuscitative measures to be carried on?

> A.6. If resuscitative measures are deemed useless and inappropriate for a certain patient in the opinion of three competent specialist physicians, then there is no need for resuscitative measures to be carried out. The opinion of the patient or his relatives should not be considered, as it is a medical decision and it is not in their capacity to reach such a decision [Albar, 2007, pp. 635–636].

In a study of physicians who worked in two neonatal intensive care units (NICUs) in India, the physicians disagreed among themselves about whether the parents of seriously ill newborns should even be involved in making decisions about withdrawing treatment from their children. In the context of poverty and low levels of education, some of those parents refused to make decisions and accepted whatever the physicians recommended. As one of the physicians asked, "How do you explain 'brain-dead' to a person who does not understand what a 'brain' is?" (Miljeteig and Norheim, 2006, pp. 28–29). Thus issues of culture and context can strongly influence the withholding or withdrawal of care.

Is it ethical for physicians and other health care professionals to consider the interests of the patient's family, other patients, or society at large in deciding whether to withhold or withdraw treatment from a particular patient? Some people would argue that the only relevant factors should be the desires or best interests of the patient. Others would disagree, and opinions on this issue appear to depend, at least in part, on culture and on limitations of health care resources. In the study of ethical issues at NICUs in India, some physicians reported that they considered the effect that continuing treatment would have on other members of the patient's family, because the high costs of treating that patient could deprive siblings of food and education (Miljeteig and Norheim, 2006, pp. 28, 30). Some of the physicians in that study also pointed out that India is different from Western countries, where financial resources and social safety nets provide a basis for guidelines that may seem unrealistic in resource-poor developing countries (p. 28). Miljeteig and Norheim (2006) explain that view as follows:

> Western doctors and literature focus on issues like the quality of life, over-treatment, the child's future and suffering in decision making in neonatology. Our informants put little weight on these considerations when encouraged to talk about ethics in neonatology. They focused less on the individual child, more on the consequences for others when treating or not treating the child. They knew their decisions would influence the family's economy and reputation, the chance of siblings receiving sufficient food and education, other children's access to the unit's equipment and resources, and all in the context of a population that was largely indigent [p. 31].

These authors offer a blanket characterization of Western ethical views; however, there appears to be a significant difference between the views of physicians in Europe and physicians in the United States. A study in ten European countries of physicians who work at NICUs found that a majority of these physicians in all these countries considered the burden on a patient's family to be a relevant factor in deciding whether to withhold or withdraw treatment from a seriously ill newborn (Rebagliato and others, 2000, p. 2454.) In contrast, in the United States, the ethical principles of the AMA do not even mention the burden on the family as a relevant factor in making these treatment decisions, saying instead that the "primary consideration for decisions regarding life-sustaining treatment for seriously ill newborns should be what is best for the newborn" (American Medical Association, 1994b). The U.S. approach thus appears to be different from the attitude in many European countries, although it may be problematic to compare self-reported attitudes in Europe with written ethical opinions in the United States. Moreover, the AMA's use of the phrase "primary consideration," which is not defined in the AMA's Code of Medical Ethics, might provide an opening in the United States for consideration of some secondary factors, such as the burden on the family, after considering the best interest of the individual patient.

ASSISTING PATIENTS IN COMMITTING SUICIDE

In evaluating the ethical arguments about helping patients to die, it is important to begin by clarifying the terminology and definitions. Different writers use the same terms to mean very different things. Moreover, as Kathryn Tucker and Fred Steele (2007) have noted, particular language, such as **euthanasia** and **physician-assisted suicide (PAS)**, can be used to influence discussion of these controversial issues (pp. 309–313). According to Tucker and Steele, the term *physician-assisted suicide* is "inflammatory," "pejorative," and "an inaccurate, value-laden term that colors the discussion" (p. 312).

Some people use the term *euthanasia* to refer to situations in which a physician actually administers a lethal drug, and use the term *physician-assisted suicide* to refer to situations in which a physician provides a drug that the patient self-administers (Pickett, 2009, p. 335). In contrast, Beauchamp and others (2008) use the term *euthanasia* to refer to causing the death of someone who is terminally ill or suffering intolerably, whether the death is caused by active means, such as lethal injection, or passive means, such as not taking action to prevent death (p. 398). Beauchamp and others also use the term *physician-assisted suicide* to refer to death with the help of a doctor, whether the patient is terminally ill or not terminal but suffering intolerably. Löfmark and others (2008), in their survey of physician experiences in six European countries and Australia, combined the terms *euthanasia* and *physician-assisted suicide* into a single category that included prescribing, supplying, or administering lethal drugs.

In light of this disagreement among experts, this chapter will try to facilitate discussion of the ethical issues by not using the term *euthanasia* at all. In addition, this chapter will use the term *physician-assisted suicide* to refer to helping a patient to die, either by administering a lethal drug or by providing a drug that the patient self-administers. Moreover, even though the term *physician-assisted suicide* refers explicitly to physicians, it is important to recognize that a request by a patient for help in dying also presents ethical dilemmas for nurses, allied health professionals, pharmacists, and the managers of health care institutions. The term *physician-assisted suicide* is used for convenience but with the understanding that the ethical issues are not limited to doctors of medicine.

Is it ethical for physicians or other health care professionals to help their patients to die? The ethical principle of autonomy supports the right of patients to make their own decisions about life and death. As Ronald Dworkin wrote, "every competent person has the right to make momentous personal decisions which invoke fundamental religious or philosophical convictions about life's value for himself" (Dworkin, 1997, p. 41). In addition, John Arras (1997) has described other arguments for PAS on the basis of mercy, the utilitarian goals of increasing happiness and reducing unhappiness, and the duty of physicians to reduce suffering (pp. 365–366). A principlist might characterize some of those latter arguments as part of the ethical duty of beneficence.

In response, some people argue that killing is simply unethical, and others argue that even if nonphysicians can ethically participate in assisted suicide, members of the medical profession should not (Arras, 1997, pp. 367–368). The World Medical Association (2005) has declared explicitly that PAS is unethical. Although some U.S. physicians disagree, the AMA has taken the position that PAS "is fundamentally incompatible with the physician's role as healer, would be difficult or impossible to control, and would pose serious societal risks" (American Medical Association, 1994a).

The difficulty of controlling PAS is often expressed as a problem of the "slippery slope" (Beauchamp and others, 2008, p. 401), and both Dworkin and Arras have described two separate slippery slope problems that might arise in the event that PAS were to be allowed (Dworkin, 1997, p. 41; Arras, 1997, pp. 368–373). These problems can be thought of as the theoretical slippery slope and the practical slippery slope (Dworkin, p. 41). The theoretical slippery slope refers to the difficulty of limiting PAS to those groups of people for whom it would be appropriate. Proponents of PAS usually argue for a right to PAS only for mentally competent and terminally ill adults. In addition, some people would add the limitation that the patient must be in unbearable pain. However, as Arras has correctly pointed out, the rationale for PAS is based on autonomy and mercy, and that rationale could be applied to other groups of patients as well (p. 369).

The practical slippery slope refers to the difficulty of enforcing any regulations that might be established in order to prevent abuse in individual cases. If PAS were to be allowed, governments would adopt regulations to make sure that each individual request for PAS was voluntary and that there was no other reasonable alternative for that patient. However, Arras (1997) expressed serious doubts that governments could really ensure that all requests for PAS would be voluntary or that all other alternatives would be explored, especially for poor and minority patients (p. 371). Arras also worried about coercion by family members, physicians, or insurance companies, as well as the inability of many physicians to diagnose and treat clinical depression (pp. 371–373). Although Arras recognized that PAS might be justified in some specific cases, he described the controversy over allowing PAS as posing a "tragic choice" in which either alternative would result in "victims" (pp. 386–387). Therefore, Arras argued in favor of retaining current prohibitions against PAS while making major changes in methods of care for dying patients (pp. 365, 387–388).

In contrast, Dworkin (1997) argued in favor of allowing PAS and reasoned that under a system of regulated PAS, with prerequisites of palliative care, poor patients would have more access to care than they have at the present time (pp. 41–42).

> More of them could then benefit from relief that is already available—illegally—to more fortunate people who have established relationships with doctors willing to run the risks of helping them to die. The current two-tier system—a chosen death and an end of pain outside the law for those with connections and stony refusals for most other people—is one of the greatest scandals of contemporary medical practice. The sense many middle-class people have that if necessary their own doctor "will know what to do" helps to explain why the political pressure is not stronger for a fairer and more open system in which the law acknowledges for everyone what influential people now expect for themselves [Dworkin, 1997, p. 41].

Finally, Dworkin (1997) has disputed the distinction between the act of performing PAS and the omission of withholding life support and passively allowing a patient to die, commenting that "such suggestions wholly misunderstand the 'common-sense' distinction, which is not between acts and omissions, but between acts or omissions that are designed to cause death and those that are not" (p. 42). If it is ethical to withhold or withdraw life support with the intent of causing death, it is also ethical to provide or administer a drug with a similar intent.

For several years, Oregon was the only U.S. state that permitted physician-assisted suicide, but the State of Washington began to permit PAS in 2009 (Yardley, 2009), and the State of Montana has taken a limited step toward permitting PAS (Johnson, 2009). Some other countries, particularly in Europe, have been more flexible about allowing PAS. These differences among countries in attitudes and practices regarding PAS facilitate cross-cultural comparisons on this complex ethical issue. In addition, these differences create an incentive for some patients to cross national borders, in order to obtain assistance in dying that they could not obtain in their home countries. For example, in a somewhat bizarre form of medical tourism, some individuals have traveled to

Switzerland for help in dying, in what has been described as *suicide tourism* (Ball and Mengewein, 2010).

The excerpt from an article by Löfmark and colleagues that follows describes a survey of physicians in six European countries and Australia that looked at their experiences with decision making at the end of life. These authors found important differences among physicians in the various countries in their experiences with and attitudes on end-of-life issues.

EXCERPT FROM "PHYSICIANS' EXPERIENCES WITH END-OF-LIFE DECISION-MAKING: SURVEY IN 6 EUROPEAN COUNTRIES AND AUSTRALIA"

BY RURIK LÖFMARK AND OTHERS

Background

...End-of-life decisions (ELDs) include decisions about withholding or withdrawing potentially life-prolonging treatment and about alleviation of pain or other symptoms with a possible life-shortening effect. In some countries it is also permissible to make decisions about euthanasia or physician-assisted suicide (EAS), defined as the administration, prescription or supply of drugs to end life at the patient's explicit request.

ELDs occur throughout the world, albeit at different rates for different actions....

Methods

In each country, a random sample of 300 physicians was drawn from the professional registers of specialties in which physicians frequently attend to dying patients... In addition to background characteristics and palliative care education, physicians were asked about: their attitudes, intended behaviour and practices concerning end-of-life care; communication with terminally ill competent patients and their families; and experiences of making ELDs. The ELDs were described as neutrally and factually as possible in order to avoid differences in interpretation. EAS, for instance,... [was] formulated as "administering, prescribing or supplying drugs with the explicit intention of hastening the end of life on the explicit request of a patient"....

For each country, the percentage of physicians who had (a) performed an ELD, (b) never performed an ELD, but would be willing to do so under certain conditions, (c) never performed an ELD and would never do so and (d) ever received an explicit request from a patient to administer, prescribe or supply drugs with the explicit intention of hastening death are presented . . . .

Discussion

There are differences between physicians in the countries under study regarding experiences with ELDs, willingness to perform ELDs and frequency with which requests for EAS are received. In general, physicians in Italy have least experience with these issues, followed at some distance by Sweden, while physicians in the Netherlands have the most experience. Foregoing treatment and alleviation of pain and symptoms by intensifying medication to a level which risks hastening death are accepted by physicians in all countries, since only a small minority have never performed them and would never do so. These are also the ELDs that were found to occur most frequently in the first EURELD (death certificate) study . . . .

Although reasons for the differences between countries can only be speculative, in the Netherlands the reason that physicians have more experience with ELDs may be a more liberal tradition and higher respect for patient autonomy. A religious influence is not evident, as Belgium, with a substantial Catholic population, has the second highest experience with ELD, and Sweden, which is a Protestant country, has the lowest together with Italy, a Catholic country. Denmark, which also has a Protestant population, is closest to Belgium. The results do indicate that a non-religious philosophy of life seems to increase the willingness to perform EAS, possibly out of respect for patient autonomy . . . .

Physicians can only perform EAS when a patient requests it. Physicians in all countries receive euthanasia requests, most often in the Netherlands, where physicians also have most experience with performing EAS.

The results show that physicians with training in palliative care are more inclined to make ELDs. While this may be expected for some of the ELDs, it is somewhat surprising for EAS. One hypothesis may be that palliative care physicians develop a higher attention to patients' wishes. Further research is needed to clarify and explain this finding.

Furthermore, the findings indicate that the legislation and medical guidelines are reflected in physicians' experiences. In all countries, physicians had the highest experiences of non-treatment decisions and alleviation of pain and other symptoms with possible life-shortening effect: kinds of ELDs, which are legal in all participating countries. The fact that experiences of continuous deep sedation, which is legal in all countries, . . . [are] relatively low, demonstrates that this ELD is more strongly influenced by situational factors such as uncontrollable pain and symptoms than by legal regulations. The different legal regulations concerning EAS are also reflected in physicians' experiences. Shortly before this study was performed, the Netherlands and Belgium changed their legislation, in 2001 and 2002, and now permit EAS under certain conditions. In the Netherlands EAS are regulated as two possible end-of-life options. In Belgium the law only regulates euthanasia. In both countries the patient involved must be a mentally competent adult when requesting help. Doctors can only proceed when they know the patient well enough to be able to assess whether their request for euthanasia is voluntary and well-considered, whether the patients' medical situation is without prospect of improvement and whether the individual's suffering is unbearable. The ability to refuse a request for euthanasia guarantees a doctor's freedom of conscience in both countries. Whether this has influenced experiences and attitudes remains to be studied in Belgium. For the Netherlands, the evaluation of the euthanasia law showed that the incidence of EAS decreased from 2.8% in 2001 to 1.8% in 2005.

In Switzerland, assistance in suicide is allowed provided that the person seeking assistance has decisional capacity and the person assisting is not motivated by reasons of self-interest; euthanasia is forbidden in all circumstances. Experiences with ELDs can be associated with two types of factors. One is the opportunity the physician has for making ELDs. The second is the attitude of the physician towards questions about philosophy of life, e.g. whether people have a right to decide to hasten the end of life and whether physicians should always aim at preserving life. Older physicians may have been practising medicine longer and thereby have an increased chance of ever having performed an ELD. Further, the number of terminal patients attended to by the physician within a given time period varies from one specialty to another. However, since having had palliative care training is positively associated with having experience with all ELDs, independent of the number of terminal patients under the physician's care, this factor probably reflects an attitude. Female physicians have less experience with ELDs, which does not seem to be related to opportunity and attitude. A similar finding comes from Italy, where male anaesthesiologists had greater experience with foregoing treatment. However, the reason is not obvious and ought to be studied in the future.

Conclusion

In conclusion, there are differences between countries in experiences with ELDs, in willingness to perform ELDs and in receiving requests for EAS. Foregoing treatment and intensifying alleviation of pain and symptoms are practiced and accepted by most physicians in all countries. Physicians with training in palliative care are more inclined to perform ELDs, as are those who attend to higher numbers of terminal patients. Thus, this seems not to be only a matter of opportunity, but also a matter of attitude....

The comparative or cross-cultural perspective on physician-assisted suicide raises one final question. Should PAS be permitted by developing countries, where health care resources are very limited and the burden of disease is very high? In an article titled "Recommending Euthanasia for a Developing Country," Bolatito Lanre-Abass (2008), a Nigerian scholar, discussed the standard arguments for and against PAS and argued in favor of permitting what she termed *physician assisted death* (PAD) in Nigeria. Lanre-Abass recognized that "[s]ome may attribute legalizing PAD to failure on the part of the government to provide the health care facilities needed by the Nigerian populace" (p. 154). In fact, that is a legitimate concern in the context of a developing county, where some patients might choose PAS because their country lacks the resources to treat their curable disease or provide appropriate palliative care for their incurable disease. Under these circumstances, permitting PAS while failing to increase the capacity of the health system would essentially be telling patients that they have no real alternative to choosing PAS.

Lanre-Abass (2008) also recognized the potential difficulty of obtaining truly voluntary consent to PAS in the context of a culture that involves the whole family in medical decisions. Another potential impediment to voluntary consent in these circumstances is a relatively low level of education for many members of the society. Finally, Lanre-Abass acknowledged the concern expressed by some opponents of PAS about potential abuse of PAS in a developing county, where economic problems might unduly influence patients and their families (p. 155). Despite these concerns, in this article Lanre-Abass favored permitting PAS in Nigeria and argued that government regulation can protect against the possibility of abuse. The counterargument, of course, is that effective regulation of PAS, or any other activity, is difficult enough in industrialized countries. It is unlikely that regulation could effectively prevent abuse of PAS in the context of a developing country.

SUMMARY

When experts from fourteen countries considered the fundamental goals of medicine, they recognized that "every society will have to work out moral and medical standards for the appropriate cessation of life-sustaining medical treatment of the terminally ill" (Callahan, 1996, p. S14). This chapter applied a comparative, multicultural approach in order to understand the diverse ways in which people in different societies are attempting to resolve these complex ethical issues of care at the end of life. People in different cultural and religious groups may have different views about brain death, withdrawal of nutrition and hydration, and prescribing or administering lethal drugs. Similarly, in making decisions to withhold or withdraw treatment from a seriously ill newborn, physicians in different countries and cultures may have different attitudes about the relevance of factors such as the needs of families, other patients, and society. Finally, these differences in attitudes and practices have created an incentive for patients to cross national borders in order to obtain services that are more consistent with their individual values.

KEY TERMS

advance directive

brain death

durable power of attorney

euthanasia

health care power of attorney

living will

palliative care

physician-assisted suicide (PAS)

withdrawing treatment

withholding treatment

DISCUSSION QUESTIONS

1. In the treatment of terminally ill patients, is it logical to permit physicians to provide palliative sedation that is given with the intent of relieving suffering but that also can be reasonably expected to make a patient die more quickly, while prohibiting physicians from using palliative sedation with the intent of causing the death of a patient?

2. Is nutrition and hydration a type of life-sustaining medical treatment, in the same category as ventilation equipment, or is nutrition and hydration part of basic care like cleaning a patient?

3. Is it ethical for health care professionals to prescribe or administer lethal drugs to help their patients to die more quickly? If so, under what circumstances would it be ethical?

4. If a country permits physician-assisted suicide (PAS), is it ethical to allow people from other countries to come to that country in order to obtain assistance in committing suicide? Would it be ethical to prohibit them from doing so?

5. Should PAS be permitted by developing countries where health care resources are severely limited?

ACTIVITY: DEVELOPING AN ETHICS POLICY ON WITHHOLDING OR WITHDRAWING TREATMENT AND PAS

Please assume that you are a physician in a Latin American country. You are an active member of the National Medical Society (NMS) in your country, and a member of that society's ethics committee. The ethics committee of the NMS is in the process of developing an ethics policy about withholding or withdrawing treatment and PAS. These issues have been discussed informally, but this is the first time that the NMS has tried to develop a written policy on these issues.

Some aspects of these topics are very controversial in your country. The population of your country is diverse and multicultural. Two religious organizations are very influential, but many people in your country take a secular approach to such issues. The membership of the NMS reflects the diversity of background and opinion in the population as a whole.

The NMS staff have prepared the following draft ethics policy. The members of the ethics committee must now evaluate it and make any changes they consider appropriate. The revised policy will then be presented to the membership of the NMS, which can approve or reject the policy by majority vote.

Please evaluate each of the seven provisions of the draft policy and analyze whether each provision is the most ethical approach to the particular issue with which it deals. If you think that another approach would be more ethical, please make the specific changes that you consider to be appropriate. Be prepared to explain your conclusions and reasoning about each provision.

Draft of the NMS Ethics Policy on Withholding or Withdrawing Treatment and PAS

1. Every competent adult patient has the right to refuse medical treatment, including life-sustaining medical treatment. Every surrogate for an incompetent patient or for a patient under the age of 18 years old has the same right to refuse treatment that the patient would have had if he or she were mentally competent or over the age of 18.

2. Ordinarily, physicians should comply with the decision of a patient or a patient's surrogate. However, a physician should not comply with the decision of a patient or surrogate if the physician concludes that the patient or surrogate lacks sufficient education or understanding to make an informed decision. Moreover, a physician should not comply with the decision of a surrogate when the physician believes that decision is not in the best interest of the patient or is not consistent with the patient's preferences as understood by the physician.

3. Artificial nutrition and hydration is a type of life-sustaining medical treatment, in the same category as ventilation equipment or chemotherapy. Therefore patients and their surrogates have the right to refuse artificial nutrition and hydration.

4. Physician-assisted suicide (PAS) is unethical, whether the physician administers the lethal drug or prescribes or supplies the lethal drug for the patient to self-administer. In other words, it is ethical to refrain from providing life-sustaining medical treatment and to passively allow the patient to die naturally, but it is unethical to take action that causes the death of a patient.

5. Physicians may prescribe or administer drugs, including palliative sedation, that can reasonably be expected to make their seriously ill patients die more quickly, so long as the physicians intend to relieve suffering and do not intend to cause death.

6. In determining whether life-sustaining medical treatment should be withheld or withdrawn from seriously ill newborns, the primary factor shall be the best interest of the newborn. Determining the best interest of the newborn includes an evaluation of the newborn's quality of life, as measured by whether the newborn's potential for happiness is outweighed by the potential for suffering. After considering the primary factor of the newborn's best interest, physicians should also consider additional factors, including the interests of the patient's family, other patients, and society at large, in deciding whether to withhold or withdraw treatment from that newborn. When specialized equipment for seriously ill newborns is scarce or limited, physicians may consider the need for that equipment by other seriously ill newborns and may withhold or withdraw that equipment from

one newborn in order to make it available to another newborn who has a more favorable prognosis.

7. It is unethical for physicians to participate in withholding or withdrawing life-sustaining treatment from a patient who is a resident of another country if the patient's country of residence would not permit treatment to be withheld or withdrawn under the circumstances of that patient's case.

CHAPTER FOUR

ETHICAL ISSUES IN REPRODUCTIVE HEALTH

LEARNING OBJECTIVES

- Understand and demonstrate an appreciation of the ways in which abortion is viewed and has been viewed in different times, places, and cultures.

- Be able to analyze the ethical issues of abortion, including whether the viability of the fetus is an ethically valid distinction.

- Learn how to evaluate whether ethical theories are really helpful in resolving the morality of abortion.

- Acquire proficiency in analyzing the ethical issues that arise in assisted reproductive technology, embryonic stem cell research, emergency contraception, and restrictions on funding that are based on the donor's ethical views about reproductive health issues.

- Be prepared to debate whether it is ethical for health care professionals and institutions to refuse to perform—or make a referral for—a service to which they object on ethical grounds.

EW aspects of human experience are influenced so strongly by culture and religion as the ethical issues of reproduction. Thus it is useful to begin analysis of this sensitive and controversial topic by acknowledging a healthy respect for the views and beliefs of others. This chapter attempts to present a range of diverse views and perspectives in an objective and nonjudgmental format. The goal of this chapter is not to try to persuade people to change their position on abortion. Rather, the goals are to analyze the ethical issues of abortion in a global context, and encourage people to think about and articulate the reasons for their positions on various ethical issues of global reproductive health.

It is also important to recognize that commonly used labels for people and groups on each side of the abortion debate can be very self-serving and misleading. People who are antiabortion like to describe themselves as being *pro-life*, as if to imply that people on the other side of the debate are *antilife*. Yet some of the people who oppose abortion because they are pro-life also support the death penalty. Meanwhile, people who support the right to abortion describe themselves as *pro-choice*, as if to imply that their opponents are against the fundamental value of freedom of choice. These labels may be used for convenience in discussion, but it is important to remember that they carry a lot of baggage and can be very misleading.

In the context of global public health, abortion and other reproductive health issues are not merely matters of abstract ethical theory. Rather, these issues have important practical consequences for the health and lives of millions of people throughout the world. In analyzing the ethics of abortion, it is particularly important to recognize the harm caused by unsafe abortions. Writing about abortion in Iran, Larijani and Zahedi (2006) acknowledged that illegal abortions are performed in Iran, as in other countries around the world (p. 130). As these authors also noted, "An estimated 68,000 women die as a consequence of unsafe abortions each year all over the world. Estimates of the World Health Organization for the year 2000 indicate that 19 million unsafe abortions take place every year and almost all of them occur in developing countries. Experience in some countries has shown that if abortion is legalized, related maternal deaths drop significantly" (p. 131, footnotes omitted). These practical consequences must be taken into account in evaluating the ethics of abortion and other reproductive health issues.

This chapter begins by describing how abortion has been viewed in different times, places, and cultures. Next, it analyzes the ethical issues of abortion, such as whether the morality of abortion really depends on the status of a fetus as a human being. The chapter also evaluates the ethical implications of assisted reproductive technology and embryonic stem cell research. Then the ethical aspects of emergency contraception are addressed in detail. That part of the chapter begins by analyzing the issues of whether the use of emergency contraception is ethical and whether it is ethical to require people to obtain a prescription from a physician before having access to emergency contraception. This leads to the further ethical issue of whether health care professionals or facilities may refuse to participate in or to provide a referral for emergency contraception—or any other health service—if the health care professional or facility objects to that service on ethical grounds. Finally, the chapter concludes by evaluating whether it is ethical for governments and other groups that are external donors to impose restrictions on funding for health services in developing and transitional countries when those restrictions are based on the donor's ethical views on reproductive health issues. An activity provides an opportunity to evaluate that specific issue in the context of emergency contraception in a developing country.

ETHICS OF ABORTION IN DIFFERENT TIMES, PLACES, AND CULTURES

Abortion has been viewed very differently in different times, places, and cultures. In some countries and cultures, abortion is practiced as a fairly common method of birth control, and many married women will have more than one abortion during their lifetimes. Other countries and cultures take a very different and more restrictive view of abortion.

When the U.S. Supreme Court considered the constitutional issue of abortion in its landmark decision in *Roe* v. *Wade* (1973), it reviewed the history of ethical views as well as legal views in other times and cultures. The Court discussed the Hippocratic Oath, which includes an explicit pledge by physicians to refrain from performing abortions. Despite its prohibition against abortion, the Hippocratic Oath did not prevent the practice of abortion in ancient times, and many modern physicians do not consider performing an abortion to violate the basic principles of medical ethics. The Supreme Court relied on the writings of Ludwig Edelstein to conclude that the Hippocratic Oath was merely the position of one school of ancient thought (the Pythagoreans) and was not followed by all physicians in ancient times. Later, the Hippocratic Oath gained in popularity, when ideas similar to those of the Pythagoreans were spread by followers of Christianity. As the following excerpt from the *Roe* v. *Wade* decision shows, the Court reviewed the development of ancient views, Christian doctrine, and the concept of "mediate animation."

> Early philosophers believed that the embryo or fetus did not become formed and begin to live until at least 40 days after conception for a male, and 80 to 90 days for a female. Aristotle's thinking derived from his three-stage theory

of life: vegetable, animal, rational. The vegetable stage was reached at conception, the animal at "animation," and the rational soon after live birth. This theory, together with the 40/80 day view, came to be accepted by early Christian thinkers.

The theological debate was reflected in the writings of St. Augustine, who made a distinction between embryo inanimatus, not yet endowed with a soul, and embryo animatus. He may have drawn upon Exodus 21:22. At one point, however, he expressed the view that human powers cannot determine the point during fetal development at which the critical change occurs.

Galen, in three treatises related to embryology, accepted the thinking of Aristotle and his followers. Later, Augustine on abortion was incorporated by Gratian into the Decretum, published about 1140. This Decretal and the Decretals that followed were recognized as the definitive body of canon law until the new Code of 1917 . . . . [Roe v. Wade, 1973, footnote 22, citations omitted].

. . . This [the point at which the embryo or fetus became "formed"] was "mediate animation." Although Christian theology and the canon law came to fix the point of animation at 40 days for a male and 80 days for a female, a view that persisted until the 19th century, there was otherwise little agreement about the precise time of formation or animation. There was agreement, however, that prior to this point the fetus was to be regarded as part of the mother, and its destruction, therefore, was not homicide [Roe v. Wade, 1973, part VI, citations omitted].

In the mid-nineteenth century a backlash against abortion in the United States was caused in large part by anti-immigrant bias (Mohr, 1979, pp. 86, 166–167, 182–184). Abortion was much more common among Protestant women who had been born in the United States than it was among Catholic women who had immigrated to the United States. Protestant clergy had not been strongly opposed to abortion. However, opposition to the practice of abortion in America grew as a result of bias against immigrants and Catholics. As James Mohr (1979) explained, "There can be little doubt that Protestants' fears about not keeping up with the reproductive rates of Catholic immigrants played a greater role in the drive for anti-abortion laws in nineteenth century America than Catholic opposition to abortion did" (p. 167).

In Latin America, abortion and other reproductive issues are strongly affected by Catholic teachings and by the authority of the Catholic Church (Diniz and others, 2007). In addition to teaching its view that abortion is unethical, the

Church has the power to excommunicate legislators, judges, and health care professionals who support the practice of abortion (Diniz and others, p. ii).

Religion also influences the views and practices of abortion in Islamic countries. In "Changing Parameters for Abortion in Iran," Larijani and Zahedi (2006) discussed the Islamic view of abortion and explained that abortion laws differ among Islamic countries. As these authors explained the Islamic view, the fetus is *ensouled* and becomes a human being at 120 days (p. 130). This does not mean that abortion is freely permitted before 120 days, but it does mean that the punishment will be less when an abortion is performed before 120 days. However, caution is required in generalizing about this or assuming the existence of a single Islamic view. There might not be a single Islamic view of abortion, just as there is not a single Christian view of abortion.

In Japan, abortion is not as controversial as it is in the United States. Nevertheless, many Japanese are Buddhists, and Buddhism opposes all killing. How can Japanese Buddhists accept—or even tolerate—abortion, in light of the Buddhist view about killing? William LaFleur (1990, 1995), a professor of Japanese studies, has described the use of Buddhist rituals in Japan to help the faithful deal with the occasional need for abortion. According to LaFleur's explanation (1990), Japanese Buddhists accept abortion as a "necessary sorrow" (p. 2). This is similar to what Westerners would call a necessary evil, but in Japan it is more a matter of sadness than a matter of sin. LaFleur's explanation is fascinating, and it describes a beautiful worldview about the process of birth and death. As LaFleur explains it, Japanese Buddhists view life as fluid or liquid. Life flows into a fetus, which becomes more dense as it progresses from the world of gods and Buddhas toward its birth in the world of humans. In contrast, death is nothing more than a process of becoming less dense and moving back to the world of gods and Buddhas. There is no specific point at which life begins or ends. In this comforting worldview, abortion is merely preventing the fetus from completing its current process of densification, and allowing the fetus to wait for densification and birth in the future. An aborted fetus is referred to as a *mizuko* ("water child").

The parents of an aborted fetus experience sadness over their decision to prevent the birth. However, according to LaFleur (1990), Japanese Buddhism provides a way for the parents to deal with their sadness by performing specific rituals for the fetus. In addition, the parents recognize that the birth of the aborted fetus has only been delayed. By performing these rituals, called *mizuko kuyo*, the parents can relieve their grief, apologize for the delay in rebirth, and wish the fetus a better opportunity for rebirth in the future.

However, professor of religion George Tanabe (1994, 1995) thinks that LaFleur is totally wrong. He writes that there is no evidence for LaFleur's conclusions about Japanese Buddhism. According to Tanabe (1995), Buddhists cannot avoid the explicit prohibition against killing by pretending that abortion is not killing. Moreover, according to Tanabe, the rituals LaFleur described are not limited to abortion and are seldom performed by Japanese women who have had abortions.

So, where does that leave us? The bottom line, and perhaps the most important take-home message from this part of the chapter, is that we need to take descriptions of abortion in other cultures and other times with a very large grain of salt. Sometimes, people see what they want to see in examining and describing abortion in other countries and at times in the past. This *observer bias* may result, at least in part, from the observer's political or social agenda. In addition, there is often a disparity between official policy and actual practice. Abortion might be officially prohibited but nevertheless tolerated as a practical matter. In other situations, abortion may be officially lawful but not available for many women as a practical matter, due to financial or geographical limitations. This does not mean that we should refrain from trying to study and understand abortion in other cultures and other times. Rather, it means that we need to keep these limitations and potential biases in mind.

CURRENT ETHICAL ISSUES IN ABORTION

This part of the chapter begins by considering why neither side in the abortion debate seems to be able to compromise. Then it considers whether the morality of abortion really depends on the status of a fetus as a human being and whether *viability* of the fetus is really an ethically valid distinction. Finally, this part evaluates whether ethical theories are really helpful in resolving the morality of abortion.

Many advocacy organizations, spokespersons, commentators, and politicians take extreme positions on one side or the other of the abortion debate. In contrast, some ordinary citizens might be willing to compromise on this issue to some extent. Some ordinary citizens who are generally opposed to abortion might be willing to tolerate abortion in some limited circumstances, even when abortion is not absolutely necessary to save the life of the mother. Some ordinary citizens who generally favor choice in abortion might be willing to tolerate restrictions on the availability of abortion in some limited circumstances. Does it have to be all one way or the other? Is there no room for compromise on this issue?

The difficulty of compromise is not limited to the issue of abortion. On many issues of public policy, advocates on each side worry about the "slippery slope." Advocates worry that if they give up a little now it will force them to give up more in the future. Some people refer to this phenomenon as "the thin edge of the wedge," or "the camel's nose under the tent." This concern over the slippery slope certainly applies to the debate over abortion. Pro-choice organizations worry that allowing any further regulation of abortion would lead us down the slippery slope to more regulation and ultimately prohibition of abortion. Opponents of abortion worry that if exceptions were made to allow abortion in some circumstances the result would be that the exceptions would swallow the rule.

However, when it comes to the debate over abortion, perhaps it is more than merely concern over the slippery slope. Maybe there is another reason that many advocates are unwilling to compromise. As discussed in the following paragraphs, it may be impossible for advocates on either side to compromise without undermining what they perceive to be the ethical basis for their position.

Imagine a scenario in which a pro-choice advocate and an antiabortion advocate talk to each other in an attempt to reach a compromise. The pro-choice advocate says to the opponent of abortion: "I know that you are opposed to abortion. I understand that you think abortion is morally wrong. But surely, *even you* would be willing to permit abortion in the very limited circumstance when a fifteen-year-old girl is raped by a member of her family?" The antiabortion advocate responds: "Oh, that's terrible. A fifteen-year-old girl was raped by a member of her family. That's just horrible. Let me think about it. Can I make an exception to permit abortion in that very limited and very terrible situation? Let me think about it. No, sorry, I cannot make an exception."

Many people who oppose abortion cannot compromise, because of their perception of what makes abortion morally wrong. Usually, opponents of abortion conclude—or assume—that a fetus is a human being who is entitled to live. If a fetus is a human being who is entitled to live, it is still a human being and is still entitled to live even if it is the product of rape and incest perpetrated on a fifteen-year-old girl. Therefore, many opponents of abortion cannot make an exception that would allow abortion in that very limited circumstance, because making an exception would undermine the perceived ethical basis for their position.

The same thing happens on the other side of the debate. Assume that an antiabortion advocate says to a pro-choice advocate: "I know that you think abortion should be available to every woman on demand. I know that you think abortion is only the choice of the pregnant woman and nobody else's damn business. But surely *even you* would be willing to prohibit the particularly gruesome procedure of so-called partial-birth abortion at a late stage of pregnancy?" After hearing the details of that procedure, the pro-choice advocate is visibly shaken, and responds: "That's just horrible. Let me think about it. Can I make an exception to prohibit that one type of abortion procedure in that one, very limited situation? Let me think about it. No, sorry, I cannot make an exception."

Like many opponents of abortion, many people who support a right to choose abortion cannot compromise, because of their perception of what makes abortion permissible and solely a matter of individual choice. Usually, supporters of choice conclude—or assume—that a fetus is not a human being who is entitled to live. Supporters of choice also argue that a woman's autonomy over her own body gives her the right to make her own decision about whether to terminate her pregnancy. If a fetus is not a human being who is entitled to live, that would even apply in cases of so-called partial-birth abortion at a late stage of pregnancy. If a woman's autonomy gives her the right to make her own decision about whether to terminate her pregnancy, her autonomy would apply even at a late stage of pregnancy. Thus, many supporters of choice in abortion are unable to make an exception that would prohibit one particular abortion procedure in one limited circumstance, because that would undermine the perceived ethical basis for the pro-choice position.

Is a fetus really a human being who is entitled to live? Pope John Paul II wrote that the fetus is a human being from the moment of conception. According to the section of John Paul's 1995 *Evangelium Vitae* headed "'Your eyes beheld my unformed substance' (Ps 139:16): the unspeakable crime of abortion," this conclusion is not based solely on religious faith or revelation but also on a "scientific" conclusion that human life begins immediately upon fertilization. Pope John Paul II also wrote that even the possibility that a fetus is a human being requires us to treat it as such. Perhaps this is a question that we simply cannot answer. We do not even have a clear understanding or consensus of what it means to be a human being. When Barack Obama was running for president of the United States, he was asked when life begins. He responded that the determination of when life begins was "above my pay grade," and later clarified that he considers this to be a theological question (Phillips, 2008).

Does it really matter whether the fetus is a human being? Does the morality of abortion really depend on whether a fetus is a human being? Some ethicists, including feminist ethicist Susan Sherwin, argue that the morality of abortion does not depend on the status of the fetus as a human being. In their view abortion may be ethical even if the fetus were a human being.

Sherwin (1992) wrote that "feminist ethics demands that the effects of abortion policies on the oppression of women be of principal consideration in our ethical evaluations" (pp. 104–105). According to Sherwin, nonfeminist arguments in favor of a right to abortion usually are based on concepts such as privacy and freedom of choice, which she describes as "masculinist" concepts that might not meet the needs of women in many cases (pp. 99–100). In contrast, feminist ethics would determine the morality of abortion primarily by considering how various policies would affect the oppression of women. Under this approach, a right to choose abortion is ethical because it would reduce the oppression of women, and it does not really matter whether the fetus is a human being.

Another ethicist, Judith Jarvis Thomson (1971), has argued that abortion may be ethical even if the fetus were assumed to be a human being. Thomson began her analysis by stating her conclusion that a fetus at an early stage is not a person. However, for purposes of argument, she then assumed that a fetus is a human being from the moment of conception, and analyzed whether abortion could still be ethical under those circumstances. Thomson concluded that abortion would be ethical in some circumstances and unethical in others (pp. 65–66). In other words, abortion might be ethical in some situations even if the fetus were a person, but abortion would be unethical in other situations.

Unfortunately, that approach raises problems as a practical matter. It is not clear how we could decide whether abortion is ethical or unethical in any particular situation. Thomson (1971) concluded that abortion would be ethical in the case of "a sick and desperately frightened fourteen-year-old schoolgirl, pregnant due to rape" (p. 65). She also concluded that in some situations abortion would be "positively indecent," such as when a late-term abortion is performed to avoid the inconvenience of rescheduling a trip (pp. 65–66). But, precisely what makes it unethical or indecent to have a late-term abortion in order to be able to go on vacation? How can we distinguish situations in which abortion would be unethical from situations in which it would be ethical? If we merely use a process of balancing all of the relevant interests, such as the interests of the pregnant woman, the fetus, and society, that could result in carte blanche to do anything we wanted in a particular case and then rationalize it as ethically correct.

Significantly, Thomson (1971) referred to "our sense" of what is appropriate and what is not (p. 65). Perhaps that is the key to the way in which people really make their decisions about the ethics of abortion. People on each side of the debate have their supposed rationale for their respective positions, which they perceive to be based on ethical rules. In fact, the views of people on each side of the debate might be based more on their "sense" of what is right and wrong, or their "gut feeling," rather than on ethical theories or principles. Perhaps people would be more willing and able to compromise if they were to recognize that their positions are based more on gut feelings than on hard-and-fast ethical rules.

Another issue on which gut feelings may have more impact than ethical principles is the concept of **viability**. Viability is often used as a dividing line in determining whether an abortion is ethical. Many people make a distinction between abortion at an early stage of pregnancy and abortion after the fetus has become viable. Viability is really a medical concept. Essentially, it refers to the time at which the fetus can survive outside of the mother. In the United States the law on abortion has adopted that distinction between the period of time before the fetus is viable and the period of time after the fetus has become viable. As a general rule, a woman in the United States may obtain an abortion prior to the time of viability, but state governments may impose certain limitations on abortion after the point of viability, subject to certain exceptions.

With advances in medical science, the time of viability has become earlier than in the past, and may become even earlier in the future. There is no indication that these scientific advancements were intended to affect the availability of abortion. However, they may have the unintended effect of reducing the window of time during which a woman has the option to obtain an abortion.

Thus, it is important to consider whether viability of the fetus is an ethically valid distinction. If an abortion would be ethical the day before the fetus becomes viable, would it really be unethical to have an abortion the next day or even the next week, when the fetus is viable? If an abortion would be unethical once the fetus has become viable, would it really have been ethical to have had an abortion the previous day or even the previous week?

If a fetus is really a human being who is entitled to live, that would seem to apply as well to the period of time before viability. If a fetus is really not a human being who is entitled to live, that would seem to make it ethical to perform a late-term abortion during the eighth month of pregnancy. The reality is that using viability as a dividing line is just a compromise, and it might not be an ethically valid distinction. Here again, people seem to make distinctions about abortion on the basis of a gut feeling about what is right, rather than on the basis of ethical theories or principles.

This leads to the final issue to be discussed in this part of the chapter, which is whether ethical theories are useful in resolving the ethics of abortion. If we try to use utilitarianism to answer questions about the ethics of abortion, we still need to decide whether the greatest good for the greatest number includes the good of fetuses. If we try to use Kantian ethics to resolve the morality of abortion, we first need to decide whether fetuses are individuals who are entitled to be treated as ends in themselves. As a practical matter, this threshold issue begs the question. Our decision on such threshold issues is likely to determine the outcome of our ethical analysis under each of those theories of ethics.

If we try to use principlism, or prima facie moral duties, we have to answer another set of threshold questions. Specifically, whose autonomy, beneficence, nonmaleficence, and justice should we consider? We could try to balance the interests of the fetus, the interests of the pregnant woman, and the interests of society. However, that would be an extremely open-ended analysis. We could probably reach any result that we wish, and then we could justify our chosen result by declaring that one moral duty outweighs all the others in this situation. The bottom line is that it does not appear that ethical theories or principles are helpful in resolving the ethics of abortion. Perhaps that is another reason why so many people seem to make their decisions on the basis of their gut feelings.

ASSISTED REPRODUCTIVE TECHNOLOGY AND STEM CELL RESEARCH

Assisted reproductive technology (ART) generally refers to a category of fertility treatments in which eggs are surgically removed from a woman's ovaries, fertilized with sperm in a laboratory by means of in vitro fertilization (IVF), and then placed in the uterus of the woman who provided the eggs or in the uterus of another woman (Centers for Disease Control and Prevention, 2010). This procedure may result in creating more fertilized eggs, or embryos, than are needed by the donors for the purposes of their assisted reproduction. Prior to implantation in the uterus, the embryos might be screened for genetic abnormalities by means of **preimplantation genetic diagnosis (PGD).** This screening process may provide an opportunity to avoid implanting a particular embryo that has an abnormality and to implant only one or more of the preferred embryos.

The creation of multiple embryos raises the issue of whether surplus embryos should be stored indefinitely, destroyed, donated to other women, or used for medical research. Medical research with **embryonic stem (ES) cells**, which have the capacity to proliferate continuously and develop into all types of human cells, might lead to treatments for conditions such as Parkinson's disease (Ethics Committee of the American Society for Reproductive Medicine, 2009).

Not surprisingly, ART and research with human ES cells are controversial and raise complex ethical issues. For those who believe, as the Catholic Church does (John Paul II, 1995), that human life begins at the time of fertilization, an embryo is a human being who is entitled to live, and its destruction is equivalent to abortion or murder. In fact, the position of the Catholic Church on ART goes further than condemning the destruction of unused embryos. Catholic teachings also oppose the use of IVF, because intercourse is replaced by a laboratory procedure and because the seminal fluid is obtained by means of masturbation (United States Conference of Catholic Bishops, 2009).

In contrast, others believe that human embryos, while deserving of respect, are not human beings with the same rights as adults or children. Under this view, research with human ES cells can be ethical "if it is likely to provide significant new knowledge that will benefit human health and if it is conducted in ways that accord the embryo respect" (Ethics Committee of the American Society for Reproductive Medicine, 2009, p. 668).

Other aspects of ART may also raise ethical concerns, even for those who believe that embryos are not human beings. Rather than using PGD to avoid genetic abnormalities, prospective parents might use PGD to create a potential organ donor or stem cell donor for an existing child (Verlinsky and others, 2001). Other prospective parents might use PGD to screen embryos for desired traits, such as gender, height, hair color, intelligence, or athletic ability (Sandel, 2004). The quest for "designer genes" raises the specter of eugenics and the possibility that some people might try to create a "master race." Even if the use of PGD and other techniques of ART were carefully regulated, these techniques would inevitably be more available to wealthy individuals and residents of wealthy countries than to everyone else. This disparity would raise concerns under the ethical principle of justice. In addition, it might be more ethical to devote limited health care resources to interventions that would have more impact on public health, in accordance with the economic concept of opportunity cost and the ethical principle of utilitarianism.

EMERGENCY CONTRACEPTION

Emergency contraception (EC), which is also known as Plan B, can be used to prevent pregnancy after unprotected sex or after failure of another method of contraception. EC is not the same as medical abortion by means of RU-486, a pharmaceutical method of terminating a pregnancy. EC does not terminate a pregnancy, and it operates before implantation. However, EC must be taken within seventy-two hours after unprotected sex.

Several ethical issues arise in connection with EC. As with abortion there is a threshold issue of whether EC itself, or the mere use of EC, is ethical. Second, is it ethical to require people to obtain a prescription from a physician in order to gain access to EC? Put another way, would it be more ethical to make EC available over the counter (OTC), that is, without a prescription from a physician? Third, may health care professionals and health care institutions refuse to provide EC—or any other health care service—if they object to that service on ethical grounds?

Just as people disagree about whether abortion is unethical, people also disagree about the ethics of using EC or any other form of contraception. In the Philippines, for example, approximately 80 percent of the population is Roman Catholic. In November of 2008, the Catholic Bishops Conference of the Philippines (CBCP) opposed some aspects of a reproductive health bill then under consideration by the Philippine legislature, on the ground that contraception is abortion:

> The current version of the Bill does not define clearly when the protection of life begins. Although it mentions that abortion is a crime it does not state explicitly that human life is to be protected upon conception as stated in the Constitution. This ambiguity can provide a loophole for contraceptives that prevent the implantation of the fertilized ovum. The prevention of implantation of the fertilized ovum is abortion. We cannot prevent overt abortions by doing hidden abortions. It is a fallacy to think that abortions can be prevented by promoting contraception. Contraception is intrinsically evil (CCC 2370, Humanae Vitae, 14) [Catholic Bishops Conference of the Philippines, 2008].

Of course, many people would disagree with the proposition that contraception is "intrinsically evil" and would dispute that contraception is the same as abortion. In fact, advocates of contraception point out that the availability and use of contraceptives can have the effect of reducing the number of abortions.

Assuming that the use of contraceptives, including emergency contraception, is ethical, is it ethical to limit access to EC by requiring people to obtain a prescription from a physician before receiving EC? In other words, would it be more ethical to make EC available over the counter? It might seem that making EC, or any other drug, available on an OTC basis should be merely a medical issue or a regulatory issue, with the outcome depending on the drug's safety and potential for misuse. Unfortunately, in the case of EC, availability without a prescription has become an ethical, religious, and political issue. In the United States the Food and Drug Administration has essentially compromised between prescription access and OTC access by allowing people over eighteen years of age (later lowered to seventeen years of age) to obtain EC over the counter but requiring younger people to obtain a prescription for EC. Moreover, the OTC EC can be obtained only from pharmacies and health care facilities and not from other OTC outlets, such as convenience stores (U.S. Food and Drug Administration, 2009). In the United Kingdom, EC is available over the counter at pharmacies to persons over the age of sixteen (U.K. National Health Service, 2009). Meanwhile, in Indonesia, some health care professionals oppose the use of EC for ethical or religious reasons, and some oppose making EC available without a prescription on the ground that it might encourage teenagers to have "free sex" (Syahlul and Amir, 2005). Writing about Iran, Larijani and Zahedi (2006) have stated that "emergency contraception is also available in family planning clinics" (p. 130). However, it is not clear whether EC is really readily available in Iran, as a practical matter.

The controversy over emergency contraception raises the broader issue of whether it is ethical for health care professionals or health care institutions to refuse to provide EC—or any other health care service—if they object to the particular service on ethical grounds. Some doctors and other health care professionals argue that they have the right to refuse to perform or to participate in performing any procedure that they consider unethical. In some jurisdictions, laws referred to as **conscience clauses** protect the right of health care professionals to make their own decisions about the procedures they are willing to perform. However, those decisions could have the practical effect of preventing patients from having access to lawful procedures that the patients consider to be ethical.

The issue of who should make this type of ethical decision is not limited to the field of health care services but affects suppliers and consumers in other areas as well. In fact, other settings may provide useful analogies. For example, at the Minneapolis-St. Paul International Airport, many travelers arrive from overseas with bags of duty-free alcohol ("Minnesota's Muslim Cab Drivers Face Crackdown," 2007). It is easy to tell what is in the bags. Many of the taxi drivers are Muslims from Somalia who have religious and cultural objections to drinking alcohol or helping others to drink it or carry it. Between 2002 and 2007, there were approximately 4,800 cases in which taxi drivers at this airport refused to accept passengers carrying alcoholic beverages in their cabs. Eventually, the Metropolitan Airports Commission took action and, in May of 2007, began to impose penalties on taxi drivers who refused to take these passengers, including a thirty-day suspension for the first offense and a two-year revocation for a second offense. In this situation no one had forced these individuals to become taxi drivers. They had agreed to serve the public as drivers of taxis and thereby gave up the right to make their own decisions about whom to serve or which ethical standards to apply in serving the public.

Similarly, when individuals join the military, they give up their right to decide on the particular wars in which they will agree to participate or the particular weapons they will agree to use. Assuming there is no draft, they made their own choice to join the military and thereby gave up their rights to make those particular decisions in individual cases.

In the health care setting, what are the rights and responsibilities of health care professionals and institutions in regard to performing procedures that they consider to be unethical? Many health care professionals believe that they should be allowed to opt out of performing any procedure to which they object on ethical grounds. In addition, many people who are not health care professionals accept the proposition that physicians should be allowed to refuse on the basis of their personal ethical views to participate in abortion. Ironically, some of the same people who support a physician's right to refuse to perform abortions are outraged by reports that pharmacists have refused on the basis of personal ethical views to dispense EC.

Health care professionals often insist that they are not merely "hired guns" who must perform any procedure requested by their patients but are instead entitled to make their own ethical decisions and are ethically responsible for their decisions. As Eike-Henner Kluge (1993) wrote, "the physician's entry into a professional relationship with a patient does not turn that doctor into a moral eunuch" (p. 289). That is also the position of the Catholic Church. As Pope John Paul II (1995) wrote, "Doctors and nurses are also responsible, when they place at the service of death skills which were acquired for promoting life.... [R]esponsibility likewise falls . . . to the extent that they have a say in the matter, on the administrators of the health-care centres where abortions are performed." Under this view a patient may have a right to obtain a particular procedure, but that does not mean that a particular health care professional or institution has an obligation to perform it. The patient may have to accept being referred elsewhere or even having to find another practitioner by himself or herself.

But what if no other health care professional is available or willing to perform the lawful procedure that is desired or needed by the patient? Under those circumstances the health care professional's refusal has the practical effect of denying treatment to the patient. This problem is not limited to abortion and EC but also arises in other situations, such as withdrawal of treatment at the end of life. Some health care professionals even insist that they should not be required to make a referral for a procedure that they consider to be objectionable. As Julie Cantor (2009) has written, "Conscientious objection makes sense with conscription, but it is worrisome when professionals who freely choose their field parse care and withhold information that patients need.... Conscience is a burden that belongs to the individual professional; patients should not have to shoulder it" (p. 1485).

An argument can be made that as an ethical matter health care professionals should not be allowed to refuse to perform lawful services requested by their patients. The health care professionals who do refuse have, like all their colleagues, been trained, at least in part, at public expense. As students or trainees, they occupied seats that could have been filled by other individuals, ones who would meet more of society's health care needs. Perhaps we should screen applicants for medical school and nursing school by asking which procedures they would not be willing to perform when they graduate, and then we could give priority in admission to those applicants who would provide the broadest range of services to the public. In hiring workers, perhaps hospitals and other health care facilities should give preference to those workers who are willing to perform all lawful procedures.

Prevailing concepts of medical ethics, however, allow health care professionals to refuse to participate in procedures on the ground of their personal beliefs. According to the *Declaration on Therapeutic Abortion* of the World Medical Association (2006), "If the physician's convictions do not allow him or her to advise or perform an abortion, he or she may withdraw while ensuring the continuity of medical care by a qualified colleague." In the United States the federal government and some state governments have adopted these concepts of medical ethics by enacting laws known as conscience clauses. As mentioned earlier these laws protect the right of health care workers to refuse to participate in any procedure to which they object on ethical grounds, and they cannot be fired or otherwise penalized for their refusal. In fact some of these laws go even further by protecting health care workers who refuse to refer patients to other providers who would be willing to perform the requested procedure.

In 2007, the American College of Obstetricians and Gynecologists (ACOG) Committee on Ethics issued a report titled "The Limits of Conscientious Refusal in Reproductive Medicine." According to that report, "Physicians and other health care providers have the duty to refer patients in a timely manner to other providers if they do not feel that they can in conscience provide the standard reproductive services that patients request" (p. 1). However, some opponents of abortion argue that a physician should not be required to violate his or her personal beliefs by making a referral for a patient who wants to obtain an abortion.

During the final months of the George W. Bush administration, the U.S. Department of Health and Human Services (HHS) (2008) issued a proposed rule to strengthen the protections for health care workers who object to performing or to assisting in the performance of specific medical procedures. In its proposed rule, HHS criticized the standards of professional organizations, such as ACOG, that might prevent individual health care providers from making their own decisions about performing or assisting in the performance of specific procedures to which they object. HHS said it was "concerned that the development of an environment in the health care field that is intolerant of individual conscience, certain religious beliefs, ethnic and cultural traditions, and moral convictions may discourage individuals from diverse backgrounds from entering health care professions" (p. 50276).

HHS was proposing to adopt a very broad definition of the term *assist in the performance*. That broad definition might include even workers who clean floors or replace light bulbs in rooms that are used for abortion, sterilization, or other procedures that a worker might consider objectionable. If adopted, such a rule might require hospital supervisors, who arrange staffing for thousands of workers, to keep track of which procedures and tasks each worker is not willing to perform or to assist in performing, such as abortion, sterilization, contraception, or removal of artificial life support from a terminally ill patient. For this practical reason it might not make sense to allow every health care worker to refuse to assist in any lawful procedure to which that worker might object (Cantor, 2009, p. 1484).

Under the new administration of President Obama, the federal government has taken a different approach to the proposed HHS rule. However, that change in government policy does not resolve the underlying issue of whether it is ethical or practical to permit every health care professional to refuse to perform or to assist in performing any health care service to which he or she objects on ethical grounds. This underlying issue also leads to a further question about the ethical practices of the governmental agencies and nongovernmental organizations (NGOs) that provide funding for health services and public health. If health care professionals and facilities may refuse to participate in activities that they consider to be unethical, does that mean that governmental agencies and NGOs may impose conditions on their funding for health services in developing or transitional countries, requiring these countries to conform with the funding organizations' ethical views about reproductive health issues? That issue of ethics in funding is addressed in the final part of this chapter.

ETHICS OF IMPOSING CONDITIONS ON FUNDING

When donors are funding health or social services, is it ethical for these donors to impose conditions based on their own ethical views? Individual taxpayers cannot refuse to pay for activities to which they object. However, governments have the power to fund activities that they consider ethical and to refuse to fund activities that they consider unethical. NGOs and other private donors also have the ability to limit their funding or impose conditions on their funding on the basis of their ethical views. Of course having the practical ability to limit funding or impose conditions on funding does not mean that it is ethical to do so. Specifically, is it ethical for governmental agencies or NGOs to impose conditions on funding in developing and transitional countries when those conditions are based on the funder's ethical views about reproductive health issues?

For many years the U.S. government imposed limits on the use of funds for activities related to abortion in other countries. Opponents of that U.S. policy have referred to it as the **global gag rule**, because it prevented NGOs from providing information about abortion or advocating for greater availability of abortion. It is also known as the **Mexico City Policy**. This policy was not a prohibition against using U.S. funds for abortion-related purposes. That prohibition is contained in a separate U.S. law. The global gag rule, or Mexico City Policy, went beyond the provisions of that law by limiting what foreign NGOs could do with their own funds if they received any USAID funds for family planning. Under that policy, if a foreign NGO received USAID money for family planning, then that NGO could not even use its own non-U.S. funds for abortion services, referrals, or lobbying.

On January 23, 2009, President Obama issued a presidential memorandum rescinding the Mexico City Policy (President, 2009). This memorandum, which explains the history and details of that policy, follows.

MEMORANDUM OF JANUARY 23, 2009

MEXICO CITY POLICY AND ASSISTANCE FOR VOLUNTARY POPULATION PLANNING

Memorandum for the Secretary of State [and] the Administrator of the United States Agency for International Development

The Foreign Assistance Act of 1961 (22 U.S.C. 2151b(f)(1)), prohibits non-governmental organizations (NGOs) that receive Federal funds from using those funds "to pay for the performance of abortions as a method of family planning, or to motivate or coerce any person to practice abortions." The August 1984 announcement by President Reagan of what has become known as the "Mexico City Policy" directed the United States Agency for International Development (USAID) to expand this limitation and withhold USAID funds from NGOs that use non-USAID funds to engage in a wide range of activities, including providing advice, counseling, or information regarding abortion, or lobbying a foreign government to legalize or make abortion available. The Mexico City Policy was in effect from 1985 until 1993, when it was rescinded by President Clinton. President George W. Bush reinstated the policy in 2001, implementing it through conditions in USAID grant awards, and subsequently extended the policy to "voluntary population planning" assistance provided by the Department of State.

These excessively broad conditions on grants and assistance awards are unwarranted. Moreover, they have undermined efforts to promote safe and effective voluntary family planning programs in foreign nations. Accordingly, I hereby revoke the Presidential memorandum of January 22, 2001, for the Administrator of USAID (Restoration of the Mexico City Policy), the Presidential memorandum of March 28, 2001, for the Administrator of USAID (Restoration of the Mexico City Policy), and the Presidential memorandum of August 29, 2003, for the Secretary of State (Assistance for Voluntary Population Planning). In addition, I direct the Secretary of State and the Administrator of USAID to take the following actions with respect to conditions in voluntary population planning assistance and USAID grants that were imposed pursuant to either the 2001 or 2003 memoranda and that are not required by the Foreign Assistance Act or any other law: (1) immediately waive such conditions in any current grants, and (2) notify current grantees, as soon as possible, that these conditions have been waived. I further direct that the Department of State and USAID immediately cease imposing these conditions in any future grants.

This memorandum is not intended to, and does not, create any right or benefit, substantive or procedural, enforceable at law or in equity by any party against the United States, its departments, agencies, or entities, its officers, employees, or agents, or any other person.

The Secretary of State is authorized and directed to publish this memorandum in the *Federal Register*.

Barack Obama, the White House, January 23, 2009.

Source: President, 2009.

Objections to the global gag rule may have been based more on the nature of the restrictions than on the concept of imposing conditions on external funding for developing or transitional countries. In fact some opponents of the global gag rule might strongly support a hypothetical policy that would require all recipients of U.S. funds to provide information or referrals for abortion. Some people would consider it ethical to impose conditions on funding that would increase access to reproductive health services, but unethical to impose conditions that would reduce access to those services.

Is it inherently unethical to impose limits or conditions on funding for global health services on the basis of the funder's religious or ethical views? To some extent the answer depends on whether we believe an ethical obligation exists to help other people and other countries, and what we see as the extent of that ethical obligation. If an obligation to provide assistance exists, it would be unethical to condition that assistance on the recipient's compliance with the donor's ethical or religious views. However, if providing assistance is laudable but not ethically required, it would not be unethical to impose limitations or conditions on that assistance. The issue of an ethical obligation to assist others is discussed in Chapter Seven of this book. In the meantime, the activity at the end of the chapter presents an opportunity for readers to further consider the issue of imposing conditions on funding, this time in the context of emergency contraception in a developing country.

SUMMARY

Rather than relying on ethical theories or principles, many people seem to base their opinion about abortion on their sense or gut feeling of what is right and what is wrong. That may be the reason that so many people have been unable to compromise on that controversial issue. This chapter analyzed the diverse perspectives on abortion and other reproductive health issues, including the ways in which abortion is viewed in other countries and cultures. In evaluating the ethics of proposed policies on abortion and other reproductive health issues, one of the most important perspectives is the practical approach of recognizing the consequences of those policies for the lives and health of real people. It is particularly important to recognize the harm that is caused by unsafe abortions, especially in developing countries.

KEY TERMS

assisted reproductive
    technology (ART)
conscience clauses
embryonic stem (ES) cells

emergency contraception
    (EC)
global gag rule
Mexico City Policy

preimplantation genetic
    diagnosis (PGD)
viability

DISCUSSION QUESTIONS

1. In making a decision about the ethics of abortion, is viability of the fetus an ethically valid distinction?
2. Is it ethical to use assisted reproductive technology (ART) and preimplantation genetic diagnosis (PGD) to screen embryos for desired traits, such as gender or intelligence?
3. Should health care professionals and facilities be required to perform or to provide referrals for all lawful health services, even if the health care professional or facility objects to a particular service on ethical grounds?

4. Is it ethical for governmental agencies and other external donors to impose restrictions on funding for health services in developing countries when those restrictions are based on a donor's ethical views about reproductive health issues?

ACTIVITY: THE ETHICS OF EMERGENCY CONTRACEPTION IN GOUANASTAN

The nation that we will call Gouanastan is a very poor country in central Asia. Millions of people in Gouanastan suffer from infectious diseases and malnutrition, and the country has extremely high rates of infant, child, and maternal mortality. There is a desperate need to improve the public health infrastructure in the country.

All the hospitals in Gouanastan are owned and operated by the Catholic Church. Most of them were established by missionaries in the late 1800s. These hospitals do the best they can with their limited resources, and they provide the only secondary and tertiary heath care services in the country.

An agency that we will call the Swedish Agency for International Development (SAID) has agreed to provide $10 billion to the government of Gouanastan. The purpose of the funding from SAID is to develop public health services and primary health care services in Gouanastan. The money cannot be used for acute-care hospital services. In addition, SAID has imposed a condition on the funding that relates to the availability of emergency contraception (EC). Specifically, SAID wants to ensure that EC, which is widely available in Sweden, will also be available at hospitals in Gouanastan to survivors of sexual assault.

In offering to provide the $10 billion to Gouanastan, SAID has stipulated that Gouanastan must adopt a law that requires all hospitals in the country to provide EC to survivors of sexual assault or, alternatively, to advise patients where they can go to obtain EC. In fact SAID has made it clear that adopting this law is a condition that must be met before the country can receive any SAID funding, and SAID is not willing to negotiate on that point. The government of Gouanastan is willing to adopt the proposed law, in order to obtain the funding from SAID.

The Catholic Hospital Association of Gouanastan (CHAG) represents all the hospitals in the country. CHAG and its members are opposed to the use of EC, which they consider to be morally equivalent to abortion and therefore morally equivalent to murder. In accordance with this religion-based policy, hospitals in Gouanastan do not provide EC to survivors of sexual assault and they do not advise patients about EC, because of the belief that human life begins at the time of fertilization. No hospital in Gouanastan currently provides EC, and CHAG is strongly against the proposed law.

In contrast, the proposed law is supported by Gouanastanians for Reproductive Rights (GFRR), which is a nongovernmental advocacy organization. According to GFRR's president, hospitals run by religious orders have no valid complaint about the proposed law because these hospitals would not be required to actually provide EC. Instead, these hospitals would have the option of advising patients where they could go to obtain EC.

Despite the arguments by GFRR, CHAG remains strongly against the proposed law. According to the president of CHAG, Sister Mary James, the government of Gouanastan should not require a religious organization to advise people on how to do something that the religious organization believes to be morally wrong. Sister Mary James recently testified at a hearing conducted by the national legislature of Gouanastan. At that hearing, she stated, "Not only do we refrain from engaging in sin; we do not advise other people where they can go to engage in sin or draw them a map!" Sister Mary James also stated that if the government enacts the proposed law, the members of CHAG will close all the hospitals in Gouanastan and move their operations to a different country, one that will not require them to violate their religious beliefs.

In order to consider the ethical issues involved in this situation from all points of view, the class members should form six teams, with each team representing one of the following groups:

A. Gouanastan Ministry of Health (MOH)
B. Swedish Agency for International Development (SAID)
C. Catholic Hospital Association of Gouanastan (CHAG)
D. Gouanastanians for Reproductive Rights (GFRR)
E. Medical Society of Gouanastan (MSOG)
F. Patients' Association of Gouanastan (PAOG)

Your task as a team member is to participate in analyzing the following ethical issues from the perspective of your stakeholder group:

1. Is it ethical for SAID to impose a condition on funding when that condition is based on SAID's views about human reproduction?
2. Is it ethical for the government of Gouanastan to adopt the proposed law? Would it be ethical for the government to refuse to adopt the proposed law?
3. Is it ethical for CHAG to close its hospitals in order to avoid being forced to do something its members consider to be morally equivalent to murder?

In analyzing these issues, please apply the ethical theories of utilitarianism, Kantian ethics, and principlism (prima facie moral duties), as well as any other theories or approaches that you think are useful. Your team should not simply choose one ethical theory. Rather, each team should apply all of these ethical theories and should try to use all of them to support the position of its stakeholder group.

In other words, the task is not simply to determine what the team thinks a utilitarian, Kantian, or principlist would say about each of these ethical issues. Rather, the task for each team is to determine how the team could use each ethical theory to support its position on these issues.

CHAPTER FIVE

ETHICAL ISSUES OF FEMALE GENITAL MUTILATION

LEARNING OBJECTIVES

- Understand and be able to explain why female genital mutilation (FGM) is a serious problem in global public health, in both developing and developed countries.

- Demonstrate an appreciation of how patterns of immigration are forcing health care providers in industrialized countries to face the clinical and ethical issues of FGM.

- Be able to analyze the ethical issues of FGM, including how health care providers in industrialized countries should respond to requests to perform FGM or to allow FGM to be performed in their facilities.

- Be prepared to debate whether there are any universal values that transcend the cultural values of societies that practice FGM.

A N interagency statement prepared by ten United Nations agencies and published by the World Health Organization (WHO) estimates that at least 100 million women and girls have been subjected to genital mutilation, and that 3 million girls are at risk of being subjected to genital mutilation every year (World Health Organization, 2008, p. 1). This statement defines **female genital mutilation (FGM)** as "all procedures involving partial or total removal of the external female genitalia or other injury to the female genital organs for non-medical reasons" (p. 4). It also declares that the practice of FGM violates human rights and should be eliminated (pp. 1, 8).

The practice of FGM has been most common in parts of Africa and the Middle East. However, as a result of widespread immigration from those regions to other parts of the world, health care professionals and facilities in industrialized countries are encountering new ethical issues as they serve an increasingly diverse patient population. In fact, many health care providers in industrialized countries are now treating patients who have undergone FGM or are requesting FGM and also minors who are at risk of having FGM performed upon them at the request of their families (Kaplan-Marcusan and others, 2009).

This chapter begins with a brief introduction to the facts about FGM, including the types of procedures that are performed, the effects of those procedures, and the reasons they are performed. In addition, the chapter presents an excerpt from an article about perceptions and experiences with FGM among health care providers in Europe. Then the chapter considers the serious challenge to multiculturalism and ethical relativism posed by FGM, and evaluates whether it is wrong to impose one nation's or region's cultural values and ethics on people from other cultures. This chapter also analyzes the ethical issue of whether FGM should be permitted for adult women, as a matter of individual autonomy and informed consent, or, alternatively, should be prohibited altogether. Finally, an activity presents an opportunity to evaluate whether health care professionals and organizations should perform FGM or allow the performance of FGM in their facilities.

THE FACTS ABOUT FGM

Here is the current four-part classification of FGM procedures that is used by WHO and other UN agencies:

> **Type I:** Partial or total removal of the clitoris and/or the prepuce (**clitoridectomy**).
>
> **Type II:** Partial or total removal of the clitoris and the labia minora, with or without excision of the labia majora (**excision**).

Type III: Narrowing of the vaginal orifice with creation of a covering seal by cutting and appositioning the labia minora and/or the labia majora, with or without excision of the clitoris (**infibulation**).

Type IV: All other harmful procedures to the female genitalia for non-medical purposes, for example: pricking, piercing, incising, scraping and cauterization [World Health Organization, 2008, p. 4, emphasis added].

These practices are usually performed on girls from birth to age fifteen, but are also performed on adults (World Health Organization, 2008). Some adult women who had been infibulated request to be reinfibulated after vaginal delivery. The severe physical and mental harms of FGM have been well documented and include extreme pain, bleeding, chronic pelvic and urinary tract infections, dermoid cysts, keloids, and problems in childbirth (Toubia, 1994). No medical benefits are known to exist (World Health Organization, 2008, p. 1). Thus, FGM is not comparable to male circumcision, which provides some health benefits, has few risks or complications, and does not interfere with normal sexual functioning.

The practice of FGM has been most common in certain parts of Africa, such as Burkina Faso, Djibouti, Egypt, Eritrea, Ethiopia, Gambia, Guinea, Mali, Mauritania, Sierra Leone, Somalia, and Sudan. It has also been practiced in some areas of the Middle East, such as Yemen (World Health Organization, 2008, p. 29). In recent years many people have migrated from those regions to Europe, North America, Australia, New Zealand, and other countries. This widespread migration has forced health care providers in industrialized countries to face ethical issues they had never expected to face.

It is important to recognize and to try to understand the cultural significance of FGM, as well as the consequences within certain cultures of rejecting FGM. As stated by Turillazzi and Fineschi (2007), "it is through the mutilation of her own genitals that every woman recognises herself and is recognised as a member of her community. Not undergoing these practices means condemning herself to exclusion and rejection and thus to a loss of the sense of belonging to a community" (p. 100). In addition, as Nahid Toubia (1994) has explained, for societies in which marriage may be the only realistic option for women, "Female circumcision is the physical marking of the marriageability of women, because it symbolizes social control of their sexual pleasure (clitoridectomy) and their reproduction (infibulation)" (p. 714). However, Fadwa El Guindi has argued that FGM increases female sexuality and female sexual enjoyment (El Guindi, 2006, pp. 27, 31–32).

Meanwhile, significant ambiguity exists as to whether FGM is a religious requirement. Some of the opponents of FGM insist that it is not required as a matter of religious belief but is only a matter of cultural practice (Center for Reproductive Rights, 2004, p. 1). The 2003 Cairo Declaration for the Elimination of FGM emphasized statements by supreme religious authorities in Egypt that no religious principle of Islam or Christianity justifies FGM (Egyptian National Council for Childhood and Motherhood, 2003). Similarly, WHO's Regional Office for the Eastern Mediterranean, in Alexandria, Egypt, published a treatise in 1996 by an Islamic scholar to demonstrate that Islam does not require the performance of FGM (World Health Organization, 1996). However, clerics still disagree about the relationship between FGM and Islam (Gibeau, 1998, pp. 87–88). For example, Sheikh Mohammed Sayed Tantawy, the Grand Sheikh of Al-Azhar, has stated that Islam does not justify FGM, but another Islamic cleric in Egypt, Yusuf El-Badry, has argued that FGM is indeed part of Islam (Fam, 2007).

In fact, when Egypt's Ministry of Health issued a decree making FGM unlawful, Yusuf El-Badry filed a lawsuit against the health minister in an attempt to overturn the prohibition. The practice of FGM had been prohibited for a long time in Egypt, but there had been loopholes in the prohibition. After a fourteen-year-old girl died during an FGM procedure, the Egyptian government strengthened the law by closing the loopholes. Then El-Badry filed a lawsuit against the government. According to El-Badry, the government was trying to criminalize a part of Islam. Eventually, the Parliament of Egypt enacted a new law, in June of 2008, to criminalize FGM (Egyptian National Council for Childhood and Motherhood, 2008).

Does the distinction between religion and culture really matter? As a practical matter, it could be more difficult to stop a practice that is required or authorized by an organized religion. As an ethical matter, however, it should not matter whether FGM is supposedly justified by religion or only by culture. If it is concluded that FGM is ethically wrong, then FGM would be wrong even if it were required or authorized by the explicit rules of an organized religion.

Some progress has been made in stopping the practice of FGM, but it is still a significant problem of public health and human rights. Agencies and organizations around the world have opposed FGM in the strongest possible terms, and have recognized February 6 of each year as the International Day of Zero Tolerance to FGM. Specifically, WHO and nine other UN agencies have declared that FGM "violates the rights to health, security and physical integrity of the person, the right to be free from torture and cruel, inhuman or degrading treatment, and the right to life when the procedure results in death" (World Health Organization, 2008, p. 1). Those international agencies also have recognized that FGM is a severe type of discrimination on the basis of gender, violates the rights of children, and is analogous to the former practice of binding women's feet in China as a method of societal control of women (World Health Organization, 2008, pp. 1, 5). Professional organizations also consider FGM to violate the principles of medical ethics. For example, the World Medical

Association (2005) has stated that it "condemns the practice of genital mutilation including the circumcision of women and girls and condemns the participation of physicians in such practices."

Many countries have enacted laws to prohibit the practice of FGM. As of February 2009, eighteen African countries had passed laws making FGM a crime, as had twelve industrialized countries to which people from Africa and the Middle East have immigrated (Center for Reproductive Rights, 2009). In addition to making the practice of FGM a crime, it is also possible to treat the practice of FGM on a minor as child abuse.

In discussing the ethical implications of a 2006 Italian law against FGM, Turillazzi and Fineschi (2007) noted that the law applies even to citizens or residents of Italy who perform FGM outside Italy (p. 100). Similarly, the 2003 law prohibiting FGM in the United Kingdom applies as well to certain actions performed outside that country by a U.K. national or by a permanent U.K. resident, and also prohibits assisting or procuring a foreign person to perform FGM outside the United Kingdom (*Female Genital Mutilation Act*, 2003, sections 3–4). Such extraterritorial provisions are extremely important because, as experts recognize, children may be subjected to FGM during holiday trips to their family's country of origin (Turillazzi and Fineschi, 2007, p. 99; Kaplan-Marcusan and others, 2009).

In the United States, under a 1996 federal law, it is a crime to perform FGM on a person under the age of eighteen (*Criminalization of Female Genital Mutilation Act of 1996*, 2006). However, FGM is permitted if the surgical procedure is necessary for the health of the patient and is performed by a licensed medical practitioner. In addition, a surgical procedure is permitted by an appropriate practitioner for medical purposes in connection with labor or delivery. It is important to note that the U.S. federal law does not prohibit the performance of FGM on a person over the age of eighteen. Meanwhile, at least seventeen U.S. states have enacted their own laws against FGM (Center for Reproductive Rights, 2009). Three U.S. states (Minnesota, Rhode Island, and Tennessee) have prohibited FGM for adults as well as for minors, which means that FGM may be performed lawfully on adult women in most of the fifty U.S. states (Center for Reproductive Rights, 2004, p. 5). Where laws prohibit FGM only for minors, we need to face the important ethical questions of whether health care professionals should perform FGM for adult women who request it, and whether health care organizations should allow FGM to be performed in their facilities. These ethical issues are discussed later in this chapter.

Legal prohibitions are important both because they can reduce the incidence of FGM and because laws have a normative function of expressing a society's strong rejection of a practice. However, laws alone are not sufficient.

The elimination of FGM will require a comprehensive strategy that combines legislation with education, social change, and greater economic opportunities for women. In addition, health care professionals and facilities need to be prepared to help their patients by preventing FGM and by treating patients who already have been subjected to those procedures.

The reading that follows comes from an article that describes the perceptions and experiences with FGM among health care providers in Spain and that also reviews previous research in two other European countries. As discussed in this excerpt, FGM poses complex ethical issues for health care professionals and organizations. For example, when health care professionals think that a child is at risk of being subjected to FGM, should they notify the police or other governmental authorities? Health care providers have an ethical obligation to notify the proper authorities about any type of child abuse, and notification might even be required by law. However, notification could also result in legal proceedings that would destabilize the family by sending a parent to prison. There are no easy answers to these dilemmas.

EXCERPT FROM "PERCEPTION OF PRIMARY HEALTH PROFESSIONALS ABOUT FEMALE GENITAL MUTILATION: FROM HEALTHCARE TO INTERCULTURAL COMPETENCE"

BY ADRIANA KAPLAN-MARCUSAN AND OTHERS

Background . . .

The substantial migratory flow of the Sub-Saharan population towards Europe in recent years is leading to increasingly more complex and diverse societies. The approach to the healthcare problems affecting this population represents a challenge to healthcare systems and the professionals working therein, who must develop their own competence to achieve transcultural care.

It is not continents or colours that emigrate but rather people and their cultures, in recent years a visible distortion has been produced in the phenomena associated with gender and immigration, especially in the case of Sub-Saharan women, their daughters and the harmful traditional practices of initiation involving mutilation of female genitals. International organisations and professional associations have made statements against FGM. Indeed, many countries have promulgated legislation against these practices. In Spain the law punishes this crime with prison sentences of 6 to 12 years for the parents, and the girls are taken into care by Social Services.

In addition to adequate laws, a preventive stand is essential which, from a perspective of knowledge and sensitization, allows healthcare professionals to approach the question of FGM and thereby avoid the conflicts produced by legal action against aspects such as those linked to the intimacy and identity of these people.

The first cases of FGM in Spain were detected and reported by healthcare professionals in 1993. Since then, new mutilations have not been reported in Spain, although it is known that some families take advantage of vacation trips to their countries of origin to carry out FGM. . . . [W]e have estimated that in our country around 9,545 women have undergone some type of FGM and approximately 3,824 girls are at an age of risk of having this done within the next few years . . . .

This emerging sociodemographic reality has led to new challenges for which healthcare professionals should be prepared to intervene from a preventive point of view. The FGM . . . [is] a problem which affects us, as healthcare professionals, in a double sense, as a violation of human rights, which we have the moral obligation to impede, and as an aggression against the health of the persons to which we have the professional obligation to attempt to prevent, to thereby avoid the consequences to the physical, psychic, sexual and reproductive well being of the women.

The cultural pressure and social structure which these practices maintain are strong since they are rooted and nourished by the tradition and the previous experience of their elders, their mothers and confusing religious messages in their communities of origin.

We believe that the receptor countries should approach the question of the FGM from any of the possible points of contact of the migrant families with Primary Health Care, advancing in the double line of:

- Training the professionals in detection and recognition and preventive intervention in the families and girls in a situation of risk of undergoing FGM.
- Identify[ing] the women and girls at risk in the population assigned to each healthcare centre.

Because of its proximity to the families and the longitudinal approach to the problems throughout the whole vital cycle, primary healthcare is one entry point for implementing a preventive intervention towards FGM.

The objectives of this study were to analyse the perceptions, degree of knowledge and attitudes of primary care professionals related to FGM, as well as explore possible trends towards a change in these perceptions and attitudes in two periods of time, 2001 and 2004.

Methods

A cross-sectional study was conducted with a self-administered questionnaire to primary healthcare professionals. In the Catalonian Healthcare System, primary healthcare professionals work in teams who attend the healthcare needs of the population assigned in a determined territory. These teams are made up of family physicians/general medicine, paediatricians, nurses and social workers. Support programs are available within the setting of sexual and reproductive health and these are mainly constituted by gynaecologists and midwives. We considered three large groups of professionals according to the characteristics of the population they attend: General Medicine (physicians and nurses) attending a population over the age of 15 years; Paediatrics (physicians and nurses) attending a population under the age of 15 years and Gynaecology (gynaecologists, nurses and midwives) attending the program of sexual and reproductive health.

Two time points were used: April-May 2001 and October-November 2004. Between the two time points the results of the first questionnaire were made public, and some educational activities were carried out (seminars, sessions and courses) in the healthcare centres, although these activities were not part of a structured training programme related to FGM. In June 2002 a "Protocol of action to prevent FGM" was edited on behalf of the autonomous Government of Catalonia and in January 2004 guidelines for professionals were presented within the framework of a European project against sexual violence.

The study was undertaken in the Maresme, a county on the Mediterranean coast north of Barcelona with a population of 412,840 inhabitants. This area was one of the first areas to receive large groups of Sub-Saharan immigrants, mainly from Gambia and Senegal during the migratory wave produced at the beginning of the 1980s. According to the census of 2005, 11.28% of the population of the county was foreigners, 30.24% of whom were from North Africa and 13.44% from Sub-Saharan Africa....

Results....

...Nurses identified the different types of FGM better than the physicians in all the professional groups in both years, except for gynaecology in 2001....

...The professionals who had attended some educative activity on FGM or were familiar with any protocol or guideline of action had up to a 5.0-fold greater probability to correctly identify the typology.

The detection of cases was mainly undertaken by female professionals...of less than 40 years in age. Females identified the FGM better than males..., developed educational attitudes from the approach to the FGM..., and declared greater interest in the subject of FGM....

The gynaecologists demonstrated better knowledge of the FGM...and a greater probability of case detection...

Discussion

This study demonstrates that the problems related to FGM are not infrequent in primary care consultations since up to 16% of the participants surveyed in 2004 declared having detected cases. Eighteen percent of the professionals declared no interest in knowing more about the subject. Less than 40% correctly identified the typology and less than 30% knew the countries in which this practice was common. There seemed to be greater sensitivity towards the subject by female nurses and midwives within the professional areas of paediatrics and gynaecology. A trend towards education and sensitisation versus the problem was observed accompanied by reporting to the authorities when these preventive approaches failed.

The percentage of professionals who declared having detected a case practically tripled from 2001 to 2004, although these values are far from the 60% declared in a questionnaire to professionals from four Swedish cities.

It should be taken into account that our questionnaire only allowed exploration of whether [they] had diagnosed or had knowledge of any child in their office that had undergone FGM. We could not determine the number of cases diagnosed. We only considered the number of professionals who, in their practice and based on their clinical practice, had diagnosed or known of any child with FGM.

In the Swedish study a very low rate of response was obtained (28%) and it cannot be ruled out that the professionals who responded had been in contact with cases of FGM and were especially motivated or sensitised with the subject. In our study the rate of response was much higher, which we believe better represents the opinion of most of the professional groups. Moreover, our study population included a lower proportion of gynaecologists and midwives than the Swedish study, which may explain the lower percent of professionals in contact with cases. Knowledge of FGM seemed to be similar in the two populations. In the Swedish survey 35% of the gynaecologists and 29% of the midwives declared having "sufficient knowledge" of the subject. In our study 45% of the participants correctly identified the typology and 24% the countries of origin. The difference...[lies] in that in our study the data was obtained from the emission of correct responses, similar to an examination, to two questions related to this subject, while the Swedish questionnaire concerned the perception of "sufficient knowledge" on behalf of the professionals.

In a study carried out in Switzerland only 8% of the 37 professionals interviewed referred [to] having developed any preventive intervention in their consultations. In our questionnaire in 2004, 31% of the professionals expressed the need to develop educational and sensitisation attitudes to avoid FGM. We believe that these differences may be due to the limited sample size, being mainly of professionals specialised in gynaecology in the Swiss study, while in our study the collective analysed included primary care professionals with a more general view of healthcare problems, being theoretically closer to preventive and educational healthcare activities.

The discrepancy between the perception of having correct knowledge (knowing in which countries FGM is performed and for what reasons) and the correct identification of the typology, the countries and the reasons for its performance, should be pointed out. This indicates that, in fact, the professionals in our environment have a significant lack of knowledge with regard to FGM. If we add the fact that 80% of those surveyed stated that they attended a population of Sub-Saharan origin and that the detection of cases tripled from 2001 to 2004, it may be deduced that we are faced with an emerging healthcare problem which we are treating with a great lack of knowledge on its social and cultural background.

Our results demonstrate that the primary care professionals surveyed declare a high interest (more than 70% answered "yes" to the question as to whether they are interested in knowing more on this subject), a low grade of knowledge (less than half correctly identified the types of FGM and less than 25% correctly identified the countries in which it is practiced) and some efficacy in the formation received (those stating that [they] had received formation had a greater probability of better identifying the typology and origin . . .). This leads to the need to prioritize strategies of sensitization and formation of professionals in relation to the identification of the population at risk and capacitation for a preventive and culturally respectful approach, to thereby avoid the families being exposed to the criminal and legal procedures linked to their socio-cultural roots and the consequent risk of familial destruction and separation.

In addition, in our country it so happens that the fertility of African women of Gambian origin doubles or triples that of women from other areas. To develop effective interventions in the immediate future it will be necessary to promote in depth knowledge of the social and cultural reality of these migrant communities which will allow these subjects to be approached with greater professional competence and thus, greater possibilities of success.

One interesting fact is the difference observed in the perception, attitudes and detection of the problem according to the gender of the professionals. The women showed greater interest, had more attitudes oriented towards education and detected most of the cases. . . .

The different perspective according to the gender of the professionals should be taken into account to avoid an increase in certain disparities in health-care based on the professionals attending the migrant women population. The challenge . . . [lies] in avoiding the creation of another barrier in the approach to problems related to FGM due to this difference in gender in the perception of the professionals in relation to FGM. The results of our study indicate that to avoid these inequities men must be sensitized, cultural stereotypes should be opposed and we must be respectful as to the preferences of the migrant women with regard to the gender of the professional they wish to be attended by, similar to what has been observed in other types of problems . . . .

Catalonia has been a receptor of Sub-Saharan immigration since the 1980s and at the end of this decade the first phenomena of family regrouping took place with the arrival of the wives and children. Legislation against FGM in Spain was promulgated in 2003 and a law allowing extraterritorial persecution of this crime came into effect in 2005. We are, therefore, before a recent and culturally alien phenomenon for which practicing physicians have not received training.

The results of this study demonstrate that the way the primary care professionals in our area confront FGM is similar to that of their colleagues in five European countries studied by Leye. It also describes important gaps in knowledge and cultural contextualisation and scarce educational measures and support for decision making, with important ethical dilemmas which make not only a clinically adequate professional approach but also [a] culturally respectful approach towards the beliefs and needs of the women.

With regard to the limitations of this study it should be indicated that the anonymity of the questionnaire does not allow paired analysis between the professionals participating in 2001 and those of 2004. It should also be mentioned that the questionnaire in 2004 did not collect exactly the same information on the knowledge, reasons and countries in which this practice is common, and therefore we could not compare this information between the two years. We believe that the lack of statistical significance in some of the trends observed on multivariate analysis was due to a lack of study power to detect these differences.

Conclusion

This study demonstrates that the problem of FGM is present in the primary care centres in our country, with the percentage of professionals detecting some case having tripled in three years. The collectives most in contact with the problem are those in paediatrics and gynaecology, with women showing greater professional sensitivity towards the subject. The professionals over-evaluated their degree of knowledge of FGM and less than half could correctly identify the typology and countries in which FGM is practiced. It is therefore necessary to promote anthropologic knowledge of the problem to develop activities of prevention and detection of family risk to avoid legal actions against these subjects. The development of positive models of intervention, with respectful transcultural attention to values and beliefs in subjects as culturally deep-rooted and sensitive as FGM, will also allow other cultural aspects linked to health and disease among immigrants to be approached more successfully. This problem has only recently appeared in Spain and should be analysed and monitored with new studies to observe in depth the attitudes of the professionals towards this situation, and to also explore the beliefs and needs of the immigrant families in our countries....

FGM AS A CHALLENGE TO ETHICAL RELATIVISM

Ordinarily, we make an effort to accept the practices and beliefs of people in other cultures, even if those practices and beliefs are different from our own. After centuries of colonialism, imperialism, and discrimination, modern intellectual life is characterized by a conscious effort to avoid criticizing the beliefs and practices of people in other cultures. In addition, many people try to refrain from characterizing any belief or cultural practice as right or wrong.

FGM, however, poses a particular challenge to multiculturalism and brings us back to the issue raised in the first chapter of this book with regard to the existence of universal values. Are there any universal values that transcend the cultural values and practices of particular societies? As Robert Schwartz (1994) has explained, it was very easy to be multicultural when the necessary accommodations were simple and inoffensive, but FGM forces us to reconsider whether we really believe in multiculturalism, and whether we are really willing to accept the autonomous choices that are made by patients from very different cultures.

As discussed in Chapter One, some people follow the approach of *ethical relativism*. Under that approach, morality exists only in the context of a particular culture, and ethics is relative to the specific culture in which people live. Whether an action is ethical depends entirely on the practices and values of the particular culture.

That approach to ethics seems to promote tolerance and multiculturalism. However, it can present serious problems in judging the morality of conduct that we consider grossly unethical but that other cultures consider perfectly appropriate. As Schwartz (1994) posed the question, "If we are so committed to multiculturalism that we are willing to entertain it even when it is inconsistent with values fundamental to the prevailing culture, are we saying that all cultural (and religious) practices are equally worthy of respect?" (p. 433). Some cultures consider slavery to be appropriate, although we consider slavery to be extremely unethical. An ethical relativist would say that the morality of slavery can be determined only in the context of the values and practices of that particular culture.

What would an ethical relativist conclude about the morality of FGM? To be consistent, a true ethical relativist would have to accept the practice of FGM as legitimate and ethical within the context of a particular culture. To a relativist, FGM would be ethical for a person in a culture that practices FGM but would not be ethical for a person in another culture. In fact, an ethical relativist would say that it is unethical to try to prevent a person from practicing FGM if FGM is part of that person's culture. Nevertheless, those ethical conclusions leave us profoundly dissatisfied. How can we reach a satisfactory conclusion about the ethics of FGM, a practice that is accepted in some cultures and vehemently rejected in others? To answer that question, we need to decide whether it is appropriate to impose the cultural values and ethics of one culture on people from another culture.

In Italy the National Bioethics Committee concluded that respect for diverse cultures does not require acceptance of FGM (Turillazzi and Fineschi, 2007, p. 99). In the United States this ethical issue was addressed by former U.S. representative Patricia Schroeder, a Democrat from the State of Colorado, who introduced the first bill in the U.S. Congress that proposed to make FGM a federal crime. That particular bill was not enacted, but the U.S. Congress eventually enacted a federal statute in 1996, as part of an immigration reform law. In a 1994 editorial about FGM in the *New England Journal of Medicine*, Schroeder argued that it is appropriate to impose U.S. values on other people when those people immigrate to the United States. As Schroeder wrote, "some may argue that prohibiting the practice within our own borders is culturally imperialistic. I cannot agree. Imposing certain values on people living in this country is our prerogative. There are a number of practices that immigrants are required to leave at home when they move here. Polygamy and slavery are two obvious examples" (p. 739).

Schroeder's approach provides a way to justify prohibiting FGM for immigrants who come to the United States or another industrialized country, and it seems very persuasive. However, this approach also opens the door to further questions. If it is appropriate to impose majority values on people who move to the United States or another industrialized country, we really cannot stop there. What about the people who do not immigrate to the United States or another industrialized country? Don't we have an ethical obligation to help people who remain in their own countries as well? On this point the issue of slavery provides a useful analogy. Because we believe that slavery is morally wrong, it is not sufficient to prohibit slavery within the boundaries of our own country. We have an ethical obligation to stop slavery in other parts of the world as well. Similarly, if we believe that FGM is unethical in our country, don't we have an ethical obligation to do everything in our power to prevent FGM in other countries? The law that prohibits FGM for minors within the United States is an important and necessary step, but it is only one step, and it does not resolve the underlying ethical dilemma.

Moreover, the suggestion that it is acceptable to impose U.S. values on new immigrants presupposes the existence of common national values. The United States is often described as a melting pot of different cultures, and other industrialized countries have become diverse societies as well. National values change over time, as a variety of people move to a country and add their distinctive cultures to the melting pot. As times have changed and as populations have changed, it is not at all clear that there is a common set of shared national values that a country should—or even could—impose on new arrivals. For all of these reasons, Schroeder's approach is helpful, but it does not fully solve the ethical problem of FGM.

ETHICS OF FGM FOR ADULT WOMEN

Some critics of FGM argue that it should be prohibited altogether. Others argue that FGM should be prohibited for minors but permitted for adult women on request, as a matter of individual autonomy and informed consent.

The Cairo Declaration for the Elimination of FGM took the position that all performance of FGM should be illegal, and that age or consent is irrelevant. According to paragraph 13 of the Cairo Declaration, "The age of a girl or woman or her consent to undergoing FGM should not, under any conditions, affect the criminality of the act" (Egyptian National Council for Childhood and Motherhood, 2003). In contrast, Toubia (1994) suggested that adult women should have the option to request and receive FGM as a matter of their own individual choice. As Toubia (1995) wrote, in the United States, "adults have the right to provide or withhold consent to any surgical procedure on any part of their bodies for cosmetic or curative reasons. In the draft bill introduced by Representative Schroeder, we recommend that 18 years be established as the age of consent for female circumcision. This would allow immigrant women from Africa the American right to make their own choice" (pp. 188–190).

In an article for the Guttmacher Institute, Frances Althaus (1997) cited Toubia's argument, saying that as "Nahid Toubia points out, Western women also subject themselves to medically unnecessary, hazardous procedures, such as cosmetic surgery and the insertion of breast implants, to increase their sexual desirability." Similarly, El Guindi (2006) compares FGM to breast enlargement and other types of dangerous and painful cosmetic surgery by which Western women alter or "mutilate" their bodies (p. 31.)

Writing in the *Canadian Medical Association Journal*, philosophy professor Eike-Henner Kluge (1993) accepted FGM for a willing adult. Kluge stated that "if there really is an informed, competent and voluntary request, then it is essentially a request for cosmetic surgery, albeit an extreme version" (p. 288). However, calling FGM cosmetic surgery does not answer the question of whether it is ethical. Most people agree that it would violate medical ethics to cut off a healthy limb or remove a healthy organ under the guise of cosmetic surgery, even if a mentally competent patient gave informed consent to the procedure. In addition, as Kluge recognized, it is a very different situation when a parent requests circumcision of a female minor. Finally, Kluge argued that even for an adult patient, a doctor is not obligated to perform a procedure that the doctor considers unethical. This is similar to the so-called right of conscience to refuse to perform abortions and other reproductive health procedures, as discussed in Chapter Four.

Kluge's analysis assumed that the adult woman asking for FGM was giving her voluntary consent to the procedure. Some people, however, argue that a woman from a culture that practices FGM cannot give a valid consent to the procedure, because her culture makes any purported consent inherently coercive. As Anne Gibeau (1998) asked, "How is choice conceptualized in a system in which profound repercussions occur when one does not make the right decision?" (p. 90). Schwartz (1994) responded to that argument by pointing out that ordinarily we do not treat a patient's culture as a reason to assume that a patient's consent is invalid on the ground of coercion (p. 436). Nevertheless, Sirrku Hellsten (2001) has noted that "social coercion easily can disguise itself as an individual's autonomous choice" (p. 104).

So, who's right? Should FGM be prohibited altogether, or should it be permitted for adult women as a matter of individual autonomy and informed consent? Should health care professionals and organizations agree to perform FGM or allow the performance of FGM in their facilities? The activity at the end of this chapter provides an opportunity to consider these ethical issues in the context of developing a hospital policy on FGM.

SUMMARY

FGM is a serious problem of global public health. The World Health Organization and other major UN agencies have estimated that at least 100 million women and girls have been subjected to genital mutilation and that 3 million girls are at risk of being subjected to genital mutilation every year. FGM has severe physical and mental consequences, and no medical benefits are known to exist. Although FGM has been most common in certain parts of Africa and the Middle East, widespread migration from those regions has forced health care providers in industrialized countries to face clinical and ethical issues they had never expected to face, in order to serve their increasingly diverse patient populations. Many health care providers in industrialized countries are now treating patients who have undergone FGM or are requesting FGM, and they are also caring for minors who are at risk of having FGM performed upon them at the request of their families. This chapter has explained the facts about FGM, including the roles of religion and culture. In addition, this chapter has analyzed the ethical issues surrounding FGM, such as whether FGM should be permitted for adult women, as a matter of individual autonomy and informed consent, or should be prohibited altogether. In both developed and developing countries, health care providers need to evaluate these ethical issues in order to respond appropriately to requests to perform FGM or to allow FGM to be performed in their facilities.

KEY TERMS

clitoridectomy

excision

female genital mutilation (FGM)

infibulation

DISCUSSION QUESTIONS

1. Is FGM a matter of religion or a matter of culture? Does this distinction make a difference in deciding whether it is ethical to perform FGM or participate in the performance of FGM?
2. When health care professionals think that a child is at risk of being subjected to FGM, should they notify the police or other governmental authorities?
3. Are there any universal values that transcend the cultural values of societies that practice FGM, and if so, what are those values?
4. Is it cultural imperialism to impose the values of the majority of the people in a country on new immigrants to that country?
5. If we think that a practice is unethical when performed in our country, do we have an ethical obligation to try to prevent that practice in other parts of the world as well?

ACTIVITY: DEVELOPING A HOSPITAL POLICY ON FGM

Jefferson County Hospital (JCH), our fictional example, is a public hospital in the United States that is owned and operated by the County of Jefferson. The hospital is located in Jefferson City, which is the largest city in Jefferson County. JCH is not a teaching hospital, but it provides most types of secondary and tertiary hospital services. It has 450 licensed beds. In addition to its inpatient operating rooms, JCH maintains an ambulatory surgery center on its campus, with four outpatient operating rooms.

Jefferson County has a large population of immigrants from Africa, including people from countries where the practice of FGM is fairly common. Many of JCH's female patients who are immigrants from Africa have already undergone FGM before immigrating to the United States. Occasionally, adult women from Africa request JCH to perform FGM on them. These requests occur most often in connection with labor and delivery. In most of these cases, women who had been infibulated in the past are requesting reinfibulation after vaginal delivery. Reinfibulating a woman after vaginal delivery may involve stitching the labia together in a way that makes intercourse impossible or difficult. In addition to requesting FGM for themselves, some adult women have requested JCH to perform various types of FGM procedures on their daughters.

JCH is located in a state that prohibits the performance of FGM on persons under the age of eighteen years. Thus, the applicable state law is similar to the U.S. federal law, which generally prohibits the performance of FGM on minors but provides for two exceptions when FGM may be performed for medical reasons. Like the U.S. federal law, the state law is silent with regard to the performance of FGM on adults.

JCH is committed to multiculturalism and wants to provide culturally sensitive care that meets the needs of its diverse community. Recently, the chief executive officer of JCH appointed a committee to consider the issue of FGM and develop a proposed policy for the hospital. The committee members include representatives of the hospital administration and medical staff, local religious leaders, and representatives of the African immigrant community in Jefferson County.

The committee's discussions resulted in heated debate. Some members of the committee argued that FGM should be prohibited altogether at JCH, even for adult women who requested reinfibulation after vaginal delivery. A second group of committee members argued that the hospital's policy should permit reinfibulation after vaginal delivery for adult patients on request, but otherwise should prohibit all FGM procedures. A third group of committee members argued that the hospital's policy should not be limited to reinfibulation after delivery, but should permit any type of FGM procedure that is requested by an adult patient. After all, argued the members of that third group, JCH performs cosmetic surgery on request for adult patients, including penis enlargement and also breast implants for purposes other than postmastectomy reconstruction. Immigrant women, that third group of committee members said, have a right to make their own decisions about FGM as a matter of individual autonomy and informed consent.

The majority of the committee members voted to accept the position of this third group and to allow FGM for adult patients, although there were strong dissents from other members. Meanwhile, one physician on the JCH medical staff has indicated that he is willing to perform FGM for adult patients, but other physicians and nurses at JCH have stated that they will refuse to participate in any FGM procedure.

Under these circumstances, the committee has developed a proposed policy for JCH that reads as follows:

1. In accordance with federal and state law, no FGM procedure may be performed at JCH on a patient under the age of eighteen years, unless the procedure fits within one of the two exceptions set forth in federal and state law.
2. For patients over the age of eighteen years (adult patients), FGM procedures (including but not limited to reinfibulation after vaginal delivery) may be performed at JCH, provided that the patient gives her informed consent for the FGM procedure.

3. For adult patients, informed consent to the performance of FGM procedures must be demonstrated and documented in accordance with the following provisions:

   a. Hospital staff shall provide the patient with written materials about the risks and consequences of FGM. The materials must be in a language that is understandable to the patient.

   b. The physician shall discuss the proposed procedure with the patient in person, while no member of the patient's family is present. If a translator is required for that discussion, the translator must be provided by the hospital and may not be a member of the patient's family.

   c. The patient must make a specific written request for the FGM procedure in a language that is understandable to the patient.

4. The proposed FGM procedure shall be reviewed by the hospital's Ethics Committee at its weekly meeting.

5. No physician, nurse, or other health care worker is required to participate in any FGM procedure that he or she considers to be unethical. The hospital shall not take any action or retaliate in any way on the ground of that refusal to participate in the FGM procedure.

Please analyze whether the proposed hospital policy is ethical. Explain your reasons for finding that it is ethical or that it is not ethical.

CHAPTER SIX

ETHICAL ISSUES OF RESEARCH WITH HUMAN SUBJECTS

LEARNING OBJECTIVES

- Understand and be able to explain the ethical problems that arise in conducting research with human subjects.

- Learn the history of the human rights violations perpetrated in the name of research.

- Acquire proficiency in analyzing the ethical principles relevant to the interests of individuals and their communities, including the principles of autonomy, beneficence, and justice.

- Demonstrate the ability to describe and evaluate the special ethical problems that arise in conducting research with human subjects in developing countries, including fairness in selecting the subjects of research and allocating the burdens and benefits of research.

BACKGROUND INFORMATION AND THE BELMONT REPORT

Perhaps more than any other issue in health ethics, the development and refinement of ethical principles for research with human subjects demonstrates a conscious effort to learn from society's past mistakes. We know about some of the unconscionable violations of human rights that have been perpetrated in the name of research, and it is reasonable to assume that many more violations remain unknown. In the infamous Tuskegee experiment, the U.S. Public Health Service conducted research for many years on the effects of not treating syphilis in African American men. The participants in that study were led to believe that they were receiving treatment, and the researchers even tried to prevent the participants from receiving treatment for syphilis from any other health care provider (Brandt, 1978). In the aftermath of World War II, the public became aware of horrendous medical experiments performed by Nazi doctors, including testing drugs for immunization against smallpox, cholera, and malaria. The postwar military tribunal found that performing medical experiments without consent of the subjects constituted war crimes and crimes against humanity. The tribunal sentenced eight doctors to prison and seven doctors to death. In addition, the tribunal issued the Nuremberg Code, which states the basic requirement of voluntary consent by human subjects of research.

More recently, the increase in the volume of research performed in developing countries and the persistence or worsening of health disparities have led to an increased concern with issues of social justice in research with human subjects. For example, Solomon Benatar (2001), a professor of medicine in South Africa, has written, "It is suggested that privileged people need to hold up a mirror to their lives, and try to see themselves from the perspective of the marginalized and weak in the world today and as historians in the future may see them in retrospect—as decadent and selfish" (pp. 338–339).

In 1979, the U.S. National Commission for the Protection of Human Subjects of Biomedical and Behavioral Research issued *The Belmont Report: Ethical Principles and Guidelines for the Protection of Human Subjects of Research*. This influential report identifies three basic ethical principles for research with human subjects: respect for persons, beneficence, and justice. In recent years the Belmont Report has been critiqued on a variety of grounds (see, for example, Childress and others, 2005), but it remains an extremely important resource in the field of research ethics. As Charles Weijer and Guy LeBlanc (2006) put it, "We have not, nor would we, suggest that the *Belmont Report* is the last word in research ethics. However, it surely is the first word" (pp. 794–795 and n. 8).

In addition, the three principles of the Belmont Report provide a convenient way to categorize and analyze the wide range of issues that arise in research on human subjects.

Thus, this chapter begins with an excerpt from the Belmont Report itself, and then separately analyzes the issues arising under each of the report's ethical principles. The **principle of respect for persons** encompasses informed consent to participation in research. The **principle of beneficence** includes balancing the benefits and risks of research. The **principle of justice** prohibits exploitation of subjects and communities and requires fairness in selecting or excluding potential subjects of research. After analyzing each of these three basic principles, this chapter will evaluate different approaches to two specific issues. The first issue is whether new drugs for serious diseases, such as HIV/AIDS, should be tested against the best existing therapy or against a placebo. The second issue is clarifying the ethical duty that researchers have to their human subjects after completion of the research, particularly when research is performed in developing countries by researchers from developed countries.

THE BELMONT REPORT: ETHICAL PRINCIPLES AND GUIDELINES FOR THE PROTECTION OF HUMAN SUBJECTS OF RESEARCH

BY THE NATIONAL COMMISSION FOR THE PROTECTION OF HUMAN SUBJECTS OF BIOMEDICAL AND BEHAVIORAL RESEARCH

Part B: Basic Ethical Principles

The expression "basic ethical principles" refers to those general judgments that serve as a basic justification for the many particular ethical prescriptions and evaluations of human actions. Three basic principles, among those generally accepted in our cultural tradition, are particularly relevant to the ethics of research involving human subjects: the principles of respect of persons, beneficence and justice.

1. Respect for Persons. Respect for persons incorporates at least two ethical convictions: first, that individuals should be treated as autonomous agents, and second, that persons with diminished autonomy are entitled to protection. The principle of respect for persons thus divides into two separate moral requirements: the requirement to acknowledge autonomy and the requirement to protect those with diminished autonomy....

In most cases of research involving human subjects, respect for persons demands that subjects enter into the research voluntarily and with adequate information. In some situations, however, application of the principle is not obvious. The involvement of prisoners as subjects of research provides an instructive example. On the one hand, it would seem that the principle of respect for persons requires that prisoners not be deprived of the opportunity to volunteer for research. On the other hand, under prison conditions they may be subtly coerced or unduly influenced to engage in research activities for which they would not otherwise volunteer. Respect for persons would then dictate that prisoners be protected. Whether to allow prisoners to "volunteer" or to "protect" them presents a dilemma. Respecting persons, in most hard cases, is often a matter of balancing competing claims urged by the principle of respect itself.

2. Beneficence. Persons are treated in an ethical manner not only by respecting their decisions and protecting them from harm, but also by making efforts to secure their well-being. Such treatment falls under the principle of beneficence. The term "beneficence" is often understood to cover acts of kindness or charity that go beyond strict obligation. In this document, beneficence is understood in a stronger sense, as an obligation. Two general rules have been formulated as complementary expressions of beneficent actions in this sense: (1) do not harm and (2) maximize possible benefits and minimize possible harms.

The Hippocratic maxim "do no harm" has long been a fundamental principle of medical ethics. Claude Bernard extended it to the realm of research, saying that one should not injure one person regardless of the benefits that might come to others. However, even avoiding harm requires learning what is harmful; and, in the process of obtaining this information, persons may be exposed to risk of harm. Further, the Hippocratic Oath requires physicians to benefit their patients "according to their best judgment." Learning what will in fact benefit may require exposing persons to risk. The problem posed by these imperatives is to decide when it is justifiable to seek certain benefits despite the risks involved, and when the benefits should be foregone because of the risks . . . .

The principle of beneficence often occupies a well-defined justifying role in many areas of research involving human subjects. An example is found in research involving children. Effective ways of treating childhood diseases and fostering healthy development are benefits that serve to justify research involving children—even when individual research subjects are not direct beneficiaries. Research also makes it possible to avoid the harm that may result from the application of previously accepted routine practices that on closer investigation turn out to be dangerous. But the role of the principle of beneficence is not always so unambiguous. A difficult ethical problem remains, for example, about research that presents more than minimal risk without immediate prospect of direct benefit to the children involved. Some have argued that such research is inadmissible, while others have pointed out that this limit would rule out much research promising great benefit to children in the future. Here again, as with all hard cases, the different claims covered by the principle of beneficence may come into conflict and force difficult choices.

3. Justice. Who ought to receive the benefits of research and bear its burdens? This is a question of justice, in the sense of "fairness in distribution" or "what is deserved." An injustice occurs when some benefit to which a person is entitled is denied without good reason or when some burden is imposed unduly. Another way of conceiving the principle of justice is that equals ought to be treated equally. However, this statement requires explication. Who is equal and who is unequal? What considerations justify departure from equal distribution? Almost all commentators allow that distinctions based on experience, age, deprivation, competence, merit and position do sometimes constitute criteria justifying differential treatment for certain purposes. It is necessary, then, to explain in what respects people should be treated equally. There are several widely accepted formulations of just ways to distribute burdens and benefits. Each formulation mentions some relevant property on the basis of which burdens and benefits should be distributed. These formulations are (1) to each person an equal share, (2) to each person according to individual need, (3) to each person according to individual effort, (4) to each person according to societal contribution, and (5) to each person according to merit.

Questions of justice have long been associated with social practices such as punishment, taxation and political representation. Until recently these questions have not generally been associated with scientific research. However, they are foreshadowed even in the earliest reflections on the ethics of research involving human subjects. For example, during the 19th and early 20th centuries the burdens of serving as research subjects fell largely upon poor ward patients, while the benefits of improved medical care flowed primarily to private patients. Subsequently, the exploitation of unwilling prisoners as research subjects in Nazi concentration camps was condemned as a particularly flagrant injustice. In this country, in the 1940s, the Tuskegee syphilis study used disadvantaged, rural black men to study the untreated course of a disease that is by no means confined to that population. These subjects were deprived of demonstrably effective treatment in order not to interrupt the project, long after such treatment became generally available.

Against this historical background, it can be seen how conceptions of justice are relevant to research involving human subjects. For example, the selection of research subjects needs to be scrutinized in order to determine whether some classes (e.g., welfare patients, particular racial and ethnic minorities, or persons confined to institutions) are being systematically selected simply because of their easy availability, their compromised position, or their manipulability, rather than for reasons directly related to the problem being studied. Finally, whenever research supported by public funds leads to the development of therapeutic devices and procedures, justice demands both that these not provide advantages only to those who can afford them and that such research should not unduly involve persons from groups unlikely to be among the beneficiaries of subsequent applications of the research.

Part C: Applications

Applications of the general principles to the conduct of research leads to consideration of the following requirements: informed consent, risk/benefit assessment, and the selection of subjects of research.

1. Informed Consent. Respect for persons requires that subjects, to the degree that they are capable, be given the opportunity to choose what shall or shall not happen to them. This opportunity is provided when adequate standards for informed consent are satisfied.

While the importance of informed consent is unquestioned, controversy prevails over the nature and possibility of an informed consent. Nonetheless, there is widespread agreement that the consent process can be analyzed as containing three elements: information, comprehension and voluntariness.

Information. Most codes of research establish specific items for disclosure intended to assure that subjects are given sufficient information. These items generally include: the research procedure, their purposes, risks and anticipated benefits, alternative procedures (where therapy is involved), and a statement offering the subject the opportunity to ask questions and to withdraw at any time from the research. Additional items have been proposed, including how subjects are selected, the person responsible for the research, etc. . . .

Comprehension. The manner and context in which information is conveyed is as important as the information itself. For example, presenting information in a disorganized and rapid fashion, allowing too little time for consideration or curtailing opportunities for questioning, all may adversely affect a subject's ability to make an informed choice.

Because the subject's ability to understand is a function of intelligence, rationality, maturity and language, it is necessary to adapt the presentation of the information to the subject's capacities. Investigators are responsible for ascertaining that the subject has comprehended the information. While there is always an obligation to ascertain that the information about risk to subjects is complete and adequately comprehended, when the risks are more serious, that obligation increases. On occasion, it may be suitable to give some oral or written tests of comprehension.

Special provision may need to be made when comprehension is severely limited—for example, by conditions of immaturity or mental disability....

Voluntariness. An agreement to participate in research constitutes a valid consent only if voluntarily given. This element of informed consent requires conditions free of coercion and undue influence. Coercion occurs when an overt threat of harm is intentionally presented by one person to another in order to obtain compliance. Undue influence, by contrast, occurs through an offer of an excessive, unwarranted, inappropriate or improper reward or other overture in order to obtain compliance. Also, inducements that would ordinarily be acceptable may become undue influences if the subject is especially vulnerable.

Unjustifiable pressures usually occur when persons in positions of authority or commanding influence—especially where possible sanctions are involved—urge a course of action for a subject. A continuum of such influencing factors exists, however, and it is impossible to state precisely where justifiable persuasion ends and undue influence begins. But undue influence would include actions such as manipulating a person's choice through the controlling influence of a close relative and threatening to withdraw health services to which an individual would otherwise be entitled.

2. Assessment of Risks and Benefits. The assessment of risks and benefits requires a careful arrayal of relevant data, including, in some cases, alternative ways of obtaining the benefits sought in the research. Thus, the assessment presents both an opportunity and a responsibility to gather systematic and comprehensive information about proposed research. For the investigator, it is a means to examine whether the proposed research is properly designed. For a review committee, it is a method for determining whether the risks that will be presented to subjects are justified. For prospective subjects, the assessment will assist the determination whether or not to participate.

The Nature and Scope of Risks and Benefits. The requirement that research be justified on the basis of a favorable risk/benefit assessment bears a close relation to the principle of beneficence, just as the moral requirement that informed consent be obtained is derived primarily from the principle of respect for persons . . . .

. . . Accordingly, so-called risk/benefit assessments are concerned with the probabilities and magnitudes of possible harm and anticipated benefits. Many kinds of possible harms and benefits need to be taken into account. There are, for example, risks of psychological harm, physical harm, legal harm, social harm and economic harm and the corresponding benefits. While the most likely types of harms to research subjects are those of psychological or physical pain or injury, other possible kinds should not be overlooked . . . .

The Systematic Assessment of Risks and Benefits. It is commonly said that benefits and risks must be "balanced" and shown to be "in a favorable ratio." The metaphorical character of these terms draws attention to the difficulty of making precise judgments . . . .

3. Selection of Subjects. Just as the principle of respect for persons finds expression in the requirements for consent, and the principle of beneficence in risk/benefit assessment, the principle of justice gives rise to moral requirements that there be fair procedures and outcomes in the selection of research subjects.

Justice is relevant to the selection of subjects of research at two levels: the social and the individual. Individual justice in the selection of subjects would require that researchers exhibit fairness: thus, they should not offer potentially beneficial research only to some patients who are in their favor or select only "undesirable" persons for risky research. Social justice requires that distinction be drawn between classes of subjects that ought, and ought not, to participate in any particular kind of research, based on the ability of members of that class to bear burdens and on the appropriateness of placing further burdens on already burdened persons. Thus, it can be considered a matter of social justice that there is an order of preference in the selection of classes of subjects (e.g., adults before children) and that some classes of potential subjects (e.g., the institutionalized mentally infirm or prisoners) may be involved as research subjects, if at all, only on certain conditions.

Injustice may appear in the selection of subjects, even if individual subjects are selected fairly by investigators and treated fairly in the course of research. Thus, injustice arises from social, racial, sexual and cultural biases institutional-ized in society. Thus, even if individual researchers are treating their research subjects fairly, and even if IRBs [institutional review boards] are taking care to assure that subjects are selected fairly within a particular institution, unjust social patterns may nevertheless appear in the overall distribution of the bur-dens and benefits of research. Although individual institutions or investigators may not be able to resolve a problem that is pervasive in their social setting, they can consider distributive justice in selecting research subjects . . . .

One special instance of injustice results from the involvement of vulnerable subjects. Certain groups, such as racial minorities, the economically disadvantaged, the very sick, and the institutionalized may continually be sought as research subjects, owing to their ready availability in settings where research is conducted. Given their dependent status and their frequently compromised capacity for free consent, they should be protected against the danger of being involved in research solely for administrative convenience, or because they are easy to manipulate as a result of their illness or socioeconomic condition.

Source: U.S. National Commission for the Protection of Human Subjects of Biomedical and Behavioral Research, 1979.

In evaluating the Belmont Report from a global perspective, it is important to consider whether its ethical concepts are universal principles of human life or merely the values of a particular culture or group of cultures. The Belmont Report, as shown in the previous excerpt, specifically refers to "[t]hree basic principles, among those generally accepted in our cultural tradition." The report authors did not reach the issue of whether principles such as individual autonomy are generally accepted in other cultural traditions, or how those principles might be understood differently in other cultures. The discussion on autonomy and informed consent later in this chapter will evaluate the cultural as well as the practical implications of making a decision to participate as a human subject of research.

In addition, the Belmont Report does not explain in detail why it is ethical to conduct experiments on human beings or why it is ethical to ask human beings to subject themselves to the risks of research. The Hippocratic Oath requires that physicians "do no harm," but the Belmont Report justifies causing some harm to human subjects on the ground that "avoiding harm requires learning what is harmful." But why is it ethical to conduct experiments on human beings in order to learn what is harmful? It is not sufficient to merely say that we always do it that way or that we need to do it that way.

From the perspective of Kantian ethics, each individual must be viewed as an end in himself or herself, and not only as a means to an end, such as advancement of scientific knowledge. On utilitarian grounds we could justify using people for the good of society, but we routinely impose limits on the extent to which society may use people, and most people reject a pure utilitarian approach. From the perspective of principlism, we could rely on the prima facie moral duty of autonomy to permit individuals to give their voluntary consent to the risks and harms of research. Nevertheless, we cannot rely solely on the fact that human subjects of research are willing to let researchers expose them to risks and harm, because society routinely imposes limits on the risks and harms to which even competent adults are permitted to subject themselves.

A principlist approach would require balancing the moral duty of autonomy with the potentially conflicting moral duties of beneficence, nonmaleficence, and justice. Under this approach some types of research with human subjects are ethically justifiable and others are not. Each proposal to conduct research with human subjects must be evaluated on its own merits. That is the approach taken by the authors of the Belmont Report, albeit without much analysis of why it is ethical for society to use individuals in this manner. The Belmont Report accepts the common assumption that the basic concept of using humans as subjects of research is ethical so long as certain conditions are met, such as voluntary informed consent and review of the study by an ethics committee.

This approach has contributed to the development of a comprehensive system of **institutional review boards (IRBs)** to review specific proposals for research with human subjects. Technically, the requirement in the United States for IRB review applies only to research that is funded by the U.S. government. As a practical matter, however, IRB review procedures—or similar procedures—are applied to a large share of global health care research, for several reasons. First, many universities in the United States use the IRB system or a similar system to review research that is funded by sources other than the U.S. government. Second, many of the largest pharmaceutical manufacturers in the world are U.S. companies. Third, countries other than the United States have adopted similar requirements for review of research with human subjects. Finally, the U.S. Food and Drug Administration (FDA) will not approve a drug for sale in the lucrative U.S. market unless the sponsor of the clinical trial meets certain requirements, even if the trial is conducted in another country or sponsored by a non-U.S. organization (U.S. Food and Drug Administration, 2009).

Under these circumstances, procedures for IRB review or similar procedures have become routine in the world of health care research, including clinical trials conducted in developing countries. These procedures include a review of the risks and benefits of the research, the fairness in selection of subjects, and the process for obtaining informed consent.

Many people consider IRB-type procedures to be a crucial safeguard for the protection of human subjects, especially for patients who are members of vulnerable groups. Others criticize IRBs as being bureaucratic organizations that elevate procedure and form over substance. In a 2009 report, the U.S. Government Accountability Office informed Congress "that the IRB system is vulnerable to unethical manipulation, particularly by companies or individuals who intend to abuse the system or to commit fraud, or who lack the aptitude or qualifications to conduct and oversee clinical trials" (p. 4). In addition, critics argue that IRBs protect themselves, their staff, and their institutions by stopping any research that might result in death or injury to identifiable subjects, while ignoring the possibly greater number of deaths or injuries to unidentifiable individuals that could have been prevented by proceeding with the research (Zywicki, 2007). In 2007, David Hyman wrote that there is "no empirical evidence that IRBs have any benefit whatsoever" (p. 756). Hyman even offered to give "\$25 to the first person who finds anything in print (as of December 14, 2006) providing empirical evidence that IRBs have any benefit whatsoever" (p. 756, n. 31).

Notwithstanding the lack of empirical evidence, most people continue to accept the value of IRB review for protection of human subjects, essentially as an article of faith. That faith in the IRB may reflect an implicit value judgment by society to err on the side of preventing research that could cause harm to identifiable subjects, regardless of the harm that might be caused to other people by preventing potentially beneficial research. As a decision-making process, the IRB review might be compared to the criminal trial, a process designed for making a decision on behalf of a society about the guilt or innocence of a defendant. It is often said that it would be better for ten guilty persons to go free than for one innocent person to be falsely imprisoned or executed. In the context of health care research, it appears that society has adopted a rule that it would be better to let ten unidentifiable people die or suffer from a disease that might possibly be prevented through research than to allow one identifiable research subject to be killed or injured in the process of research.

AUTONOMY AND VOLUNTARY INFORMED CONSENT

The Belmont Report explains that the basic principle of respect for persons includes the two concepts of individual autonomy and protection for individuals with "diminished autonomy." **Autonomy** requires that individuals have the opportunity to make their own decisions about whether to participate in research, after they receive appropriate disclosure of the risks through the process of informed consent. Chapter Two of this book analyzes the ethical issues of informed consent in the context of clinical practice, where health care professionals and their patients might disagree about the adequacy of disclosing the risks. In contrast, this chapter analyzes the ethical issues of informed consent in the context of research with human subjects. In this context as well, researchers and their subjects might disagree about whether the disclosure of risks was sufficient, and whether the consent to participate was truly informed.

One important example of a dispute about informed consent involves a 1996 study by Pfizer, Inc., of the use of the antibiotic trovafloxacin mesylate (trade name Trovan) in children in Kano, Nigeria, during an epidemic of bacterial meningitis (Stephens, 2006). Some children and some guardians of children who participated in the study alleged that Pfizer had failed to obtain informed consent for the children's participation. This dispute was the subject of complex legal proceedings in Nigeria and the United States. The plaintiffs in the U.S. litigation made the following allegations:

> [They] claim that Pfizer, working in partnership with the Nigerian government, failed to secure the informed consent of either the children or their guardians and specifically failed to disclose or explain the experimental nature of the study or the serious risks involved. Although the treatment protocol required the researchers to offer or read the subjects documents requesting and facilitating their informed consent, this was allegedly not done in either English or the subjects' native language of Hausa. [They] also contend that Pfizer deviated from its treatment protocol by not alerting the children or their guardians to the side effects of Trovan or other risks of the experiment, not providing them with the option of choosing alternative treatment, and not informing them that the nongovernmental organization Médecins Sans Frontières (Doctors Without Borders) was providing a conventional and effective treatment for bacterial meningitis, free of charge, at the same site [*Abdullahi* v. *Pfizer, Inc.*, pp. 169–170, footnote omitted].

In response, Pfizer, Inc. (2009), insisted that the "1996 Trovan clinical study in Kano was conducted with the approval of the Nigerian government, and consent of the participants' parents or guardians, and was consistent with both international and Nigerian laws." During the process of the litigation, a U.S. appellate court recognized the extreme importance of informed consent to international peace, security, and public health, as follows:

> Over the last two decades, pharmaceutical companies in industrialized countries have looked to poorer, developing countries as sites for the medical research essential to the development of new drugs . . . . Life-saving drugs can potentially be developed more quickly and cheaply, and developing countries may be given access to cutting edge medicines and treatments to assist underresourced and understaffed public health systems, which grapple with life-threatening diseases afflicting their populations.

The success of these efforts promises to play a major role in reducing the cross-border spread of contagious diseases, which is a significant threat to international peace and stability. The administration of drug trials without informed consent on the scale alleged in the complaints directly threatens these efforts because such conduct fosters distrust and resistance to international drug trials, cutting edge medical innovation, and critical international public health initiatives in which pharmaceutical companies play a key role. This case itself supplies an exceptionally good illustration of why this is so. The Associated Press reported that the Trovan trials in Kano apparently engendered such distrust in the local population that it was a factor contributing to an eleven-month-long, local boycott of a polio vaccination campaign in 2004, which impeded international and national efforts to vaccinate the population against a polio outbreak, with catastrophic results. According to the World Health Organization, polio originating in Nigeria triggered a major international outbreak of the disease between 2003 and 2006, causing it to spread across west, central, and the Horn of Africa and the Middle East, and to re-infect twenty previously polio-free countries.

The administration of drug trials without informed consent poses threats to national security by impairing our relations with other countries [*Abdullahi* v. *Pfizer, Inc.*, pp. 185–187, footnotes and citations omitted].

In addition, the Belmont Report explains that consent must be voluntary in order to be valid. For it to be voluntary, researchers must avoid **coercion**, which refers to an intentional threat to secure the individual's agreement to participate, and **undue influence**, which refers to an inappropriate or excessive reward or payment to secure the individual's agreement.

The traditional view has been that researchers should not ordinarily pay individuals to participate in research, but may provide reimbursement to compensate individuals for their costs of participating in the study. "Inducement payments for research subjects are thought to be 'undue' when they distort the judgment of potential research subjects and undermine the voluntariness of the subject's consent" (Ballantyne, 2008, p. 184, footnote omitted). But if offering money can be an undue influence that interferes with voluntary consent, what about offering potentially life-saving medical care to individuals, on condition that they agree to participate in the research? Why is that not undue influence and a lack of truly voluntary consent? The majority of research subjects participate as a way to receive medical care (Ballantyne, p. 190). Especially in developing countries, where most people lack access to medical care, individuals often agree to enroll in a clinical trial as the only way to obtain services that they desperately need (Schüklenk, 2004, p. 197). Under those circumstances, researchers offer potentially life-saving care to those patients, and only those patients, who voluntarily agree to participate in their clinical trial.

The Belmont Report recognizes that undue influence would include "threatening to withdraw health services to which an individual would otherwise be entitled." If the individuals were not otherwise entitled to the services, however, the conventional wisdom seems to be that offering to provide life-saving treatment is not an undue inducement for participation in research. In other words, most people take the position that the desperate situation of the patient is not the researchers' fault, and it is not the researchers' problem. As Angela Ballantyne (2008) wrote:

> Potential research participants in developing countries are often particularly vulnerable to the anticipated therapeutic benefit of research because of the limited availability of affordable therapies or accessible healthcare . . . . Presumably the primary source of potential undue influence resides in the hope of therapeutic benefit from the trial. If this motivation is "undue", it is a function of the background conditions of poverty against which the trials take place, rather than a function of any additional benefits offered during the trial. The chance that the trial will result in therapeutic benefit for trial participants is an irreducible part of clinical medical research [p. 187, footnote omitted].

One could argue to the contrary, of course, that the conventional view is both too limited and too convenient. As Benatar (2001) wrote, "Medical research, health care, conditions of life around the world and how humans flourish may seem separate, but they are all interdependent" (p. 337). It may be a radical proposition to suggest that there is a potential ethical concern in offering life-saving medical care to poor people in developing countries on condition of participating in a clinical trial. However, it is difficult to see how offering money is undue inducement but offering a chance for survival is not. At the very least, more consideration and analysis of this important issue is needed.

Meanwhile, questions arise about obtaining informed consent from subjects whose cultures and worldviews are very different from those of the industrialized West (Hyder and Wali, 2006, p. 34; Frimpong-Mansoh, 2008). As discussed in Chapter Two of this book, about informed consent for treatment, individuals in some cultures see themselves as integral parts of their families and communities, rather than as the autonomous decision makers on whom the Western concept of informed consent is based. As Nicholas Christakis (1988) explained, "signing or even thumbprinting a consent form may be deemed highly suspect in certain societies, as may a physician's 'excessive' explanation of the purpose of the research (which may be taken as indicative of some hidden, detrimental purpose)" (p. 35). Others believe that informed consent from the human subjects of research is a universal principle (Hyder and Wali, 2006, p. 34). Harold Shapiro and Eric Meslin (2001) have taken the position that informed consent is applicable to research conducted anywhere in the world, although they acknowledge that procedures to obtain consent might need to be adjusted to the cultures of developing countries (p.140). In an empirical study on the views of developing country health researchers, Adnan Hyder and Salman Wali (2006) concluded that those researchers strongly support the concept of informed consent but favor a flexible approach to the procedures for consent (p. 40).

In evaluating consent procedures, some experts have suggested that consent should be sought from leaders of the subject's community. According to Christakis (1988), "It may be necessary to secure the consent of a subject's family or social group instead of or in addition to the consent of the subject himself." That is, Christakis took the position that in some cases of essential research, consent by a leader of the community might be an alternative to consent by the individual subject (pp. 34–35). However, what the guidelines of the Council for International Organizations of Medical Sciences (2002) state is this: "In no case . . . may the permission of a community leader or other authority substitute for individual informed consent." In the United States, individual consent to research may be waived in unusual circumstances, such as a research study on emergency treatment in which individual or family consent is impractical. In those situations, community consultation and education have been used, but some of those studies have been questioned on ethical grounds (Dalton, 2006). With regard to research conducted in Africa, Augustine Frimpong-Mansoh explained in 2008 that consent by community leaders is a "customary African communitarian practice," and is merely a first step before obtaining informed consent from the individual subject of research (pp. 111, 113).

Even if the consent of community leaders is seen as an additional requirement rather than as an alternative to individual consent, several ethical and practical questions remain. It may be unrealistic to think that an individual could refuse to participate in a study that had been approved already by the leader of his or her community, especially where individuals see themselves as part of a group rather than as autonomous decision makers. In addition, there may be social pressure for individuals to go along with a study that provides some benefits to the community. Moreover, is it ethical to deprive individuals of the right to say yes because the leader of their community has said no? Individuals should not only have the right to refuse to participate in research but should also have the right to participate if they choose to do so.

Frimpong-Mansoh (2008) has argued that prior approval by African community leaders is analogous to the requirement in Western countries to seek approval from administrators of nursing homes or principals of schools before seeking individual consent from residents or students (pp. 110–111). However, there are two problems with that analogy. First, nursing home residents and students might have ways outside the institutional context to participate in clinical trials, but members of an African community might not have such opportunities. Second, it seems inappropriate to treat every member of a community in a developing country as having inherently diminished capacity to make his or her own decisions, as though he or she were comparable to a child or an elderly resident of an institution.

Of course, even in Western countries, individuals do not have the option to give their consent unless and until the applicable IRB has agreed to allow the research to proceed. Perhaps the African communitarian practice of consent by community leaders should be viewed as analogous to approval of proposed research by an IRB. In the next section of this chapter, on beneficence and cost-benefit analysis, we will evaluate the criticism that the system of IRB review may be unduly paternalistic, in that it deprives individuals of the opportunity to make their own choices after full disclosure of the risks.

At the end of this chapter, an activity provides an opportunity to analyze the ethical issues in using prisoners as subjects of research.

BENEFICENCE AND COST-BENEFIT ANALYSIS

As set forth in the Belmont Report, the basic ethical principle of beneficence is not limited to the traditional concept of helping other people. It also includes the related concept of nonmaleficence, which refers to not causing harm to other people. Thus, the traditional precept in medical ethics to "do no harm" is included within the basic principle of beneficence. In addition, the concept of beneficence, as used in the Belmont Report (as shown in the previous excerpt), includes an obligation to "maximize possible benefits and minimize possible harms."

Reasonable people may differ in their evaluation of the possible benefits and harms of a particular proposal. In fact, some people have argued that the acceptability of a specific risk will depend on the health conditions and resources of a particular society. More than twenty years ago Christakis (1988) wrote that "AIDS may be so widespread and deadly a disease in Africa that a higher degree of research risk must perforce be tolerated to deal with the problem, and this may well be socially sanctioned" (p. 36). Of course, others may disagree with the proposition that greater risks should be tolerated in that type of situation.

From a libertarian perspective, Richard Epstein (2008) has criticized the Belmont Report's inclusion of risk-benefit analysis within the concept of beneficence, because it effectively undercuts the principle of individual autonomy: "This report . . . starts off with a paean to individual autonomy. Yet by the time it is finished, it ends up with paving the way for the creation of centralized planning boards with complete authority to make decisions on what studies may be conducted and how . . . . The *Report* invokes an off-kilter account of individual beneficence . . . in the *Report* beneficence includes the ability to make decisions for others by means of a cost/benefit analysis and deprive individuals of the right to make it for themselves" (pp. 580–581). Should individuals have the opportunity to make their own decisions to participate in clinical trials, after full disclosure of the risks, even without approval by an IRB? Epstein argues that the IRB system is too paternalistic, and believes that we should focus instead on providing information to potential subjects. As he put it, we should "use the IRB process as a bulletin board, not a barricade" (p. 582). A contrary argument, of course, is that many potential subjects of research do not have the scientific knowledge, language skills, or education to evaluate the serious risks involved in many research projects. Even if potential subjects had those abilities, their medical conditions might impair their ability to make objective and carefully reasoned decisions about undergoing particular risks.

ISSUES OF JUSTICE AND FAIRNESS FOR HUMAN SUBJECTS

The Belmont Report explains the basic ethical principle of justice as a matter of fairness in distributing the burdens and benefits of research, including fairness in selecting participants. In particular the Belmont Report cautions against using members of vulnerable groups, such as institutionalized persons, poor persons, and minorities, merely because they are convenient or more easily manipulated. When the Belmont Report was issued in 1979, the primary concern in selection of subjects was unfairly imposing the burdens of research on vulnerable persons or groups by improperly selecting them to serve as research subjects. The authors of the report gave little attention to the potential unfairness of excluding people from participation in research, except for the brief admonition that researchers "should not offer potentially beneficial research only to some patients who are in their favor."

In recent years more attention has been paid to the need to provide fair access to participation in research for members of traditionally underserved groups. Rather than viewing medical research as an evil to be avoided whenever possible, many people now view participation in a clinical trial as a way—and perhaps the only way—to obtain a beneficial or life-saving drug, especially in the case of "last-chance" therapies for cancer. In addition there is now greater recognition of the disparities in health status and in utilization of specific treatments on the basis of race, gender, national origin, age, and other characteristics. In addition to recognizing the unfairness of excluding particular individuals and groups from participation in clinical trials, experts now also understand that they do not have sufficient data on the ways in which particular treatments may have differential effects on women, children, and other categories of patients. This information gap may have resulted from discrimination in the system of recruiting subjects for clinical trials and, to some extent, from additional regulatory requirements for conducting research on children and women of childbearing age. Although such requirements are intended to protect women and children from the harms of research, they may also be having the unintended effects of discouraging their inclusion in clinical trials and thus limiting the usefulness of results. Recently, regulatory authorities have made efforts to encourage or require the sponsors of research to include women, children, and other groups as appropriate when selecting the subjects of research.

When research is conducted in developing countries, the selection of subjects raises even more ethical issues. As explained by Shapiro and Meslin (2001), "If the intervention being tested is not likely to be affordable in the host country or if the health care infrastructure cannot support its proper distribution and use, it is unethical to ask persons in that country to participate in the research, since they will not enjoy any of its potential benefits" (p. 139). That concern, among others, caused commentators to criticize a proposal by a U.S. company to study a new surfactant drug to treat premature infants with respiratory distress syndrome in Latin America, because poor patients in Latin America were very unlikely to have access to expensive surfactant drugs for the foreseeable future (Shapiro and Meslin, 2001, pp. 140–141; Hawkins, 2006, p. 471). This does not mean that all poor residents of developing countries should be categorically excluded from participation in research. As a group of researchers in Ghana has written, "the objective[s] to generate generalizable results and to fairly distribute risks and benefits of research, oblige researchers not to bar underprivileged persons as participants without cause" (Oduro and others, 2008). The principle of justice requires not only that individual subjects of research should have access to drugs tested in the study but also that the drugs selected for study should be relevant to the medical problems in the community in which the subjects reside. In other words, there are ethical implications for researchers and funding organizations in what they choose to study and support.

Another ethical issue of justice is presented by the use of placebo controls in research with human subjects. In essence the issue is whether a potential treatment should be tested against a placebo or against the best existing method of treatment, if any. Sometimes, this issue is referred to as the **standard of care debate**, with the existing, proven treatment being the applicable standard of care. By failing to use the appropriate standard of care, the use of placebos may unfairly raise the burden on research subjects and thereby violate the ethical principle of justice.

In an influential 1997 article, Peter Lurie and Sidney Wolfe criticized some clinical trials in developing countries for a treatment to limit perinatal (mother-to-child) transmission of HIV. Researchers had already found an effective treatment to reduce perinatal transmission of HIV, but it was very expensive and was difficult to administer in developing countries. Therefore, it was important to determine if a less expensive and more practical treatment regimen would be effective in preventing transmission of HIV. Lurie and Wolfe criticized the clinical trials that tested the proposed new treatment by comparing it to a control group that received only a placebo and therefore was at risk of transmitting HIV. They argued that the trials were unethical and that the proposed treatment should have been tested against the existing treatment, which was already known to be effective.

The issue of placebo controls has generated substantial debate among experts in ethics and research. On this issue the World Medical Association (WMA) has made a series of changes to its Declaration of Helsinki, but those changes have resulted in even more confusion and disagreement. Initially, the Declaration of Helsinki essentially stated that it is ethical to test a proposed treatment against a placebo only if no proven method of treatment exists (World Medical Association, 2000, para. 29). Some people objected strongly to this formulation. In addition to being based on ethics, the dispute may also have been driven by apparently conflicting requirements from, on the one hand, scholarly journals that might refuse to publish papers from researchers who violated the Declaration of Helsinki and, on the other hand, government regulatory authorities that would not approve certain new drugs unless they were tested in a placebo-controlled trial.

The WMA essentially backed down and adopted what it described as a "note of clarification." This note said that it might be ethical to use a placebo in a clinical trial when a proven method of treatment already existed, if "for compelling and scientifically sound methodological reasons its use is necessary to determine the efficacy or safety of a prophylactic, diagnostic or ther-apeutic method" (World Medical Association, 2001, para 29, note). Although characterized as a clarification, the note really changed the result by declaring, in effect, that a placebo-controlled trial is ethical whenever the researchers really need to do it. Commentators strongly criticized the WMA (Lie and others, 2004, p. 190), and some argued that the WMA had "lost any moral authority in the hotly contested standards of care debate" (Schüklenk, 2004, pp.194–195). In particular, commentators objected to the WMA's position that a scientific necessity should override all ethical considerations (Schüklenk, p. 194; Lie and others, p. 190.) Moreover, Schüklenk (2004) has argued persuasively that what are often described as matters of scientific necessity are really matters of economic concern (pp. 196–197). Meanwhile, Hawkins (2006) has taken a creative and potentially useful approach by distinguishing the obligations that researchers owe their subjects from the obligations that treating physicians owe their patients, and concluding that some placebo-controlled trials are ethical and others are not.

In the 2008 version of the Declaration of Helsinki, the note of clarification is gone and the statement has been revised as follows:

> The benefits, risks, burdens and effectiveness of a new intervention must be tested against those of the best current proven intervention, except in the following circumstances:
>
> - The use of placebo, or no treatment, is acceptable in studies where no current proven intervention exists; or
> - Where for compelling and scientifically sound methodological reasons the use of placebo is necessary to determine the efficacy or safety of an intervention and the patients who receive placebo or no treatment will not be subject to any risk of serious or irreversible harm. Extreme care must be taken to avoid abuse of this option [World Medical Association, 2008, para. 32].

This 2008 version of the Declaration of Helsinki is not likely to contain the last word on the ethics of placebo-controlled clinical trials.

Finally, a separate issue of justice involves the duty of researchers to provide care to subjects and their communities after completion of the research. As discussed previously, the principle of justice includes fairness in distributing the burdens and benefits of research. Ballantyne (2008) has explained that the research population must receive a larger share of the benefits than it has traditionally received, in order to avoid exploitation (p. 179).

The Belmont Report states that it would be an injustice to deny someone a benefit without good cause if it is a benefit to which the person is entitled. Thus, the question is whether subjects of research and their communities are entitled to posttrial treatment as a matter of reciprocity, by virtue of having subjected themselves to the risks of research and having made a contribution to scientific progress. The principle of beneficence is also applicable to this issue in the sense of minimizing harm, because a failure to continue treatment could lead to drug resistance for both the individual subjects and their communities.

Here again, the WMA's Declaration of Helsinki has been less than helpful. As originally phrased, the statement on this issue provided that at "the conclusion of the study, every patient entered into the study should be assured of access to the best proven prophylactic, diagnostic and therapeutic methods identified by the study" (World Medical Association, 2000, para. 30). Apparently, some people objected to that obligation for practical or financial reasons. The WMA again backed down considerably by adding a "note of clarification" that required researchers merely to identify posttrial access to some appropriate care and allow the applicable ethics committee to consider the arrangements for posttrial care. Interestingly, the WMA did not admit that it was changing its position, but rather described its clarification as a reaffirmation of its previous position (World Medical Association, 2004, para. 30, note).

In the 2008 version of the Declaration of Helsinki, the statement on this issue provides that at "the conclusion of the study, patients entered into the study are entitled to be informed about the outcome of the study and to share any benefits that result from it, for example, access to interventions identified as beneficial in the study or to other appropriate care or benefits" (World Medical Association, 2008, para. 33).

One example of a dispute over responsibility for posttrial care arose from a proposal to test Tenofovir on female sex workers in Cambodia. The purpose of the proposed trial was to determine if Tenofovir would be effective in preventing HIV infection. However, some of the sex workers in Cambodia protested against the trial. In addition to requesting additional information and better compensation, they requested long-term health insurance for participants in the study (Cha, 2006). In the following excerpt from an article by Kao Tha and colleagues, this controversy is described from the perspective of the potential subjects of research.

EXCERPT FROM "THE TENOFOVIR TRIAL CONTROVERSY IN CAMBODIA: CAN A TRIAL BE CONSIDERED ETHICAL IF THERE IS NO LONG-TERM POST-TRIAL CARE?"

BY KAO THA AND OTHERS

The Women's Network for Unity (WNU) was established in June 2000 by a group of sex workers for sex workers. It provides a foundation for support and builds solidarity and self-empowerment among sex workers....

The first ever Cambodian sex worker–planned and run press conference was held in Phnom Penh on March 29, 2004. The network expressed its opposition to an experiment which is recruiting healthy female sex workers to test an anti-HIV drug, Tenofovir DF, and find out if it is safe to use on HIV-negative women and whether it would reduce the risk of HIV infection. Similar drug trials are starting soon in Ghana, Cameroon, Nigeria and Malawi . . . . The researchers are looking for 960 Cambodian sex workers who are HIV-negative to take a pill once a day for one year in exchange for free medical services, counseling and $3 per month. Testing is due to start in the summer of 2004.

The WNU is against the use of sex workers for experimentation in a poor country like Cambodia, especially when the drug has only been tested on healthy monkeys—never on healthy humans. Side-effects of the drug when given as AIDS treatment are diarrhoea, nausea, tendency to major liver and kidney failure and "brittle bone" disease (osteoporosis). According to WNU President Kao Tha, many sex workers worry about being the first healthy humans to test the drug and are worried about the side-effects of taking a drug for prevention purposes: "They said they don't want to try the drug because they are poor and they are sex workers . . . . If they fall ill, who will look after their mothers, children, sisters or brothers? If the researchers are so sure that this drug is safe for HIV-negative women to take, in the short and long term, why won't they commit to insurance for us and our families? If we get sick or can't work it can be the difference between life and death for our families".

What WNU wants

The network wants insurance against possible side-effects of Tenofovir for 30 or more years and not just health care for the duration of the trial. When the researchers are finished and leave Cambodia who will take responsibility for sex workers and their families who may be suffering longer-term side-effects?

WNU believes that all sex workers who participate in the trial have the right to ask questions and be fully informed about the risks and to demand better medical and financial protection. Must poor sex workers in Cambodia take the risk of taking Tenofovir, withstand the side-effects, sacrifice health and income for $3 month and no longer-term guarantees?

If our members agree to take the risk, which may one day benefit people in richer countries and the drug company, then we deserve adequate protection for our future lives and our families. The high cost of this drug means that, even if it is successful in preventing HIV, Cambodian sex workers will never be able to afford it . . . .

Source: Excerpted from "The Tenofovir Trial Controversy in Cambodia: Can a Trial Be Considered Ethical If There Is No Long-Term Post-Trial Care?" by Kao Tha and others, 2004. *Research for Sex Work, 7,* 10–11. Copyright 2004 by Vrije University Medical Centre in the Netherlands. Reprinted by permission.

The foregoing article was published in June of 2004. After the protests by some of the potential subjects of research, the trial was canceled by the prime minister of Cambodia in the fall of 2004 (Cha, 2006). Ironically, protests that were intended to obtain more protection for human subjects had the unintended effect of slowing down the rate of research on HIV/AIDS. One AIDS activist criticized others for alleged "ethical imperialism" by insisting that poor residents of a developing country should receive the same level of benefits that would be received by residents of a rich Western country (Cha, 2006).

SUMMARY

The increase in the volume of research performed in developing countries has heightened the need to recognize and respond to ethical issues, and has raised ethical concerns not usually considered in the past. This chapter has analyzed the ethical principles of autonomy, beneficence, and justice and has evaluated the application of these principles to meet the needs of individuals and communities in developing countries. With regard to the ethical principle of autonomy, questions arise about obtaining informed consent from subjects with diverse cultures and worldviews. Nevertheless, informed consent is a crucial requirement for protection of autonomy and human rights. This chapter has analyzed in detail the ethical principle of beneficence, which includes an ethical obligation to ensure a favorable risk-benefit ratio. Finally, this chapter has analyzed the ethical issues arising under the principle of justice, including fairness in selecting the subjects of research and allocating the benefits and burdens of research. In the context of developing countries, this ethical principle prohibits using poor people to test drugs that they could never realistically afford, and requires researchers to provide appropriate care to subjects and their communities after the completion of research. Many of these ethical problems remain unresolved, thereby creating an exciting opportunity to participate in influencing their solutions in the future.

KEY TERMS

autonomy

coercion

institutional review
boards (IRBs)

principle of beneficence

principle of justice

principle of respect for
persons

standard of care debate

undue influence

DISCUSSION QUESTIONS

1. Are the ethical concepts identified in the Belmont Report universal principles of human life, or are they the values of a particular culture or group of cultures?

2. Is it ethical to offer potentially life-saving medical care to individuals on condition of their participating in a clinical trial, or does that constitute undue influence to participate?

3. As an ethical matter, should a potential treatment be tested against a placebo or against the best existing method of treatment?

4. At the conclusion of a study, do researchers have an ethical duty to provide subjects and their communities the best proven methods identified by the study?

ACTIVITY: THE USE OF PRISONERS AS SUBJECTS OF RESEARCH

In October of 2001 there were several cases of anthrax in humans in the United States, in connection with letters deliberately contaminated with anthrax that were sent through the mail, resulting in at least three fatalities. Since that time, governmental agencies and health care researchers have been actively looking for ways to detect, prevent, and treat anthrax and other types of illness associated with of bioterrorism.

For purposes of this activity, please assume that there is no effective vaccine to prevent anthrax. In addition, assume that researchers at a well-known medical center have developed a vaccine that might protect a person from anthrax. Although the vaccine has been tested on animals, it has not yet been tested for effectiveness in humans. The potential vaccine looks promising, but at this time researchers simply do not know whether the vaccine will be effective in preventing anthrax in humans.

Researchers have proposed to evaluate the effectiveness of the vaccine in humans by means of a double-blind, randomized trial with 2,000 research subjects. The research subjects will be assigned randomly to one of two groups, and neither the subjects nor the researchers will know the group to which a particular individual has been assigned. The researchers will give the potential vaccine to 1,000 people and simultaneously give a placebo to 1,000 other people. Then the researchers will expose all 2,000 people to envelopes containing anthrax. Any research subject who contracts anthrax will be treated immediately and without charge with the best available treatment.

According to the researchers, it is necessary to use a randomized trial with a placebo for this study, because otherwise it would not be possible to determine the effectiveness of the potential vaccine. The researchers had considered the possibility of merely giving the potential vaccine to 1,000 people and then exposing only those 1,000 vaccinated people to envelopes contaminated with anthrax, without any control group. However, under that scenario, if 200 out of 1,000 vaccinated subjects (20 percent) contracted anthrax from the envelopes, there would be no way of knowing whether (a) the vaccine is effective 80 percent of the time, because only 20 percent of the vaccinated people contracted anthrax; (b) the vaccine has no effect whatsoever, but only 20 percent of a population will contract anthrax from exposure to contaminated envelopes even in the absence of a vaccine; or (c) the vaccine has an effect somewhere between those two extremes. Therefore, according to the researchers, it is necessary to compare the number of subjects that contract anthrax from contaminated envelopes with and without the benefit of the potential vaccine.

All of the 2,000 research subjects will be inmates at the state penitentiary. Participation in the study will be voluntary, and no prisoner will be forced to participate. However, if a prisoner volunteers for the study, the prisoner will receive a 50 percent reduction in his or her remaining sentence, regardless of whether he or she is given the vaccine or a placebo and regardless of whether he or she contracts anthrax. In selecting subjects the researchers will not discriminate on the grounds of race, gender, or national origin, but a disproportionate percentage of prisoners in the state penitentiary are members of minority groups.

Please analyze the ethical issues involved in the proposed research study. In analyzing each of those ethical issues, please apply the ethical theories of utilitarianism, Kantian ethics, and principlism (prima facie moral duties), as well as any other theories or approaches that you think are useful. Be sure to state your own conclusion on each of those ethical issues, and explain the reasons for your conclusion.

CHAPTER SEVEN

THE RIGHT TO HEALTH CARE AND ETHICAL OBLIGATIONS TO PROVIDE CARE

LEARNING OBJECTIVES

- Demonstrate proficiency in analyzing the ethical basis for a right to health care.

- Understand and be able to explain the issues in evaluating the ethical obligations of doctors and other health care professionals to provide care for people who cannot afford to pay for their care.

- Be prepared to debate whether health care professionals have a duty to provide services during a pandemic or other public health emergency, even at a risk to the professionals' own health and safety.

- Learn how to evaluate the ethical obligations of private companies that provide health care goods and services.

- Be able to analyze the ethical implications of preserving patent rights to life-saving drugs, with regard to sales of those drugs in developing countries.

R IGHTS and obligations can be described as two sides of the same coin. As explained in this chapter, if an individual has an ethical right to something, some other individual or group has an ethical obligation to satisfy that right (O'Neill, 2005, pp. 430–431). Therefore, the ethical right to health care should be evaluated in conjunction with the ethical obligations of various parties to ensure that the right is satisfied.

This chapter begins by analyzing the ethical arguments about the right to health care, as well as the practical consequences of concluding that the right exists. Some people assume, without much ethical analysis, that a right to health care exists. Meanwhile, many writers have argued for or against the existence of the ethical right to health care, on various grounds. Even writers who support the existence of the right often disagree about the ethical basis for that right. Moreover, some writers have argued that it really does not matter whether there is an ethical right to health care. This lack of consensus has complicated efforts to clarify the extent of the right or the entities that have the duty to satisfy the right.

Next, this chapter evaluates the ethical obligations of doctors and other health care professionals to provide services to patients. This part of the chapter begins by analyzing the ethical duty of health care professionals to provide care to indigent patients, either for free or at a discount. Then it analyzes the ethical obligation of doctors and other professionals to treat patients during a public health emergency, despite the risk to the life or health of the professional. An activity at the end of this chapter provides an opportunity to develop a policy for a community health center regarding the obligations of employees to report for work and provide services during a pandemic or other public health emergency.

Finally, this chapter evaluates the ethical obligations of for-profit companies that provide health care goods and services. This part of the chapter addresses the business ethics of private companies in the health sector, such as the duty to comply with fair marketing practices. This part of the chapter also analyzes the issues in the ongoing dispute over preserving patent rights to life-saving drugs, in light of the desperate need for those drugs in low-income countries.

IS THERE AN ETHICAL RIGHT TO HEALTH CARE?

In establishing the World Health Organization (WHO) in 1946 and writing that agency's constitution, the participating nations declared the basic principle that "the enjoyment of the highest attainable standard of health is one of the fundamental rights of every human being" (World Health Organization, 1946). Similarly, in the Universal Declaration of Human Rights (UDHR), promulgated in 1948, the General Assembly of the United Nations provided that "everyone has the right to a standard of living adequate for the health and well-being of himself and of his family, including . . . medical care . . . and the right to security in the event of . . . sickness, disability, . . . old age or other lack of livelihood in circumstances beyond his control" (United Nations, 1948). Neither of these documents, however, provides an explanation of the ethical basis for concluding that health is a right or, even more, a fundamental right.

Like these international organizations, many writers and advocates have simply assumed—or taken for granted—that individuals have a right to health or at least a right to health care services. The failure to identify the ethical basis for such a right has made it difficult to specify the scope of the right or the parties responsible for ensuring that the right has been satisfied. As Onora O'Neill (2005) has explained, to say that an individual has an ethical right to something requires us to say also that some person or entity has an ethical obligation to satisfy that right. That is, "there cannot be a claim to rights that are rights against nobody, or nobody in particular" (p. 430). Thus, if there is an ethical right to health, a failure to satisfy that right for any member of society would not merely constitute bad public policy. It would mean that some person or entity has acted in an unethical manner. Under these circumstances it is important to consider the ethical basis for a proposed right to health, the scope and limitations of that right, and the persons or entities that would have an ethical obligation to ensure that the right has been satisfied.

Some individuals and organizations have tried to rely on international agreements or declarations as the ethical basis for a right to health. Those agreements and declarations include the Universal Declaration of Human Rights and the Constitution of the World Health Organization, as discussed previously, as well as the right to health put forth in article 12 of the International Covenant on Economic, Social and Cultural Rights (Toebes, 1999). Unfortunately, those international agreements are extremely vague. In addition, the right to health under international agreements is generally considered to be nonjusticiable, because it cannot be enforced through procedures at the United Nations and would not be binding on the courts of any nation, unless that particular nation had adopted a similar law or constitutional provision of its own (Toebes, 1999, pp. 661–662, 670–673). Therefore, this type of right has been described as "aspirational" (Giesen, 1995, p. 289). Nevertheless, the fact that international agreements and declarations are not enforceable as legal rights does not necessarily mean that they could not provide a moral basis for a right to health. The problems with relying on those agreements and declarations as foundational sources of moral authority lie elsewhere. The first problem is that it would constitute circular reasoning to declare that a certain right is fundamental and then to conclude that there must be such a fundamental right because it has been declared to be so. The second problem with relying on international agreements and declarations as sources of ethical rights is that doing so would undercut the argument that those rights are universal. As O'Neill (2005) has written, "Declarations and Covenants cannot show that some particular configuration of institutional rights and obligations is universally optimal or desirable, or even justifiable" (p. 432). Finally, if the right to health exists by virtue of international agreements and declarations, then that right would cease to exist if, at some time in the future, those agreements were to be amended, repealed, or dissolved. For all of these reasons the ethical basis for a right to health must be sought elsewhere.

Some people have relied on the concept of human rights as the ethical basis for supporting the existence of a right to health. Under this approach a human right to health existed long before it was described in any international agreement or declaration, and that right to health exists independently of any such agreement or declaration. One problem with this approach is that it begs the question as to the ethical basis for a right to health by characterizing it as a human right to health. It is not enough to assert that health is a fundamental human right. It is necessary as well to identify the basis for the very existence and definition of human rights as a whole.

Although we have an intuitive sense that human beings are entitled to certain human rights, there is little consensus as to the basis and scope of those rights. In fact, John Arras and Elizabeth Fenton (2009) have described the conventional wisdom among scholars of global human rights that it makes sense to consciously avoid the difficult and divisive questions about the underlying ethical basis for those rights in order to avoid undercutting support for the human rights movement (p. 28). An additional problem with relying on the concept of human rights as an ethical foundation is that all rights, including the right to health, must have corresponding obligations, as discussed previously. Thus, it would be necessary to identify the specific persons or entities that could be held responsible for the unethical conduct of failing to satisfy legitimate claims under the proposed human right to health (Arras and Fenton, 2009, p. 34; O'Neill, 2005, pp. 430–433).

Other ethical theories or approaches have been used in an effort to support the existence of a right to health. For example, utilitarianism can provide support for a right to health for all members of a society, because a healthy population would promote the common good and because a safety net of health insurance or public health care services would promote a sense of security and social solidarity. However, as a basis for an ethical right to health care, utilitarianism raises difficult problems, such as requiring the denial of long-term care to individuals who will never be socially productive (Daniels, 1998, p. 318). Other writers, such as Elaine Fox (2006), have used religious principles to support an ethical basis for a right to health (p. 13).

Relying on John Rawls's theory of justice, Norman Daniels (1998) used the concept of equality of opportunity as the basis for his approach to the right to health (pp. 319–320). According to Daniels, illness and disability limit the opportunities that individuals would have were they not ill or disabled. Equality of opportunity is also limited by other factors such as education and money, as well as by the unequal distribution of talent for performing various functions. However, Daniels rejected the notion that equality of opportunity requires society to use health care resources to increase the capacities of individuals whose normal functioning leaves them at a disadvantage compared to healthier or more physically able individuals. Instead, Daniels concluded that individuals have a right to health care that can help them to "function as 'normal' competitors, not strictly equal ones" (p. 319).

Under Daniels's approach, the right to health care is a positive right, one that provides an entitlement for each individual to receive a fair share of health care services. In addition, the right to health care imposes an obligation on society to provide a sufficient percentage of its resources for purposes of health (Daniels, 1998, p. 317). Daniels argues that

> there are social obligations to design a health-care system that protects oppor-
> tunity through an appropriate set of health-care services. If social obligations
> to provide appropriate health care are not met, then individuals are definitely
> wronged. For example, if people are denied access because of discrimination or
> inability to pay to a basic tier of services adequate to protect normal functioning,
> injustice is done to them. If the basic tier available to people omits important cat-
> egories of services without consideration of their effects on normal functioning,
> for example, whole categories of mental health or long-term care or preventive
> services, their rights are violated [p. 320].

However, not everyone agrees that there is a right to health or a right to health care. O'Neill (2005) has criticized the succession of claims about various rights, claims that are vague or poorly defined and that fail to specify the persons or entities that could be held responsible for violating those rights (p. 428). According to O'Neill, the goals of the human rights movement are not limited to protecting vulnerable populations but also include extending governmental power over individuals and installing mechanisms of governmental control (p. 439).

Other writers have criticized the entire concept of **positive rights** to goods and services, such as a right to health care, by arguing that the only real rights are **negative rights** to be left alone (Epstein, 1997). Moreover, Robert Sade has argued that medical services are produced by the work and thought of individual doctors and those services are the property of the doctors who produced them

(Sade, 2007, p. 1430; 2000, pp. 181–182). According to Sade, patients have no more of a right or entitlement to those medical services than they have a right or entitlement to the bread produced by a baker, the food grown by a farmer, or the house constructed by a builder. Moreover,

> The concept of medical care as the patient's right is immoral because it denies the most fundamental of all rights, that of a man to his own life and the freedom of action to support it. Medical care is neither a right nor a privilege: it is a service that is provided by doctors and others to people who wish to purchase it. It is the provision of this service that a doctor depends upon for his livelihood, and is his means of supporting his own life. If the right to health care belongs to the patient, he starts out owning the services of a doctor without the necessity of either earning them or receiving them as a gift from the only man who has the right to give them: the doctor himself [Sade, 2000, p. 182].

The problem with Sade's analysis is his underlying assumption that medical care is produced solely by the work and thought of individual doctors. In reality, society contributes greatly to the education and training of doctors. In addition, society provides substantial resources to assist doctors in treating their patients, such as the use of hospital facilities and equipment, payments for treating patients who are enrolled in various government payment programs, and use of tax revenues to support medical and scientific research. Finally, society grants doctors an exclusive and lucrative franchise to provide services to other members of the community. Under these circumstances it is specious to argue that medical services are produced solely through the effort of individual doctors, or to imply that doctors do not have an affirmative obligation to give back some portion of their time and services to other members of the community.

Other people have taken a very different approach by arguing either that it is simply impossible to answer the question of whether a right to health care exists, or that it really does not matter whether there is an ethical right to health care. That is the approach taken by the President's Commission for the Study of Ethical Problems in Medicine and Biomedical and Behavioral Research when it issued its report on access to care in 1983. The commission took no position on the issue of whether there is a right to health care, but rather focused on the uniqueness of health care and the moral obligation of society:

> As long as the debate over the ethical assessment of patterns of access to health care is carried on simply by the assertion and refutation of a "right to health care," the debate will be incapable of guiding policy. At the very least, the nature of the right must be made clear and competing accounts of it compared and

evaluated. Moreover, if claims of rights are to guide policy they must be supported by sound ethical reasoning and the connections between various rights must be systematically developed, especially where rights are potentially in conflict with one another. At present, however, there is a great deal of dispute among competing theories of rights, with most theories being so abstract and inadequately developed that their implications for health care are not obvious. Rather than attempt to adjudicate among competing theories of rights, the Commission has chosen to concentrate on what it believes to be the more important part of the question: what is the nature of the societal obligation, which exists whether or not people can claim a corresponding right to health care, and how should this societal obligation be fulfilled? [President's Commission . . . , 1983, pp. 34–35, footnote omitted].

Does it really make sense to argue, as does the President's Commission, that society has a moral obligation to provide health care services to which no individual necessarily has any right? According to O'Neill (2005), it is possible to have "imperfect" moral obligations, which are not paired with any rights of particular claimants (p. 430). However, Baruch Brody (1991) argued that the commission's reasoning is illogical. Brody conceded that the moral obligation of a single individual to help other people in society does not give any potential recipient a right or entitlement to the assistance of that particular donor. However, Brody distinguished that situation of individual donors and recipients from the commission's position because the commission supported a more general obligation of society as a whole to every individual in need. "If, as the Commission believes, society has an obligation to provide some level of health care to all of the indigent, then it would seem that, as a correlative to that obligation, the group of the indigent have a right, which they hold against society as a whole, that that health care be provided" (p. 117). Thus, Brody reasoned that the commission was incorrect in its analysis, although he recognized that the commission and its advisers might have decided to avoid relying on a right to health care in order to make the commission's report more politically acceptable (pp.117–118).

In addition, Brody argued that the proposed right to health care is not helpful in resolving the most significant policy issues, which concern the volume of care and types of care that society should provide for people who cannot afford to pay the cost of their care (pp. 113, 120–126). Brody did not take a position on whether there is, in fact, a right to health care (p. 14). Rather, Brody argued that the answer to that question does not really matter, because it does not help us to answer the questions that need to be answered. Similarly, Arras and Fenton (2009) agreed that the difficult decisions about which types of care to provide for specific types of patients cannot be made by concluding that individuals have a right to health care (p. 33). Even Norman Daniels (1998) acknowledged that the existence of a right to care does not avoid the need to determine, by fair procedures, the particular services to which patients would be entitled in light of the available resources, technological capacity, effectiveness of treatments, and the impact of various treatments on equality of opportunity (pp. 320–323). Countries that have adopted a right to health care for their residents by implementing universal systems of coverage, such as Norway, still face the difficult problem of rationing limited resources (Norheim, 2005). These issues of rationing care and allocating limited resources are discussed in detail in Chapter Eight.

Other writers have agreed that efforts to prove the existence of a right to health care would not solve the most important problems faced by modern societies. For example, writing from a feminist perspective, Susan Sherwin (1992) noted that a right to health care would not necessarily meet the needs of various groups of women. Even if a society were to provide greater access to health care by means of universal health insurance coverage, that would not solve health problems that result from systemic oppression of women, such as violence and insufficient resources for proper nutrition (pp. 227–228).

So, where does that leave us? Some people take for granted that a right to health care exists. Other people argue, on various ethical grounds, that a right to health care does or does not exist, and yet other people respond that it really does not matter whether there is an ethical right to health care. On balance it is reasonable to conclude that there is at least some minimum level of health care to which every member of a decent society is entitled, merely by being a member of that society, even if we cannot specify the precise limits of that entitlement. Admittedly, this conclusion leaves many difficult questions unanswered. However, under this approach, proposals for health care reform and expansion of coverage would be recognized as being supported by moral authority, rather than merely by arguments about policy, politics, or economics. As Arras and Fenton (2009) have stated, a right to health care "removes the issue of access to a basic level of health care from the vagaries of the free market" (p. 32). In Chapter Nine the importance of values and ethics in health system reform is discussed in greater detail.

ETHICAL OBLIGATIONS OF HEALTH CARE PROFESSIONALS

Obviously, providing health care services to indigent patients is beneficial and laudable. But is providing indigent care merely a gift, or is it an ethical obligation? Do doctors and other health care professionals have an ethical duty to provide some amount of free or discounted services, such that failure to do so would constitute unethical conduct?

As discussed earlier, Sade (2000) argued that patients do not have a right to health care, but Sade acknowledged that a physician could choose to provide his or her services as a gift (p. 182). Sade did not mention any ethical obligation that would require a physician to make a gift or otherwise provide services without charge. However, accepted principles of professional ethics recognize an ethical obligation to provide some amount of indigent care, as discussed later. Sade also insisted that the physician's highest professional value is the best interest of his or her patients (p. 185). What Sade failed to address is the ethical obligation of physicians to those individuals or groups who are not fortunate enough to be patients of those physicians or of any other physicians.

In analyzing the underlying values of health systems in the United States and other countries, Reinhard Priester (1992) noted that one of the dominant values in the U.S. health system is the autonomy of physicians to select their patients. Physicians in the United States generally recognize an ethical duty to provide charity to the poor, but they reserve the power to select the particular recipients of their charity (p. 89). Moreover, physicians make their own decisions about the volume of charity care to provide. Prevailing standards of medical ethics in the United States include an obligation to provide some amount of uncompensated care, although the appropriate amount is left to the discretion of the individual physician. Priester recommended that physician autonomy should be subordinated to the higher value of providing fair access to care (pp. 103–104). According to Priester, "if fair access cannot be assured without imposing restrictions on a provider's freedom to choose patients, then provider autonomy may be restricted, for example, by requiring providers to see a minimum number of Medicaid enrollees or other underserved people" (p. 104).

The organized medical profession in the United States, which determines its own standards of medical ethics, has not adopted Priester's recommendation that autonomy of physicians should be subordinated to the higher goal of promoting access to care. Instead, the standards of medical ethics in the United States generally allow physicians to accept or deny new patients, unless a medical emergency exists. The Principles of Medical Ethics of the American Medical Association (AMA) (2001) provide that a "physician shall...except in emergencies, be free to choose whom to serve." According to the AMA, physicians ordinarily have the right to decide whether to enter into a physician-patient relationship with any particular patient. The AMA has recognized, however, that this prerogative of physicians is limited by the obligation to "respond to the best of their ability in cases of medical emergency" (American Medical Association, 2003). In addition, a physician's prerogative may be limited by that physician's prior agreement in a contract to treat certain patients, and physicians may not refuse to enter into a physician-patient relationship for a discriminatory reason (American Medical Association, 2003).

In situations that do not constitute a medical emergency, the AMA has taken the position that "physicians have an obligation to share in providing charity care . . . but not to the degree that would seriously compromise the care provided to existing patients" (American Medical Association, 2003). The AMA's approach emphasizes that physicians bear some of the obligation for care of the indigent, but not the sole responsibility, because society also bears the obligation to provide sufficient resources (American Medical Association, 1993). The AMA has not specified an appropriate volume of indigent care, which would depend on the circumstances, but it has stated, "Caring for the poor should be a regular part of the physician's practice schedule" (American Medical Association, 1994). One specific aspect of this issue, involving the duty to provide care for undocumented aliens, is addressed in detail in Chapter Ten.

Aside from the ethical obligation to provide indigent care, health care professionals have a duty to provide services during a pandemic or other public health emergency, even at some risk to the professional's own health and safety. However, the basis and scope of that duty has been subject to dispute. In 166 AD Galen apparently left Rome at the time of a plague, and most physicians who encountered the Black Death in fourteenth-century Europe ran away (Emanuel, 2003, p. 590). In contrast, when the AMA developed its first ethical code in 1847, the code explicitly required physicians to continue to treat patients during times of "pestilence," regardless of their own risk of death. One hundred and ten years later, in 1957, the AMA shortened its ethical code and eliminated that section (Zuger and Miles, 1987, p. 1926). A 2004 AMA ethics opinion recognizes the ethical duty of physicians to provide services during a disaster, despite the personal risks, but encourages physicians to balance the need to help patients during the disaster with the need to preserve the physician's availability to serve other patients in the future (American Medical Association, 2004).

Some writers have argued that by entering into their profession, doctors and other health care professionals voluntarily assume the risk of infectious disease (Ruderman and others, 2006). However, in a 2002 survey of U.S. physicians, only 55 percent agreed with the statement that "physicians have an obligation to care for patients in epidemics even if doing so endangers the physician's health" (Alexander and Wynia, 2003, p. 195). A separate survey in 2005 of workers at local health departments in the State of Maryland found that almost half of those workers would probably not be willing to work during an influenza pandemic (Balicer and others, 2006). Canadian researchers have reported that some hospital staff members were fired for failing to work during the SARS epidemic (Ruderman and others, 2006). However, in a survey of workers at a large teaching hospital in the United Kingdom, only about one-fifth of the workers responded that they would not work if the risk of infection were high and personal protection were limited (Barr and others, 2008, p. 50). Of course, that type of survey measures only self-reported statements of future intent. In an emergency, people might act differently from what they had predicted.

In 2007, the World Health Organization published a report on the ethical issues in preparing for pandemic influenza. That report recognized that one important aspect of preparing a public health response is ensuring that health workers will be willing to perform their functions during a pandemic, despite the personal risks (p. 13). The WHO report also recognized that the extent of the ethical obligation to provide services during a pandemic is unclear and that the obligation of the health professional to provide services during a pandemic must be balanced against the professional's other ethical obligations:

> A strong case can be made for recognizing a moral obligation to provide care during an outbreak of communicable disease, especially a disease of pandemic proportions . . . . However, even for workers with specialized skills, the moral obligation to work during an influenza pandemic is not unlimited. Judgments about the scope of any particular worker's moral obligations must take into account factors such as the urgency of the need for that individual's services and the difficulty of replacing him or her, the risks to the worker and indirectly to his or her family, the existence of competing moral obligations, such as family care-giving responsibilities, and his or her duties to care for other (present and future) patients [World Health Organization, 2007, p. 13].

Writing about pandemic planning in Australia, Adrienne Torda (2006) agreed that the ethical duty to provide services must be balanced against other ethical duties (p. S74). Moreover, under the principle of reciprocity, society has an obligation to provide support for health workers who undertake the risk of infectious disease, including appropriate protective equipment, assistance to these health workers and their families, and possibly even priority in receiving vaccinations and other limited medical resources (Barr and others, 2008, p. 51).

As Caleb Alexander and Matthew Wynia (2003) have explained, ethical theories do not provide clear answers about the duty to provide services during a pandemic, "and none can provide specific guidance as to the exact degree of risk to be undertaken" (p. 195). Under these circumstances, the 2007 World Health Organization report takes a very practical approach by recommending that the obligations of health workers in a pandemic should be set forth in policies that are developed in a transparent and open manner and with the participation of workers and professional organizations (pp. 13–15). According to that report, policies should consider the roles and risks for different categories of workers and should "accommodate legitimate exceptions regarding assignment of individuals with fragile health status to risky situations (e.g., individuals who are immunodeficient or pregnant)" (p. 14). The WHO report also emphasizes that policies developed in this manner can influence the behavior of health workers, even if the policies are not legally enforceable, because workers would probably view those policies as legitimate (p. 15). Considering Toronto's experience with the SARS epidemic, Alison Thompson and others (2006) also emphasized the importance of fair processes for making hard decisions during a pandemic, in part because those decisions would then be perceived as more legitimate. However, these writers also acknowledged that compared to the experience of SARS in Canada, the experience of SARS in China might demonstrate the importance of a different set of ethical values. The activity at the end of this chapter provides an opportunity to use a transparent, participatory process in developing a policy for a community health center about the obligations of employees to work during a pandemic or other emergency.

ETHICAL OBLIGATIONS OF FOR-PROFIT HEALTH CARE PROVIDERS

In the case of nonprofit health care organizations, the primary purpose for their existence is to provide services to people in their communities. In contrast, for-profit organizations in the health sector exist primarily for the purpose of earning money for their owners. All health care facilities, regardless of their ownership or governance, must impose some limitations on their services in order to remain financially viable and continue in operation. Nonprofit and publicly owned health care facilities often have their own institutional agendas and do not necessarily operate at all times in the best interest of their local communities. Nevertheless, it is fair to distinguish nonprofit and public facilities from those facilities that exist primarily for the purpose of making a profit.

Is it inherently unethical to provide health care on a for-profit basis? In many countries the vast majority of physician practices are operated on a for-profit basis, either as sole proprietorships or in some form of group practice. In addition, private enterprise can be a method of generating resources for the construction and operation of health care facilities, when sufficient funds cannot be raised from taxpayers or donors.

Many people criticize pharmaceutical manufacturers and medical device companies for charging high prices for their products in an effort to increase their profits. However, it may have been their drive to earn a return on investment that resulted in creating many of the life-saving drugs and technologies that currently exist. If for-profit companies fail to operate in the best interest of society, that might indicate a problem of inadequate regulation of those companies by the government rather than a problem with the ownership structure of those companies. Under these circumstances this chapter will not attempt to resolve the question of whether it is inherently unethical to provide health care for profit. Instead, for purposes of discussion, this chapter will assume that it is ethical to provide health care for profit and will analyze the ethical obligations of for-profit companies that sell health care goods and services. In other words, what are the proper business ethics of for-profit companies in the health sector?

In any sector of the economy, and especially in health care, business organizations must use fair marketing practices. One aspect of fair marketing is honesty in describing the advantages and risks of the organization's products. In addition, it would be unethical for sellers of health care goods and services to try to convince a patient to purchase or accept treatments that the patient does not really need. The concept of **supplier-induced demand** refers to "misleading a patient into agreeing to inappropriate or ineffective treatment" (Ensor and Duran-Moreno, 2002, p. 111). Direct-to-consumer (DTC) advertising by pharmaceutical companies also raises potential problems of supplier-induced demand. Other important issues of business ethics arise in the relationships between companies that manufacture or sell drugs and physicians who prescribe drugs or conduct research on drugs. These relationships can create conflicts of interest that have the potential to influence a physician's professional judgment (Steinbrook, 2009).

Finally, is it unethical for business corporations to insist on preserving their patent rights to life-saving drugs, particularly with regard to sales of those drugs in developing countries? This issue raises the ethical conflict between intellectual property rights and access to desperately needed medications. As a general rule, most countries in the world have bound themselves to recognize patent rights, under the World Trade Organization's Agreement on Trade-Related Aspects of Intellectual Property Rights, commonly known as the **TRIPS Agreement** (Abbott and Van Puymbroeck, 2005, p. 2). However, the World Trade Organization member countries reached a specific agreement in 2001, known as the **Doha Declaration**, with regard to the effect of TRIPS on public health (Abbott and Van Puymbroeck, pp. 2, 8). The Doha Declaration recognizes that TRIPS does not prevent member countries from taking necessary actions to protect the public health and that governments of member countries may grant **compulsory licenses**, by which those governments permit the production or importation of a patented drug without permission of the company that holds the patent (Abbott and Van Puymbroeck, pp. 7–8).

Public health advocates argue that compulsory licenses are necessary in order to provide essential medicines to patients in developing countries. In response, pharmaceutical manufacturers argue that compulsory licenses will reduce investment in research and development of new drugs, although that is a factual issue that remains in dispute (Cohen, 2007). According to Volker Heins (2008), "at the most fundamental level, we do not know to what extent pharmaceutical companies need to recoup their R&D expenditures through TRIPS-style patent monopolies to develop new drugs. If such a link could be proven, attending to those who are worst-off *today* by suspending intellectual property protections might have the effect of reducing the available resources of those who will suffer *tomorrow*" (p. 227, footnote omitted). Thus, the issue of compulsory licenses for essential drugs in developing countries seems to be caught in a factual dispute about whether reducing protection for intellectual property rights would, in fact, reduce research and development of new medicines.

Perhaps people have been asking the wrong question. Rather than arguing about the factual question of whether reducing or eliminating patent protection would actually reduce research and development of new drugs, we could simply assume that as a fact for purposes of discussion. For the purposes of argument, we could concede that research and development for new drugs would be significantly reduced. We could go further and concede that some of the drugs that would have been developed with intellectual property protection would not have been merely duplicative (so-called me-too drugs), but rather would have been beneficial to some patients by being more effective, easier to administer, or having fewer side effects for those patients. Finally, we could go even further and concede that, without intellectual property protection, some patients would indeed die as a result of the failure to develop those new drugs. However, even if we assumed that all these results would come to pass, that still would not necessarily mean that intellectual property protection should be preserved.

Societies do allow people to suffer or die because of competing values and priorities, especially when those people are merely abstract and not identifiable. A society can accept the fact that some unidentified people will suffer or die as a result of its unwillingness to make cars even more safe or food even more pure, because the high marginal cost of further improvement is considered to outweigh the low marginal benefit from that improvement. Moreover, that additional improvement would use up resources that could be spent much more effectively on other needs of the society. By refusing to permit medical research that might harm a small number of identifiable human subjects, society routinely forgoes potential benefits to a large number of unidentified patients, whose lives might be significantly improved or even saved through development of new drugs or treatments (Zywicki, 2007). Therefore, the assumed fact that some patients would die without intellectual property protection for drugs does not really answer the question of whether intellectual property protection should be retained.

The more relevant question is whether reducing or eliminating intellectual property protection for drugs would have a significant adverse effect on public health. Our current knowledge of what affects public health suggests that the unavailability of some new advanced medicines would probably not have a significantly adverse effect. As pointed out by the World Health Organization (2000), some interventions may help specific individuals without making much of a contribution to improving the health status of the population (p. 52). Moreover, compulsory licenses could significantly improve population health, by making essential medicines available to large numbers of people in developing countries. Udo Schüklenk (2004) has suggested that we should devote more effort to making existing drugs available, rather than emphasizing the development of new drugs (p. 197). In evaluating the ethics of intellectual property rights, the most important question is whether the potential lack of new drugs would really have an adverse impact on population health in developing countries and developed countries.

SUMMARY

This chapter has analyzed the arguments about the existence, basis, and extent of an ethical right to health care. Although writers disagree, there must be some minimum level of health care to which every human being is entitled and that every decent society is ethically obligated to provide. Despite uncertainty about the extent of the right, the effect of concluding that the right exists is to change debates over health reform from matters of politics to matters of ethics.

This chapter has also evaluated the ethical obligations of doctors and other health care professionals to provide services to patients, including the duty to provide care for indigent patients and the duty to provide services during a pandemic or other public health emergency. Finally, this chapter has evaluated the ethical obligations of private companies that provide health care goods and services, such as the duty to comply with fair marketing practices. If reducing intellectual property protection for drugs would not have a significant adverse effect on population health, the interests of private drug companies in preserving their patent rights would be outweighed by the need for life-saving drugs in low-income countries.

KEY TERMS

compulsory licenses   negative rights   supplier-induced demand

Doha Declaration   positive rights   TRIPS Agreement

DISCUSSION QUESTIONS

1. Is there an ethical right to health care? If so, what are the practical consequences of concluding that this ethical right exists?

2. Do doctors and other health care professionals have an ethical obligation to provide some amount of care for indigent patients, either for free or at a discount?

3. In the event of a pandemic or other public health emergency, should each health care professional be allowed to make his or her own decision about whether to report for work and provide services to patients?

4. Is it unethical for private companies to insist on preserving their patent rights to desperately needed medications, particularly with regard to developing countries?

ACTIVITY: DEVELOPING A POLICY ON THE OBLIGATIONS OF HEALTH CARE EMPLOYEES TO WORK DURING AN EMERGENCY

The local public health and primary care facility that we will call the East River Community Health Center (CHC) is owned and operated by East River County. As an agency of local government, it must have all its policies approved by the elected board of county commissioners. All meetings of the board are open to the public, and all its written policies are available to the public and the news media. All CHC staff members are public employees; there are ten doctors, twenty nurses, thirty allied health professionals, twenty administrative and clerical workers, and twenty maintenance and facilities personnel.

The CHC provides a wide range of public health and primary care services, including immunization, screening, health education, preventive care, and family medicine. In the event of an outbreak of communicable disease, such as an epidemic or pandemic, the CHC would be responsible for surveillance, disease control, distribution of medications for prevention and treatment, and referral of patients to a hospital as needed.

In order to prepare for a possible pandemic, the board has directed the CHC staff to develop a written policy about the responsibilities of the CHC and its employees in the event of a public health emergency. The CHC's executive director has appointed a committee to develop a draft policy for consideration by the board. This committee is composed of CHC employees. Several subcommittees have been appointed to analyze specific issues in detail, including a subcommittee on the obligations of CHC employees to report for work and perform their jobs during a pandemic or other emergency. Please assume that you have been appointed to the subcommittee on the obligations of CHC employees.

As discussed in the text of this chapter, several experts have emphasized the importance of developing policies for pandemic planning in a transparent manner, with participation of all stakeholders (World Health Organization, 2007, pp. 13–15). It is also important to explicitly address ethical issues, including ethical aspects of the duty to provide services during a public health emergency. According to experts in Canada, "as the SARS experience in Toronto taught health care organisations, the costs of not addressing the ethical concerns are severe: loss of public trust, low hospital staff morale, confusion about roles and responsibilities, stigmatization of vulnerable communities, and misinformation" (Thompson and others, 2006).

The recommendations of experts can be categorized as either procedural or substantive. Procedural issues can be divided further into (1) processes for the development of policies in advance of a pandemic and (2) processes for making exceptions and resolving disputes during a pandemic. These procedural and substantive aspects are described here in detail in outline form.

Procedural Issues in Workforce Planning for a Pandemic

1. Processes for the development of policies in advance of a pandemic
   - Arrange for the participation of stakeholders who would be affected directly (World Health Organization, 2007, p. 14).
   - Discuss the policies before implementation (World Health Organization, 2007, p. 14).
   - Educate workers about the possible scenarios and the importance of each worker's role in those scenarios (Balicer and others, 2006).
2. Processes for making exceptions and resolving disputes during a pandemic
   - In assigning individual workers, make exceptions as appropriate for individuals whose health condition poses additional risks, such as workers

who are pregnant or immunodeficient (World Health Organization, 2007, p. 14).
- Establish dispute resolution mechanisms (including procedures for grievances and appeals) that are accountable, fair, and developed in a collaborative manner. These mechanisms are particularly important for disputes over exemptions from work and the vaccination or treatment of workers (Thompson and others, 2006, Table 2).

Substantive Issues in Workforce Planning for a Pandemic

- Address the different roles and responsibilities of various categories of health workers (including any traditional healers or other nonconventional providers who might be involved) (World Health Organization, 2007, p. 14). Also, consider the roles and responsibilities of volunteers.
- Decide whether to allow changes in job functions between professionals and nonprofessionals, including allowing workers to perform tasks for which they have no formal training or licensure (World Health Organization, 2007, p. 14). Also, decide whether to require highly trained and licensed professional staff to perform functions usually performed by nonprofessional workers.
- Fairly distribute the risks among categories of workers and among individuals, while recognizing that some workers might need to face higher risk as a result of their functions (World Health Organization, 2007, p. 14).
- Request workers to accept risks only when their involvement would be likely to affect the outcomes for individual patients and the community (World Health Organization, 2007, p. 14).
- Acknowledge the existence of limits on the duty to provide services when a worker's health is at risk (World Health Organization, 2007, p. 14).
- Establish a strong role for the organization's leadership in the event of a pandemic, with an emphasis on "leading by example" (Torda, 2006, p. S74).
- Satisfy the reciprocal obligations of the employer, including supplying protective equipment to workers and possible priority in receiving scarce drugs and treatment (World Health Organization, 2007, p.14). Workers must have confidence that the employer will meet its obligations to the workers, including the provision of truthful information in a timely manner (Balicer and others, 2006).
- Ensure that workers have confidence that they are well prepared to handle a public health emergency (Balicer and others, 2006).

The task of your subcommittee is to develop a draft policy on the obligations of CHC employees to report for work and perform their jobs during a pandemic or other emergency. Please begin by specifying the process that your subcommittee will use in developing its draft policy, including identification of all stakeholders and an explanation of how those stakeholders will be involved in developing the draft policy. Then develop your draft policy, using the list of substantive issues supplied here as a checklist of the elements to include in your draft policy. Please list the specific conditions under which employees will be exempt from the obligation to report for work during a pandemic, and describe the process by which individual requests for exemption will be granted or denied. Finally, please include a specific, step-by-step process for the fair resolution of disputes, including procedures for handling grievances and appeals.

CHAPTER EIGHT

ETHICAL ISSUES IN RATIONING AND ALLOCATION OF LIMITED RESOURCES

LEARNING OBJECTIVES

■ Understand and be able to explain how the rationing of health care fits within a broader set of issues about allocating the resources of society.

■ Be able to analyze the ethical implications of allocating limited health resources to specific types of health services.

■ Understand and be able to explain the issues involved in evaluating various explicit and implicit methods of rationing health resources and the ethical considerations involved in each method.

■ Be able to analyze the ethical implications of comparative effectiveness research and cost-effectiveness analysis, including the use of those methods in countries with universal health insurance.

IS it really necessary to ration care? Or would there be enough health resources for all if only we could rid the health care system of all of the waste, fraud, abuse, administrative overhead, profits, bureaucrats, bean counters, and lawyers? Eliminating unnecessary expenses would indeed increase the amount of money available for needed health care services. However, as recognized by the President's Commission for the Study of Ethical Problems in Medicine and Biomedical and Behavioral Research (1983), "there is virtually no end to the funds that could be devoted to possibly beneficial care for diseases and disabilities and to their prevention" (p. 19). Because needs for care are infinite and resources are finite, some beneficial care must be denied to some patients on some basis (Morreim, 1989, p. 1014).

For any good or service, rationing becomes necessary when the demand is greater than the available supply. A **rationing system** is defined as a method of limiting consumption of some good or service, in order to limit the demand to the level of supply (Rosen and others, 2005, p. 1098). "Rationing takes place when an individual is deprived of care which is of benefit . . . and which is desired by the patient" (Maynard, 1999, p. 6).

Is it ethical to ration beneficial health care services? In its World Health Report 2000, the World Health Organization (2000) recognized "the ethical principle that it may be necessary and efficient to ration services but . . . it is inadmissible to exclude whole groups of the population" (p.16). Thus, the ethical issue of rationing is not whether it is ethical to ration but rather how the rationing is done. Which methods of rationing are most ethical, and which should be avoided on the ground that they are unethical? One way of limiting the demand for a good or service is by rationing on the basis of the ability to pay (Maynard, 1999, p. 6). With regard to health care, however, most people believe it is extremely unethical to ration scarce resources on the basis of an individual's ability to pay. Therefore, other criteria must be developed and applied to limit demand to the level of supply.

This chapter begins by putting the issues of rationing in context, explaining how rationing of medical care fits within a broader set of issues about different ways to allocate the resources of a society. Decisions about allocating societal resources present a series of questions with important ethical implications. Then the chapter evaluates the various methods of rationing and the ethical considerations in each method. For example, should we ration scarce health care resources on the basis of the age of the individual patient, social worth of the patient, or some other explicit or implicit criterion? This discussion includes an excerpt from an article about rationing of scarce antiretroviral therapy for HIV/AIDS in Africa, and the various ways in which those rationing decisions could be made. This chapter concludes with an analysis of comparative effectiveness research and cost-effectiveness analysis, including the use of those methods in countries with national health systems and universal health insurance. At the end of this chapter, an activity provides an opportunity to evaluate the ethical implications of cost-effectiveness analysis from several different perspectives.

LEVELS OF ALLOCATING RESOURCES

Most discussions about rationing and allocation of health resources focus on specific situations involving denial of care for patients with cancer or other terminal diseases. For example, when people in the United States think about rationing, they might think about a for-profit health maintenance organization (HMO) that refuses to pay for a bone marrow transplant or similar procedure for a patient with cancer, on the ground that the treatment is experimental or "not medically necessary." Similarly, many people in the United Kingdom are concerned about guidelines for the National Health Service (NHS) that declare certain new drugs for cancer to be not sufficiently "cost effective" for use in the NHS. These types of decisions not to provide or pay for specific drugs or treatments are really part of a much broader set of issues about how to allocate the resources of a society. These broader issues, as set forth in the remainder of the chapter and in Figure 8.1, present a series of decisions that proceed from the most general to the most specific, and these decisions have important ethical implications.

First, a society must decide how much of its resources it wants to devote to health as opposed to other societal needs. Money, personnel, and other resources that are devoted to health will not be available for other needs of the population, such as food, housing, or education, and resources that are devoted to those other purposes will not be available for health (Brock, 2004, p. 201). For example, if current trends in the United States continue, health care spending could use up 35 percent of the nation's income by 2040, which would severely reduce the money available for other national priorities (Aaron and others, 2005, p. 1).

The second step in this process is to decide on the appropriate balance between public health interventions for the population as a whole and clinical treatment for individuals in the society. For a health system to use its available resources in a cost-effective manner, it needs to give priority to those interventions that have the most effect on population health for each dollar of spending, rather than to interventions that help only individuals and do not make a significant contribution to overall population health (World Health Organization, 2000, p. 52). Allocating resources in ways that best improve population health would be

FIGURE 8.1   Decision Tree for Allocating the Resources of a Society

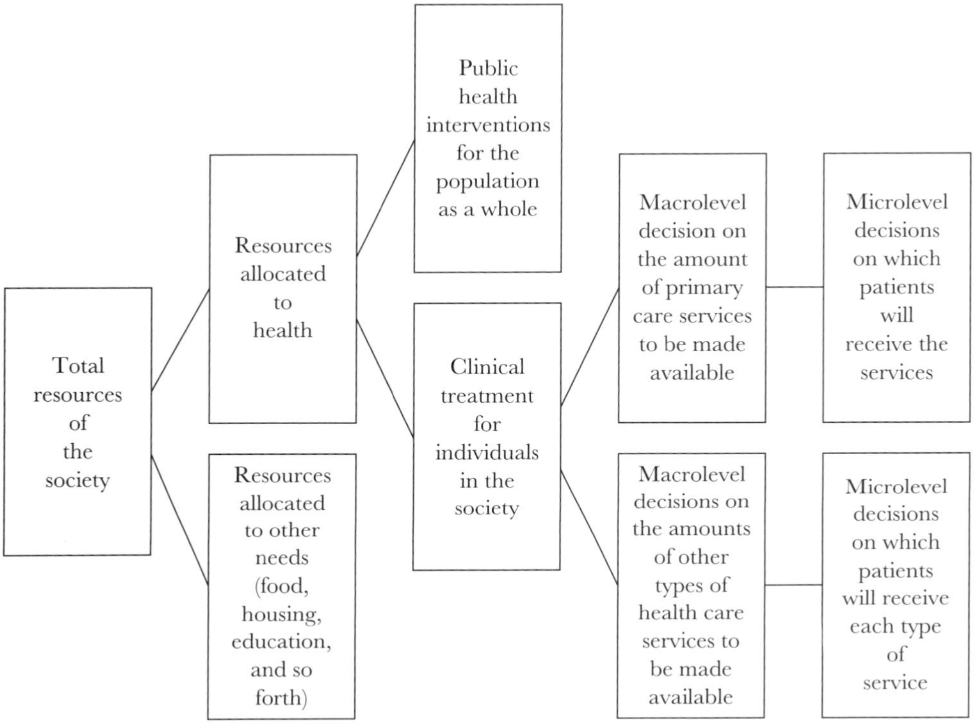

consistent with the utilitarian principle of doing the greatest good for the greatest number, and would also promote the ethical principles of justice and beneficence.

Once a society decides how much of its resources it will devote to the category of treatment for individual patients, the next step is to decide on the amount of each type of care that will be made available. Specific levels of resources can be devoted to primary care, secondary care, and tertiary care, as well as other types of health care services, such as mental health and long-term care. Resources can be allocated to specific types of care by making decisions in the process of government budgeting about the amounts of money that governmental entities will spend to provide various categories of health care facilities and services. In some places, governmental entities also have the authority to control the types of health care facilities and services that are available in the private sector. They can impose regulatory barriers to market entry by passing certificate of need laws, for example. In addition, public and private health insurance systems can allocate their resources to specific types of care by making decisions about covered and noncovered services in the process of insurance plan design.

At this level of decision making, ethical principles of utilitarianism, beneficence, and justice militate in favor of devoting as many resources as possible to primary care services. Primary care has more impact on health than other types of care (Starfield and others, 2005). In addition, primary care is less expensive than other services, because it employs lower technology and workers with less extensive training. So primary care is both more effective and less expensive. Therefore, it is not necessary in this situation to make a trade-off between cost and effectiveness. Moreover, primary care provides more benefit for poor people and residents of rural areas, whereas hospital services are used disproportionately by people who are rich, or at least relatively rich. As the World Health Organization (2000) has recognized, the "distribution of primary care is almost always more beneficial to the poor than hospital care is, justifying the emphasis on the former as the way to reach the worst-off" (p. 16).

Determining the total volume of a health care service that will be made available to the public, by methods such as government budgeting, could be described as a **macrolevel decision**. After making that macrolevel decision, society can address the **microlevel decision** of which patients will receive the service. As explained by John Kilner (1984), "Microallocation focuses on determining who gets how much of a particular lifesaving medical resource, once budgetary and other limitations have determined the total amount of the resource available" (p. 18). These microallocation decisions can be made in several different ways, and each of those ways has significant ethical implications.

METHODS OF RATIONING HEALTH RESOURCES

As discussed earlier, it is possible—although not desirable—to ration health care on the basis of ability to pay. That is one of the primary ways in which health care is rationed in the United States, in contrast to the health systems of Europe and other developed countries (Maynard, 1999, p. 6). Although U.S. hospitals have a limited obligation to provide emergency care, and many health care facilities and professionals provide some amount of charity care, inability to pay poses a major barrier to access for millions of people in the United States. More than forty-six million people in the United States are uninsured in the sense that they have no health insurance whatsoever, and many more are severely underinsured. Even people who have health insurance may be unable to pay for necessary care, because their insurance imposes limitations on coverage and requires the patient to pay deductibles and copayments. The system of rationing health care on the basis of ability to pay has been justly criticized on ethical grounds (Persad and others, 2009a). Clearly, it is necessary to find a better way to ration or allocate medical resources.

Another method that has been strongly criticized is rationing care on the basis of the social worth of the individual patient. In the early days of kidney dialysis for end-stage renal disease, anonymous hospital committees chose patients for that life-saving technology by evaluating criteria such as the potential patient's occupation, education, income, net worth, dependents, and record of public service (Sanders and Dukeminier, 1968, pp. 371–378). Members of those secret committees, individuals such as ministers, lawyers, and bankers, could apply these vague criteria in light of their own values and biases in deciding who would live and who would die. People may have very different views about social worth, and it is clearly inappropriate to permit secret committees to make rationing decisions on the basis of their personal views of the social value of particular individuals. Nevertheless, it may be appropriate in some circumstances to allocate resources to individuals who perform certain functions in society, as a way of promoting the overall good of society. For example, during a pandemic flu, it would be ethical to allocate scarce flu vaccine to public health workers and essential medical personnel, so that they would be able to help other members of society (Persad and others, 2009b, p. 426).

Why not simply ration scarce health care resources to those patients who need them the most or can benefit the most, on the basis of explicit medical criteria? In fact that is the assumption on which many governments rely when they limit available resources and force health care professionals or others to perform the rationing (Aaron and others, 2005, p. 143). In many countries, governments limit their total expenditures for health care services by appropriating a maximum sum of money to provide or pay for care. Those budgetary limitations, such as are found in global budgeting, are not in themselves methods of rationing. However, they create the need for rationing by limiting the available funds, equipment, facilities, and staff. This forces the "budget-holder" to make the difficult rationing decisions (World Health Organization, 2000, p. 58). Governments and their citizens might assume that limited resources are being allocated on the basis of explicit medical criteria. Unfortunately, rationing care on the basis of medical criteria is not straightforward, typically runs into many difficulties, and raises ethical problems in several ways.

First, in some situations, far too many patients will meet the medical criteria for needing particular treatments, such as antiretroviral therapy for HIV/AIDS in Africa, even if the medical criteria are extremely conservative (Rosen and others, 2005, p. 1098). Therefore, medical criteria alone will not solve the problem of deciding who will receive treatment and who will not. Second, medical criteria can be manipulated by health care providers to obtain resources, such as organ transplants, for their patients, even if their patients are not really eligible for those resources (Persad and others, 2009b, p. 427). In the United States, for example, data indicate that some physicians are willing to lie about a patient's medical condition so that the patient can receive care that the physician considers necessary (Freeman, 1999). Another way in which medical criteria can be abused is by mischaracterizing a patient's personality, behavior, or social situation as a failure to meet the medical criteria for access to limited resources. For example, patients who lack a stable home or income might be excluded from a list of potential recipients of organ transplants on the "medical" grounds that they have not demonstrated a sufficient likelihood of compliance with posttransplant care or a sufficient network of family or community support. Even without manipulation or mischaracterization, medical criteria do not tell us how to allocate limited resources between people with the same degree of medical need. For example, a young person and an old person might have the same severity of medical need for a transplant. Finally, medical criteria are not purely scientific; they include value judgments. As Persad and others (2009b) have explained, "There are no value-free medical criteria for allocation" (p. 423).

Similarly, rationing care on the basis of first-come, first served, waiting lists, queues, or lotteries would present various ethical complications. These methods of rationing seem to be fair, but in fact they would unfairly benefit certain groups of people (Rosen and others, 2005, p 1102; Persad and others, 2009b, pp. 423–424). For example, people with money, education, and influence would have an unfair advantage in finding out about waiting lists and putting their names on those lists. The use of queues would give an advantage to people who are able to travel to a health care facility and spend long periods of time waiting in line. Lotteries would result in decisions to allocate care on a random basis, without the need to make value judgments among potential recipients. Although that would seem to be fair in the abstract, lotteries could lead to absurd results, such as giving scarce life-saving resources to someone who is already extremely old (Persad and others, 2009b, p. 423). Thus, we might actually prefer to incorporate some value judgments into the process for making allocation decisions, such as including or excluding potential recipients on the basis of age.

Some people have suggested that we should indeed ration care on the basis of age, by denying expensive treatments to patients who already have reached a particular age. In the early part of the 1980s, Great Britain essentially rationed kidney dialysis on the basis of age (Aaron and others, 2005, pp. 36–38). Almost no patients over the age of fifty-five received dialysis in Britain at that time, although dialysis is now provided to patients who are much older. In regard to age, Daniel Callahan has argued that "one fundamental goal of health care and medicine is to help young people become old people, but it is not to have old people become infinitely older" (Sage Crossroads, 2003, p. 4). Therefore Callahan recommended replacing the current "infinity model" of unrestricted obligation with a democratically determined age beyond which expensive treatments would not be provided. Callahan recognized that many people would object to his proposal to ration care on the basis of age, but argued that it is the least bad alternative, because all of the demands for care in society cannot be met. In contrast, Christine Cassell strongly objected to rationing care on the basis of age, because it is impossible to set a particular age for appropriate life expectancy, life expectancy differs for men and women, and patients at a particular age are not uniform in their medical condition or their ability to benefit from additional treatment (Sage Crossroads, 2003, pp. 5–6). Persad and others (2009b) have acknowledged "the public preference for allocating scarce life-saving interventions to younger people," but have argued that it is inappropriate to sacrifice a young adult in order to save an infant (p. 425).

Most important, both the current public preference to allocate scarce resources to young people and the controversial proposal to restrict allocation for older people are based on value judgments that might be made differently in different countries and cultures. In his research on the Akamba people of Kenya, for example, Kilner (1984) identified several ways in which age-related preferences for rationing scarce health care resources differed from the usual preferences in the United States.

> For instance, where only one person can be saved, many Akamba favor saving an old man before a young, even where the young man is first in line. Whereas in the United States we tend to value the young more highly than the old because they are more productive economically, these Akamba espouse a more relational view of life . . . . Another Akamba priority documented by the study is: where only one person can be saved, save a man without children rather than one with five . . . . A third surprising (by U.S. standards) priority acknowledged by numerous Akamba is the insistence that it is better to give a half-treatment to each of two dying patients—even where experience dictates that a half-treatment is insufficient to save either—than to provide one patient with a full treatment which would almost certainly be lifesaving [Kilner, 1984, p. 19].

Even within Kenya the Akamba are only one group of people among others, and each group may have its own set of preferences for rationing health care resources. The point is not that one set of preferences is preferable or more ethical than another, but rather that any preferences may be limited to a particular culture. Therefore, preferences of any one culture should not be used as a uniform system of rationing in global health or even within a multicultural society.

The following discussion of various ways of rationing scarce antiretroviral therapy (ART) for HIV/AIDS in Africa is excerpted from an article that evaluated explicit and implicit methods of rationing life-saving medical treatment and noted the conflict between social equity and economic efficiency. The article authors concluded that explicit methods of rationing are more likely to maximize the welfare of society and are more likely to promote accountability and transparency in making decisions on public policy.

EXCERPT FROM "RATIONING ANTIRETROVIRAL THERAPY FOR HIV/AIDS IN AFRICA: CHOICES AND CONSEQUENCES"

BY SYDNEY ROSEN AND OTHERS

...The message...is clear: rationing of ART is already occurring and will persist for many years to come. The question facing African governments and societies is not whether to ration ART, but how to do so in a way that maximizes social welfare, now and in the future.

Inevitably, the social and economic consequences of rationing a scarce and valuable resource—treatment for a life-threatening illness—will vary widely depending on the rationing system chosen.... In this paper, we...use an expanded set of criteria to evaluate several rationing systems that already exist in sub-Saharan Africa.

Systems for Rationing

In economic terms, any policy or practice that restricts consumption of a good is a rationing system.... Non-price rationing of health care has a long history and is widespread and accepted in many parts of the world, reflecting the widely held view that access to health care should be based on some notion of need, and not determined solely by ability to pay. At the same time, non-price rationing is inherently political. It can be, and often is, used to channel resources toward or away from particular groups for reasons unrelated to their absolute or relative need for the resource.

In this paper, we define an ART rationing system as any allocation of public resources that prioritizes access to HIV/AIDS treatment on the basis of any geographic, social, economic, cultural, or other nonmedical factor. This is important, as virtually all programs will set a medical threshold for access to treatment, in most cases having a CD4 count lower than 200 cells/μl or an AIDS-defining illness. A less conservative medical eligibility threshold, such as that of the United States Department of Health and Human Services, which recommends that ART be started at a CD4 count of 350 cells/μl, would dramatically increase the number of eligible patients and intensify the need for rationing. Even with the more conservative eligibility threshold now being applied, however, the figures . . . indicate that demand for treatment will exceed supply. In the remainder of this paper, we will focus our attention on the nonmedical bases for rationing.

Explicit Rationing Systems

In many cases, governments will set explicit criteria for which types of patients should be eligible for ART first or at lowest cost. The criteria can target selected subpopulations directly, or they can set eligibility requirements that intentionally give some patients better access than others. Possible subpopulations for direct targeting of treatment include:

Mothers of new infants. Rather than face an ever-increasing burden of orphan support, many countries are making ART preferentially available to HIV-positive mothers through testing and treatment at antenatal clinics . . . .

Skilled workers. African countries face the loss of vast numbers of educated or trained workers, whose skills are vital to maintaining social welfare, sustaining output, and generating economic growth. Human capital can be conserved by giving treatment priority to nurses, teachers, engineers, judges, police officers, and other skilled workers whose contributions are important to economic development or social stability . . . .

Poor people. The social justice agenda pursued by some governments and many nongovernmental organizations argues that the poorest members of society, who are least likely to be able to afford private medical care, should have preferential access to publicly funded treatment programs. Means-testing, which can be applied at the level of the household or the community and calibrated to achieve the desired number of patients, is a common way to ration social benefits.

High-risk populations. The extent to which ART can curb HIV transmission is a subject of current debate in the literature. If treatment reduces the probability of transmission by suppressing viral load, then a public health argument can be made for giving preferential access to high-risk populations, such as commercial sex workers, truck drivers, or intravenous drug users.

Governments can also intentionally create eligibility requirements that result in rationing, without specifying particular target populations. Rationing systems of this type include:

Residents of designated geographic areas. One obvious way to limit access to treatment is to offer it only to those who reside in specified geographic catchment areas. These areas can be distributed around the country, centered in regions of high HIV prevalence, or concentrated in urban centers or politically important regions. Excluding patients who do not live within the designated areas may not be feasible, but most patients will not be able to afford the cost of regular transport or permanent relocation.

Ability to co-pay. If patients are required to contribute even a small share of the cost of treatment, the number who can access therapy is likely to fall dramatically. Governments could in principle match supply and demand by setting and adjusting the level of co-payment required. The obvious outcome is a rationing system that favors the upper socioeconomic tiers of patients, who likely include the majority of skilled workers. In some societies men will also have preferential access when a cash payment is required. A drawback of requiring co-payment is that poorer patients may stop therapy because they run out of funds. This is the reason for stopping cited by nearly half of all non-adherent patients in a recent study in Botswana.

Commitment to adherence to therapy. Adherence to treatment regimens has been found to be the most important determinant of the success of ART at the individual patient level. One way to improve the success of a large-scale treatment program, while at the same time limiting access, could therefore be to restrict therapy to patients who are judged to have the ability and willingness to adhere or who demonstrate high adherence after initiating therapy . . . .

Implicit Rationing Systems

The alternative to specifying explicitly who will have priority access to resources is to allow implicit rationing systems to arise. These can be thought of as the default conditions that will prevail in the absence of explicit choices.

Access to HIV testing. Voluntary counseling and HIV testing (VCT) is typically the entry point into an HIV/AIDS treatment program. If some subpopulations, such as youth or particular occupational groups, are targeted for HIV education and VCT services or promotion campaigns, they will have an advantage over others in seeking treatment, as will those who simply live closer to VCT facilities.

Patient costs. Most countries will scale up their treatment programs incrementally, at first offering services at only a few facilities before gradually adding more . . . . For most patients, bus or taxi fare will be required for regular trips to the clinic, and each trip will take up a good deal of time. Previous research has found that indirect costs due to travel time and transport play an important role in limiting access to medical care. Unless transport is subsidized, limiting the number of service sites will effectively ration treatment to those who live nearby and to better-off households that have the resources to travel.

First come, first served. In the absence of any other requirements, most facilities are likely to treat everyone who is medically eligible, until the supply of drugs, diagnostics, or expertise runs out. Patients who arrive after that happens may be put on a waiting list, sent to another facility, or simply sent away. This approach, which reflects an absolute shortage of treatment "slots," is likely to favor three groups of patients: those who are already paying privately for antiretroviral drugs and shift over to publicly funded treatment once it is available; those who develop AIDS-related symptoms first, in most cases because they were infected earliest; and the few HIV-positive individuals who do not yet have AIDS but have taken the initiative to go for a test and know their own status.

Queuing. One of the most common ways to ration scarce resources is the time-honored, time-consuming tradition of queuing. While it is possible to create a waiting list that keeps track of individuals' places in line, in many African countries the queue is a literal line outside the clinic door. Such queuing will favor patients whose opportunity cost of time is low. This group is likely to be dominated by unemployed men and by women who can bring their small children with them. It may penalize employed persons and farming households that face a high seasonal demand for labor.

No matter what system is used, informal and/or illicit arrangements can often be made that give preferential access to treatment to those with social, economic, or political influence. In all of the implicit systems, and in some of the explicit ones, there will very often be a high degree of queue jumping. Elites capture a disproportionate share of resources in all countries; in developing countries, where enforcement of rules tends to be weak and informal arrangements common, it is safe to assume that members of the elite who are medically eligible for therapy will find a way to get it. De facto rationing on the basis of social or economic position will thus occur. It is the phenomenon of queue jumping that turns what appear to be equitable, if inefficient, rationing systems, such as first-come, first-served, into an inequitable and inefficient approach.

Many other potential criteria for rationing ART have been proposed or are in use. Treatment access could be targeted, for example, to young people (because they respond best to the therapy and have their most productive years ahead of them); families of current patients (to promote adherence); those with debts (so that the loan default rate does not increase); patients with tuberculosis (to suppress transmission of tuberculosis); or children (who are least able to protect themselves).

Evaluating the Systems

The different approaches to rationing ART described above will inevitably have very different social and economic consequences for African populations. In this section, we assess the rationing systems' probable outcomes using criteria that capture most of the principles that governments use to evaluate policies and social investments. They are by no means the sole criteria of interest, nor should they necessarily be given equal weight. We propose them only as a starting point for thinking about the consequences of alternative approaches.

Effectiveness. Does the rationing system produce a high rate of successfully treated patients? . . .

Cost savings. Is the cost per patient treated low, compared to other approaches? . . .

Feasibility. Are the human and infrastructural resources needed for implementation available? We define an approach as feasible if there are no obstacles to carrying it out that appear to be insurmountable under typical conditions in sub-Saharan Africa.

Economic efficiency. To what extent does the system mitigate the long-term impacts of the HIV epidemic on economic development? . . .

Social equity. Do all medically eligible patients, including those from poor or disadvantaged subpopulations, have equal access to treatment? . . .

Rationing potential. Will the chosen system sufficiently reduce the number of patients? . . .

Impact on HIV transmission. To what extent does treatment reduce HIV incidence? Preferentially treating those who are likely to transmit the virus could reduce HIV incidence more than treating those who are not likely transmitters.

Sustainability. Can the system be sustained over time? This criterion pertains to the durability of the source of funding . . . .

Effect on the health care system. How does the system for allocating ART affect the country's health care system as a whole? The choice of rationing strategies could influence whether expanding treatment access will strengthen general health services for poor communities or drain resources from non-HIV health care to meet the demand for ART, further crippling general health services . . . .

There are several limitations to the analysis presented . . . Cost and feasibility are clearly related, for example; at some level of cost, any system could be considered feasible . . . .

Conclusions...

Rationing of medical care is not a new phenomenon, nor is it by any means limited to developing countries. Waiting lists, whether for specific procedures, organs for transplant, or experimental treatments, are common in North America and Europe. Many state governments in the US are explicitly limiting access to more expensive AIDS drugs. The HIV/ AIDS crisis in Africa is simply bringing the need for rationing into stark relief.

There is no single rationing system, or combination of systems, that will be optimal for all countries at all times . . . . [All systems make a] trade-off between economic efficiency and social equity: rationing systems that rate high in terms of efficiency generally rate low in terms of equity. African societies will place different weights on the values inherent in goals such as equity and efficiency . . . .

Because access to antiretroviral drugs is a matter of life or death for patients with AIDS, the choice of rationing systems matters deeply. African governments can take one of two courses: ration deliberately, on the basis of explicit criteria, or allow implicit rationing to prevail. Implicit rationing is not likely to maximize social welfare, nor does it allow for transparency and accountability in policy making. We believe that the magnitude of the intervention now underway and the importance of the resource allocation decisions to be made call for public participation, policy analysis, and political debate in the countries affected. Several proposals have been made for how such processes could be carried out. In the absence of such processes, decisions about access to treatment will be made arbitrarily and will, most likely, result in inequity and inefficiency—the worst of both worlds. Governments that make deliberate choices, in contrast, are more likely to achieve a socially desirable return from the large investments now being made than are those that allow queuing and queue-jumping to dominate. Countries that promote an open policy debate have the opportunity to ration ART in a manner that sustains both economic development and social cohesion—in the age of AIDS, the best of both worlds.

Source: Excerpted from "Rationing Antiretroviral Therapy for HIV/AIDS in Africa: Choices and Consequences," by Sydney Rosen, Ian Sanne, Alizanne Collier, and Jonathon L. Simon, 2005. *PLoS Medicine*, *2*(11), 1098–1104 (references, tables, and some text omitted). Copyright: 2005 Rosen et al. This is an open-access article distributed under the terms of the Creative Commons Attribution License, which permits unrestricted use, distribution, and reproduction in any medium, provided the original work is properly cited.

COMPARATIVE EFFECTIVENESS RESEARCH AND COST-EFFECTIVENESS ANALYSIS

Every health system must develop a method of making the difficult decisions about allocation of resources and rationing of care. Even countries with national health systems and universal health insurance coverage, such as the United Kingdom and other European countries, need to find their own ways of limiting care. Some of those countries use methods that are based, at least in part, on comparative effectiveness research and cost-effectiveness analysis.

Comparative effectiveness research (CER) is the analysis of different groups of patients to evaluate the relative effectiveness of different treatments. This research provides information on which to base clinical treatment and health policy (Garber and Tunis, 2009, p. 1925). For example, researchers might evaluate whether surgery, radiation therapy, or chemotherapy is most effective in treating patients with a particular form of cancer. Alternatively, researchers might evaluate whether a new drug is more effective than an existing drug in treating a particular condition. CER is different from the analysis used for approval of a new drug product by a regulatory agency, such as the U.S. Food and Drug Administration, which might evaluate the safety and potential effectiveness of a new drug by comparing it to a placebo rather than to an existing drug (Avorn, 2009, p. 1927). However, the evaluation of effectiveness for CER is similar to the evaluation of effectiveness for regulatory approval in at least one important respect. Like the analysis for regulatory approval, CER does not include consideration of the cost of a particular method of treatment.

In contrast to CER, **cost-effectiveness analysis (CEA)** evaluates the improvement in health in relation to the different cost of each alternative treatment (Jamison and others, 2006, pp. 42, 56). If the same amount of money were devoted to each alternative, which alternative would produce more improvement in overall health status? Thus CEA identifies the way to obtain the greatest benefit to health from the use of limited funds (Brock, 2004, p. 202).

CEA is not the same as **cost-benefit analysis (CBA)**, which puts a financial value on human life or years of human life. According to Cutler (2007), one year of life is usually valued at approximately U.S.$100,000 (p. 1099). CBA compares the financial cost of a proposed intervention with the financial gain of human lives that would be saved or extended by that intervention. Jamison and others (2006) contrast the two methods this way: "One of the advantages of using cost-effectiveness ratios is that they avoid some ethical dilemmas and analytical difficulties that arise when attempting cost-benefit analyses. Applying the alternative analytical technique of cost-benefit analysis requires assigning a monetary value to each year of life. By foregoing this step, cost-effectiveness analysis draws attention exclusively to health benefits, which are not monetized" (p. 44). For these reasons, CEA has become the primary tool in health policy for comparing the costs of alternative interventions and determining the most effective use of finite resources.

Jamison and others (2006) also explain how cost-effectiveness analysis can be used to help make decisions at various levels of a health system (pp. 48–51). At the macrolevel, CEA can be used to compare alternative uses of limited funds to address different diseases or conditions. For example, spending U.S.$1 million to expand immunization coverage for children would improve health status between 1,000 and 10,000 times more than spending the same amount of money to provide open-heart surgery in certain high-risk cases (p. 49). CEA can also be used to compare alternative ways of treating the same disease, such as drug therapy versus surgery for treatment of the same medical condition. Finally, CEA can be used to compare two different drugs for treatment of the same medical condition, such as comparing a new drug to an existing drug. At that level of analysis, however, it is important to consider whether the methodology is sufficiently accurate to compare relatively small differences in effectiveness. In fact, Jamison and others (2006) recommend using CEA to identify interventions that differ by orders of magnitude, rather than interventions that differ by smaller amounts that could be affected by methodological issues (p. 48). At that level of analysis it is also important to remember that CEA indicates only the average effectiveness for a group of patients, or even a subgroup of patients with certain characteristics, and does not necessarily indicate the most effective treatment for any particular patient. Moreover, there may be complications in using data from clinical trials to evaluate the relative effectiveness of different drugs when the clinical trials were not originally designed to collect data for that purpose (McGuire and others, 2008, p. 4).

The use of cost-effectiveness analysis also raises important ethical issues in making health policy and allocating limited health resources. Those who serve as stewards of scarce health care resources have an ethical obligation to use those resources in the most cost-effective manner. CEA can help to determine the best ways to meet that ethical obligation. However, using CEA means that some treatments will not be provided, even if they would be effective, because they are less cost effective than other uses of society's limited funds. According to the President's Commission for the Study of Ethical Problems in Medicine and Biomedical and Behavioral Research (1983), "some health services (even of a lifesaving sort) will not be developed or employed because they would produce too few benefits in relation to their costs and to the other ways the resources for them might be used" (p. 19). Although that statement seems to be reasonable in the abstract, many people would object strenuously if the same statement were to be made by a for-profit insurance company or HMO.

In terms of ethical theory, CEA is utilitarian. It uses quantitative analysis in an attempt to determine the greatest good for the greatest number of people. CEA not only considers the number of people who would be benefited or harmed by a particular intervention but also incorporates methodologies to consider the degree to which people would be benefited or harmed. Specifically, CEA measures the number of years of life that would be gained or lost, and makes adjustments to that number of life years on the basis of quality of life (**quality-adjusted life years [QALYs]**) or on the basis of disability (**disability-adjusted life years [DALYs]**).

However, CEA does not consider the degree of equity in distribution of these benefits or harms. As Brock (2004) has explained, "Cost effectiveness and utilitarian standards require minimising the aggregate burden of disease and maximising the aggregate health of a population without regard to the resulting distribution of disease and health, or *who* gets what benefits" (p. 215, italics in original). Therefore, experts in CEA caution that it should not be used alone to make rationing decisions, but rather should be used in conjunction with an analysis of equity in the distribution of benefits (Brock, 2004, p. 221; Persad and others, 2009b, pp. 427–429; Jamison and others, 2006, p. 52). As Jamison and others (2006) have written, "cost-effectiveness should not be the exclusive basis for making health-related public policy decisions and should be complemented with information about distributional consequences" (p. 52). Several methods exist for complementing CEA with consideration of other social values (Drummond, 2008).

In addition to its failure to consider equitable distribution, cost-effectiveness analysis requires making certain assumptions and methodological decisions. Each of those assumptions and methodological decisions is based on a value judgment with significant ethical implications (Brock, 2004, pp. 221–222). For example, CEA requires making a value judgment about whether to give the same weight to years of life for patients of different ages or, alternatively, to weight years of life more heavily for young people, elderly people, or people of working age. The QALY system treats one year of life equally for patients of all ages, subject to adjustment for quality of life. That value judgment can lead to the irrational and unfair result of treating one year of additional life for a seventy-year-old as being the same in value as one year of additional life for a twenty-five-year-old, provided there was no difference in the quality of life (Brock, 2004, p. 207; Persad and others, 2009b, p. 428). The DALY system is also problematic from an ethical perspective, because it gives more weight to an additional year of life for a person of working age than it gives to an additional year of life for a person who is too young to work or too old to work, assuming similar states of disability (Brock, 2004, p. 207; Persad and others, 2009b, at 428). Jamison and others (2006) chose to use the DALY system, but decided not to provide greater weight on the basis of age (p. 41). As discussed earlier, people in different countries and cultures have very different views on the issues of rationing by age and the value to be given to individuals at different stages of life. Therefore it seems inappropriate to apply the quantitative methodology of CEA as a uniform framework for health care allocation decisions in all countries and cultural groups.

Another value judgment with ethical implications is the definition of life expectancy. Should cost-effectiveness analysis use a uniform life expectancy for all human beings in determining the benefits of a proposed treatment, or should CEA use different life expectancies for people in various countries or for people of different races, genders, and economic status? Technical accuracy in calculating the actual benefits of a proposed treatment would seem to require recognition that some people have lower life expectancies and will continue to have lower life expectancies, even after receiving the proposed treatment. However, that approach to CEA would make it appear more valuable in terms of QALYs or DALYs to save a rich person in North America who has a long life expectancy than it would be to save a poor person in Africa with a shorter life expectancy. Under these circumstances the developers of the DALY system elected to apply a uniform life expectancy, based on the long life expectancy of Japan, except for that portion of the difference in life expectancy by gender that is based on biological factors (Brock, 2004, p. 211–12). In contrast, Jamison and others (2006) elected to use regional averages of life expectancy, which tends to lower the cost effectiveness of proposed treatments in developing countries with shorter life expectancy, but facilitates more appropriate comparison of proposed treatments within a region (p. 41). The point here is not that one approach or the other is correct, but rather that there is no single approach that resolves all of the ethical problems of using CEA.

Ethical problems also arise in making adjustments for disability or quality of life for purposes of cost-effectiveness analysis (Persad and others, 2009b, p. 427). In considering the benefit of a proposed intervention, it is logical to adjust the additional life years that would be gained by the applicable level of disability or quality of life that would result from the proposed intervention. For example, most people would agree that ten additional years of life in a persistent vegetative state would be worth much less than ten additional years of life in a fully functional condition. Moreover, adjusting for various levels of disability helps to recognize the cost effectiveness of valuable treatments that would prevent more serious disabilities (Jamison and others, 2006, pp. 43–44). The ethical problem is how to weigh various levels of disability or differences in quality of life without imposing our value judgments or discriminating against persons with disabilities. Some of the adjustments for disability that are used in CEA are based on the opinions of health professionals, although persons who actually have those disabilities might reach very different conclusions because of coping, adaptation, and cultural or socioeconomic differences (Brock, 2004, pp. 203–206). Moreover, quantitative methods of CEA give less weight to treatment of persons with disabilities than they do to treatment of persons without disabilities, which led Brock (2004) to conclude that CEA may unfairly discriminate, in violation of the basic ethical principle of justice (pp. 218–220).

For all these reasons, policymakers should not make rationing decisions simply on the basis of numerical calculations derived by means of CEA. They should remember the caveats from experts in CEA about focusing on interventions that differ by orders of magnitude and about using CEA in conjunction with an analysis of equity in the distribution of benefits. They should also remember that the numbers generated by CEA are affected by certain assumptions and methodological decisions, each of which is based on a value judgment with ethical and cultural implications. The real danger is that politicians, health officials, media, and the public will ignore all these caveats and give far too much credence to numbers that appear unassailable because they are based on a scientific methodology and generated by computer.

At the present time, several countries use cost-effectiveness analysis in an attempt to identify the most effective treatments, obtain the best value for their money, and limit their health care expenditures (Chalkidou and others, 2009). Some European countries that have national health systems and universal insurance coverage use CEA to limit the costs of the benefit package they have undertaken to provide to their residents. In the United Kingdom, for example, the National Institute for Health and Clinical Excellence (NICE) provides guidance for the NHS about the use of new medicines, treatments, and technologies (Owen-Smith and others, p. 1936; Newdick, 2005). One of the goals of NICE has been to create uniformity in the adoption of new treatments, rather than allow each local health authority to make its own decision, which would lead to differences in availability of particular treatments on the basis of "post-code" (Newdick, 2005, p. 665). NICE uses the cost per QALY to decide whether a new treatment is a cost-effective use of NHS resources. As in every system of CEA, the methodology used by NICE is based on certain value judgments (Rawlins and Culyer, 2004). For example, NICE modified its analysis to consider the additional value that society in the United Kingdom places on life-extending treatments (National Institute for Health and Clinical Excellence, 2009). In fact NICE has demonstrated its willingness to permit use of some expensive drugs that can prolong life for a minimum of three months, provided the drugs are used for treatment of diseases that affect a small enough number of patients to prevent budgetary problems (Cheng, 2009).

Compared to European countries, the United States has made much less use of CEA. In 2009, the U.S. Congress provided more than $1 billion for comparative effectiveness research (CER) to evaluate the effectiveness of various treatments, but not for CEA to evaluate the costs of alternative treatments. Nevertheless, opponents of the legislation have argued that the funding will lead to rationing of care and payment limitations on the basis of cost effectiveness (Avorn, 2009). Proponents of CER, both inside and outside the U.S. government, have denied that CER will lead to rationing and have insisted that CER will simply help doctors and patients to have more informed conversations about their options for treatment. However, many proponents of CER are also hoping that it will help to reduce the increasing costs of care in the United States (Connolly, 2009). The U.S. Congressional Budget Office (2009) has acknowledged that research alone would probably not have a significant effect on health care costs and that reducing costs would probably require changes in the payment policies of insurance companies and public programs, in order to alter the incentives for patients and their doctors (p. 15). In Germany, France, and Australia, organizations that were established to perform CER, without a mandate to consider the cost of treatment, later experienced "mission creep" to include explicit consideration of costs (Chalkidou and others, 2009, p. 353). Under these circumstances the debate is continuing in the United States about the appropriate scope and likely effect of the more than $1 billion in newly funded research on comparative effectiveness.

SUMMARY

Every health system, including national health systems with universal insurance coverage, must develop some method of making difficult decisions about the allocation of resources and rationing of care. This chapter has evaluated the various methods of rationing limited health resources, both explicit and implicit, and has analyzed the ethical implications of using each method. As explained in this chapter, decisions about the most appropriate way to ration scarce health resources are based on value judgments that differ across countries and cultures. Thus, we should not impose the values of any particular country or culture as a uniform method of rationing in global health or within multicultural societies.

Experts agree that there is no single best method of rationing (World Health Organization, 2000, p. 59; Brock, 2004, pp. 202–203). Some experts recommend combining ethical principles into complex systems for making allocation decisions (Persad and others, 2009b, p 426). Some stress the importance of procedural fairness in making these difficult decisions, including accountability, transparency and public participation (Rosen and others, 2005,

p. 1103). Others argue that procedural solutions are insufficient, that societies also need to consider substantive ethical principles such as equity and justice (Persad and others, 2009b, p. 429; Brock, 2004, p. 203). Ultimately, developing an effective and ethical system of rationing may require significant cultural change. People need to accept the fact that they are simply not going to get all of the health care services that they want, or even all of the services that are potentially beneficial. What people can get is a sense of comfort and social solidarity from knowing that significant improvements are being made in the public health and welfare of their country.

KEY TERMS

comparative effectiveness research (CER)

cost-benefit analysis (CBA)

cost-effectiveness analysis (CEA)

disability-adjusted life years (DALYs)

macrolevel decision

microlevel decision

quality-adjusted life years (QALYs)

rationing system

DISCUSSION QUESTIONS

1. From the most general to the most specific, what are the decisions that each society must make in allocating its resources for health?
2. In your opinion, are explicit or implicit methods of rationing more ethical? Why?
3. What are the differences among cost-effectiveness research (CER), cost-effectiveness analysis (CEA), and cost-benefit analysis (CBA)?
4. What are the ethical implications of using cost-effectiveness analysis to make rationing decisions?

ACTIVITY: COST-EFFECTIVENESS ANALYSIS IN A COUNTRY WITH UNIVERSAL HEALTH CARE COVERAGE

The Republic of Arborea (a fictional example) is a democratic country that provides universal coverage for its residents through a system of tax-supported, national health insurance. The Ministry of Health (MOH) provides funding to local health authorities (LHAs), in the form of a fixed annual budget for each

LHA, calculated on the basis of population in each area. LHAs are required to provide all the health services authorized by MOH to all residents of their areas, but LHAs may not spend more than their annual budget from MOH. If an LHA runs out of money before the end of a year, MOH will not provide any additional funding to the LHA for that year. Thus, LHAs need to use their resources in ways that will meet all their obligations to their area residents without exceeding their annual budgets.

Three years ago the government of Arborea created a national-level agency known as the Center for Quality Assessment (CQA). CQA provides guidance to MOH about the use of new medicines, treatments, and technologies in order to identify the most effective treatments and help MOH obtain the best value for its money.

If CQA determines that a new drug is not cost effective, that drug will not be provided to patients through the national health insurance system. However, if CQA recommends a drug, all patients in the country will have the right to receive that drug through the national health insurance system, provided that drug is prescribed by their physicians. Neither CQA nor MOH will provide any additional funding to the LHAs to pay for new drugs that CQA has recommended. Therefore LHAs need to use their existing funds for this purpose, and might need to eliminate the use of other drugs or treatments that have not been recommended—or even evaluated—by CQA.

In evaluating new drugs and technologies, CQA uses the cost per QALY to decide whether a new treatment is a cost-effective use of MOH resources. Ordinarily, CQA will not find a treatment to be cost effective if it costs more than U.S.$50,000 per QALY. However, CQA has made exceptions in some situations. For example, CQA has recommended some drugs for use by small numbers of patients with very rare diseases, even though the cost per QALY for these drugs exceeds the usual threshold of $50,000. Such drugs are often referred to as *orphan drugs*. They cost a lot of money for each patient, but they are used by so few patients that they do not present a problem for MOH's budget. Nevertheless, the cost of providing orphan drugs can present budgetary problems for LHAs.

Recently, CQA recommended the use of a new orphan drug (drug no. 1), which has a cost per QALY of $75,000. The LHA in the town of Littlehaven notified the people in its area that it would begin providing that orphan drug to patients as prescribed by their physicians. However, the Littlehaven LHA also announced that in order to pay for drug no. 1 within the limit of its fixed annual budget, it would no longer provide an existing drug (drug no. 2) to patients in its area. Drug no. 2 has been used by many patients in Littlehaven for years but has never been evaluated for cost effectiveness by CQA. Therefore, the cost per QALY for drug no. 2 is unknown.

Several patients who have been taking drug no. 2 have formed the Littlehaven Patient Advocacy Group in order to protest the LHA's action in refusing to provide drug no. 2. These patients argue that it is unfair to deny them access to an existing drug, which has been used for many years and which CQA has not had the opportunity to evaluate, in order to provide a very expensive orphan drug to a small number of patients.

This advocacy group has been joined by another group of patients, people who want the Littlehaven LHA to provide drug no. 3. Drug no. 3 has a cost per QALY of $60,000, which exceeds the usual threshold of $50,000. Therefore CQA found drug no. 3 not cost effective. However, drug no. 3 is more cost effective than drug no. 1 (the orphan drug), which has a cost per QALY of $75,000. This group of patients argues that it is unfair to provide drug no. 1 though the national health system while refusing to provide drug no. 3. However, drug no. 3 could be used by a large number of patients and could have more budgetary impact than drug no.1.

Please analyze the ethical issues presented by this scenario. Apply the perspectives of patients who are current or potential users of drugs 1, 2, and 3, as well as the perspectives of MOH, the Littlehaven LHA, and the taxpayers of Arborea.

CHAPTER NINE

ETHICAL ISSUES OF HEALTH INSURANCE AND HEALTH SYSTEM REFORM

LEARNING OBJECTIVES

■ Acquire proficiency in analyzing the ethical issues in raising money for health services and designing a fair health insurance system.

■ Understand and be able to explain the meaning of fairness in the context of health financing, and be able to evaluate which method of financing is the most fair.

■ Learn how to analyze the ethical issues raised by employment-based insurance coverage.

■ Understand and demonstrate an appreciation of the fundamental values on which the health systems of various countries are based.

■ Demonstrate the ability to evaluate the trade-offs that people in various countries have made—or need to make—in the process of health system reform, in light of the fundamental values of their health system and their society.

ROM an ethical perspective, which method of raising money for health services is the most fair? Health services can be financed in several different ways, such as private insurance, government insurance, social or community systems, and payment out of pocket at the point of service. The World Health Organization (WHO) has considered the fairness of various methods of financing, and developed a framework to evaluate the fairness in financial contribution to the health system of a particular country. This chapter begins by describing WHO's concept of fairness in health system financing and by analyzing WHO's framework for evaluating the level of fairness in any given country. Then the chapter compares the fairness of the health financing system in the United States to that of other countries, such as Canada, the United Kingdom, and Germany. In all countries—developing, transitional, and high-income—designing a fair health insurance system requires trade-offs, and those trade-offs have ethical implications.

An activity at the end of this chapter provides an opportunity to evaluate the most ethical way to establish a new system of health insurance for a developing country that has a finite sum of money for this purpose. Finally, the chapter analyzes the fundamental values on which various countries have based their health systems, including the important value of solidarity found in countries of Western Europe and local communities in Africa.

ETHICAL ISSUES IN FINANCING HEALTH SERVICES AND DESIGNING INSURANCE SYSTEMS

Financing refers to the methods of raising money for health services (Roberts and others, 2008, pp. 26, 153). A variety of mechanisms exist to finance health services, such as general taxation, employee health insurance or other private coverage, social insurance, community-based health insurance, and payment out of pocket at the point of service (Roberts and others, p. 153). As an ethical matter, which system of financing health services is the most fair? The answer to that question requires consideration of the meaning of fairness in the context of health financing.

The World Health Organization considers fairness in financing to be one of the three objectives of every health system (2000, p. 25). In its World Health Report 2000, WHO described this concept as follows:

> *Fair financing* in health systems means that the risks each household faces due to the costs of the health system are distributed according to ability to pay rather than to the risk of illness . . . A health system in which individuals or households

are sometimes forced into poverty through their purchase of needed care, or forced to do without it because of the cost, is unfair . . . .

Paying for health care can be unfair in two different ways. It can expose families to large *unexpected* expenses . . . Or it can impose *regressive* payments, in which those least able to contribute pay proportionately more than the better-off . . . .

. . . [F]inancial fairness is best served by more, as well as by more progressive, prepayment in place of out-of-pocket expenditure . . . . [T]he ideal is largely to disconnect a household's financial contribution to the health system from its health risks, and separate it almost entirely from the use of needed services [World Health Organization, 2000, pp. 35–36, emphasis in original].

WHO's framework for determining the fairness of financial contribution to a health system can be broken down into several principles, each of which can be used to evaluate the fairness of financing in particular countries. These principles are as follows:

1. Protection from the financial risks of illness should be universal, so that no individual or family is prevented from access to care or driven into poverty as a result of illness (World Health Organization, 2000, p. 35).
2. People should be protected from high, unexpected, and out-of-pocket costs at the point of service. Therefore, prepayment of costs by means of taxes or insurance is fairer than out-of-pocket payment (World Health Organization, 2000, pp. xviii, 35).
3. Payment for health services should be progressive rather than regressive. Therefore prepayment should be based on the ability to pay, instead of on the risk of illness or utilization of necessary services (World Health Organization 2000, pp. 35–36). As explained by Christopher Murray and Julio Frenk (2000), who developed the conceptual framework for the WHO report, poor people have less disposable income, in part because they must spend a larger percentage of their income on necessities like shelter and food (p. 720). If prepayment were to be based on the risk of illness, each individual would be charged a rate that reflects his or her individual risk, and no individual would be required to subsidize anyone else (Light, 1992, pp. 2506–2507). As Donald Light (1992) has pointed out, payment on the basis of risk may satisfy the libertarian principle that no person should be required to pay for any other person, but such "actuarial fairness is morally unfair, because it reduces access to life opportunities and increases suffering for those disadvantaged by risk, pain, and illness" (p. 2507). Thus WHO, and others, take the position

that prepayment should be based on the ability to pay, rather than on the risk of illness.

4. Fairness requires the pooling of risks, whereby healthy people subsidize sick people and rich people subsidize poor people (World Health Organization, 2000, p. xviii). **Risk pooling** refers to combining risks for individuals, which are uncertain and potentially unaffordable, into one risk for a large group, which is calculable and manageable (Gottret and Schieber, 2006, pp. 4–5).

5. Risk pools should be as large as possible, in order to minimize the risk to individuals and their families (World Health Organization, 2000, p. xviii). Prepayment on an individual basis, such as occurs in a medical savings account, does not ensure fairness of financing, because it does not spread the risk or subsidize the elderly or the sick (World Health Organization, 2000, p. 99).

In terms of the principles used by WHO, the health financing system of the United States is less fair than the systems of other industrialized countries, such as Canada and the United Kingdom, for several reasons. First, the U.S. system of health financing is not universal, although the U.S. government is undertaking some reforms toward a long-term goal of universality. The U.S. system fails to provide universal protection and access to care, with more than 46 million people in the United States uninsured in 2009. Millions of people in the United States have been prevented from having access to care or have been driven into bankruptcy as a result of medical bills. Even those U.S. residents who have health insurance may need to pay high, unexpected costs out of pocket at the point of service because of high deductibles, copayments, and charges for noncovered services.

The U.S. system is based to a large extent on employment-based insurance coverage, which, under the principles used by WHO, is arguably less fair than tax-supported, national health insurance. In fact Victor Fuchs (2008) has argued that a tax-financed system, which is unrelated to employment status, is not only the most equitable method of providing universal coverage but is also the most efficient (p. 1751). Employment-based coverage is unfair to those people who are unemployed or who work for employers that do not provide health insurance for their employees. As the World Health Organization (2000) put it, employment-based systems limit coverage to "their privileged membership" (p. xviii). Nancy Jecker (1993) argued that the employment-based insurance system found in the United States is inherently unethical because of unjust discrimination in the distribution of jobs that provide insurance and because, even if jobs were distributed fairly, the reasons for distributing jobs are not valid reasons for distributing health care. Therefore, Jecker argued that rather than mandating all employers to offer health insurance for their employees, health reform efforts in the United States should be directed toward "uncoupling health insurance and jobs" (p. 671.)

In addition to being less inclusive than other health insurance systems, employment-based health insurance is also less portable, and it can be difficult for individuals to retain coverage after termination of employment. Employment-based coverage is also less uniform than the coverage of national health systems, because the benefits, coverage levels, and degree of cost sharing can vary considerably among employers. The financing of employment-based coverage is not transparent, as a direct tax for health care would be. Many workers mistakenly believe that most of the cost for their health insurance is borne by their employers, but actually that cost is borne, one way or another, by the workers (Fuchs, 2008, p. 1750). Moreover, employment-based coverage can encourage employers to discriminate against people who are less healthy when those employers are making decisions on hiring and promotion, and this kind of coverage raises serious risks of disclosing medical information to supervisors and coworkers.

The U.S system of employment-based insurance coverage is also regressive. First, an individual employee's share of contributions for health insurance is not based on his or her level of income. Therefore, low-wage workers are required to pay the same amount as workers or managers who earn much more money, even though that amount represents a larger percentage of the low-wage worker's earnings and a larger percentage of disposable income. This system violates the principle of **vertical equity**, which requires fair treatment for groups of people with different levels of income (Roberts and others, 2008, p. 103).

In addition, U.S. federal tax laws make the system of health financing even more regressive. The U.S. government provides a significant tax break to those employees who receive health benefits from their employers (Carey and others, 2009, pp. 25–26). As a general rule, employees must pay income tax on the compensation that they receive from their employers. Wages and salaries are considered to be part of an employee's taxable income. However, an employer's contribution for an employee's health insurance is not considered part of the employee's taxable income. This tax break is unfair in many ways because it does not benefit all taxpayers or all employees equally (Emanuel and Fuchs, 2005, pp. 1255, 1257). It gives the most tax advantages to those employees who have the most expensive insurance benefits or the highest incomes, or both. This violates the principle of vertical equity by treating high-income workers more favorably than low-income workers (Carey and others, 2009, p. 27). This tax break provides no advantages whatsoever to those employees who receive no health insurance from their employers. Therefore, this system also violates the principle of **horizontal equity** by providing differential treatment for people with the same level of income (Roberts and others, 2008, p. 104; Carey and others, 2009, p. 27). Meanwhile other taxpayers are forced to pay more taxes than they would otherwise, in order to make up for the revenue not collected by the government.

The employment-based insurance system in the United States also violates WHO's principle that risk pooling should be as broad as possible. As discussed previously, fairness requires the pooling of risks so that healthy people subsidize sick people and rich people subsidize poor people. Risk pools should be as large as possible, in order to minimize the risk to specific individuals. To the contrary, employer-based coverage is an attempt to limit each company's risk pool to people associated with that company, such as current employees, retirees, and their dependents.

Many employers in the United States complain about the high and rapidly increasing costs for their employee health plans. Some employers would like to be relieved of the obligation to pay the cost for their employees' health insurance, and some say that they would like someone else, such as the government, to pay for those costs. However, many U.S. employers prefer the current system, under which they are primarily responsible for their own employees, retirees, and dependents, to a system of national health insurance, under which they could be required to pay higher taxes in support of a broader risk pool. To some extent this attitude reflects the uncertainty about the relative costs to employers of shifting from an employment-based system to a tax-supported system, as well as employers' concern about relinquishing control of the health insurance system while continuing to be largely responsible for its costs (Galvin, 2008). Under the current U.S. system, employers in the private sector have substantial flexibility to design their own employee benefit plans, determine the levels of benefits and cost sharing, and change their plans prospectively, quite possibly to the detriment of their employees.

Moreover, the reluctance of many employers to support a national health system may also reflect a desire to limit their risk pool to people who are likely to be healthier on average than other groups of people. That is, a company's employees, retirees, and dependents may be healthier than the population at large. That parochial attitude may be understandable from a purely financial perspective. However, it is questionable from an ethical perspective because it bases the entire system of health financing on selfish efforts to keep other people out of one's risk pool. It would be fairer to include everyone in the society in the same risk pool, including people who are poor, elderly, disabled, chronically ill, unemployed, or working for other companies.

Some supporters of the U.S. system argue that private health insurance is more likely to encourage the development and use of new medical technology and drugs, whereas systems of national health insurance might try to control health care costs by limiting the use of expensive new treatments and not providing incentives for their development. However, access to new technologies and drugs in a system of private health insurance can be extremely inequitable and unfair.

For all of these reasons, from the standpoint of the WHO principles, the U.S. system of employment-based health insurance, which is both regressive and inequitable, is less fair than methods of health financing used by other industrialized countries. Of course, fairness is not the only ethical value to consider. Under the ethical theory of principlism, one might argue that the U.S. system of employer-based coverage promotes the ethical duty of autonomy, by maximizing the choices for employers and employees. However, other ways of preserving choice are available, even in systems that provide universal coverage. For example, the social insurance system of Germany provides universal coverage but permits individuals to choose among competing, nonprofit sickness funds (European Observatory on Health Systems and Policies, 2004, p. 4). Moreover, under the theory of principlism, any gain in autonomy under the U.S. system of insurance is outweighed by the system's unfairness as well as its failure to promote beneficence. The U.S. system also fails to treat each individual as an end in himself or herself, as required by Kantian ethics, and it is not a system that we could wish to be universally applied to the distribution of other things on which we are similarly dependent. Perhaps most telling, the U.S. system of employer-based health insurance fails even the test of utilitarianism. The United States outspends other industrialized countries but ranks poorly on some important measures of health (Davis, 2008), and thereby fails to provide the greatest good for the greatest number of people.

According to Julio Frenk and Octavio Gómez-Dantés (2009), discussions in Mexico about the ethical deficiencies of that country's previous health system had helped to build consensus for reform (p. 1406). It is to be hoped that people in the United States and other countries can learn from their example.

Designing a fair health insurance system requires trade-offs, not only in high-income countries but also in developing and transitional countries. The activity at the end of this chapter provides an opportunity to consider the most ethical way to employ a finite sum of money in establishing a new system of health insurance for a developing country.

FUNDAMENTAL VALUES OF HEALTH SYSTEMS

As economists frequently remind us, there is no such thing as a free lunch. Every country that has accomplished the goals of universal access to care and financial security for its people had to give up something. Most people in those countries firmly believe that the trade-off was worth it.

How can people decide what they and their society are willing to forgo? The way to make those decisions in a politically acceptable and morally defensible manner is to begin by identifying the fundamental values of a country's health care system (Priester, 1992, pp. 85–86, 105–106). As Frenk and Gómez-Dantés (2009) have explained, "every health system reflects value assumptions, which are expressed in the distribution of benefits and the organisation of its institutions" (p. 1406). After identifying those basic values, people will be able to judge whether particular proposals for reform are consistent with their values. Moreover, those values will guide people in making the difficult decisions about what they are willing to forgo.

In Mexico the health reform of 2003, which created a public insurance system, was based on specific values and on the principle that health care is a social right, rather than a privilege or a commodity (Frenk and Gómez-Dantés, 2009). Other countries that have succeeded in developing universal health systems, such as Canada and the United Kingdom, have also explicitly identified the values that form the basis for their respective systems. What did the people in those countries really care about as a society, and what were they willing to give up as the price of health reform?

The heath care system of Canada is based on five fundamental values, which are set forth in the Canada Health Act. These five principles are universality, public administration, comprehensiveness, portability, and accessibility (Jecker and Meslin, 1994, p.189). In order to obtain federal government funding for its health program, each province in Canada must meet specific criteria, including compliance with those five principles (European Observatory on Health Systems and Policies, 2005, pp. 2–3, 8). Canada has a single-payer system, in which universal health coverage is financed primarily by taxation. Under these circumstances the role of private insurance companies is strictly limited. Private health insurance that duplicates public coverage is prohibited, although Canadians may have private insurance for services that are not covered by the public plan. In effect Canadians have given up the option to choose basic insurance coverage from any organization other than the government, in exchange for universal insurance coverage and comprehensive financial security. Although Canadians gave up the individual freedom to choose their health insurance plan and they accepted waiting lists for nonemergency services, they retained the freedom to choose their health care providers. The Canadian health insurance system operates on a single-payer model, but the health care delivery system is pluralistic. Most hospitals are not-for-profit organizations, and most doctors are in private medical practice. Generally, Canadians have the option to choose their health care providers, although some Canadians have complained about long waiting lists.

In the United Kingdom the government and the people support the values of a national health system that is funded by taxation and free at the point of service. About 12 percent of the population also has private health insurance, for avoiding queues, better amenities, and choice of specialist, but purchasing private insurance does not relieve those people of the obligation to pay taxes in support of the public health insurance system. On January 21, 2009, Prime Minister Gordon Brown signed a new constitution for the National Health Service (NHS). This new constitution sets forth the basic principles that guide the NHS, including provision of comprehensive service to all patients without discrimination, access on the basis of need rather than ability to pay, quality of services, respect for patient preferences, and accountability to the public (U.K. Department of Health, 2009). All patients in the United Kingdom have the right to services free of charge, unless specific exceptions have been authorized by Parliament. Patients have the right to choose their general practitioner (GP) practice, unless there is a reasonable basis for refusal. Patients do not have the right to see a particular doctor within their GP practice, but patients may express their preference and the GP practice must try to comply. Ordinarily, if patients want their care to be covered by the NHS, they are limited to choosing a GP practice within the NHS and must obtain their inpatient services at an NHS hospital, although the NHS may arrange for care to be provided by private hospitals or surgery centers in some situations.

Thus, people in the United Kingdom have given up some freedom to choose their health care providers in exchange for universal access to care and comprehensive services without regard to the ability to pay. Moreover, the NHS constitution explicitly recognizes that resources are limited, and that hard decisions need to be made in operating the system. "The NHS is committed to providing best value for taxpayers' money and the most effective, fair and sustainable use of finite resources" (U.K. Department of Health, 2009, p. 4). Under these circumstances, patients have the right to new drugs if those drugs have been prescribed by their doctor and if those drugs have been recommended by the National Institute for Health and Clinical Excellence (NICE), on the basis of its evaluation of cost effectiveness (p. 6). However, as discussed in Chapter Eight of this book, patients of the NHS might not receive a new treatment if NICE does not consider that treatment to be a cost-effective use of limited NHS resources.

In contrast to the systems in the United Kingdom and Canada, the health care system of the United States is based on very different fundamental values. However, this does not mean that the U.S. health care system lacks values. In a 1992 article, project director Reinhard Priester summarized the analysis of the "New Ethic" research project, cochaired by Sheila Leatherman and Arthur Caplan at the Center for Biomedical Ethics at the University of Minnesota, Minneapolis. As Priester explained, the U.S. health care system is based on the values of individualism and physician autonomy, with much less concern than other systems have for the values of universal access to care, social solidarity, and the good of the community as a whole (pp. 86–87, 91). The values of U.S. health care are based instead on the underlying values of U.S. society, including "strong faith in individualism, distrust of government and preference for private solutions to social problems, belief in American exceptionalism, a standard of abundance as the normal state of affairs, the power of technology, and the uniquely American frontier orientation" (p. 87). Thus, the United States allows individual physicians the freedom to choose their patients, and allows individual patients the freedom to choose expensive treatments of little marginal benefit, even though both these types of individual choice can result in denial of care to other patients and undermine efforts to achieve universal access to care (pp. 89–90, 103–104).

In addition to having a unique view about the paramount importance of individual choice, the United States has a unique attitude about the poor. First, U.S. culture distinguishes between the so-called worthy poor, who deserve to be helped, and other poor people who are supposedly less deserving of aid. As Priester (1992) explained, "The concept of the worthy poor derives from the peculiarly American notion that for many poor people, poverty is somehow deserved" (p. 89, footnote omitted). Generally, persons who have major disabilities or are over sixty-five years of age are considered to be more *worthy* of assistance than able-bodied adults who are unemployed. Thus, federal and state governments in the United States operate medical assistance programs for the poor, called Medicaid, but keep those programs separate from the public health insurance program for people who are elderly or disabled, called Medicare. The U.S. approach to the problem of poverty has been described as a "poor law system" that attempts to alleviate the effects of poverty, as opposed to a "welfare system" that provides a guarantee of necessary services to every member of the community (Jecker and Meslin, 1994, pp. 190–191). Another unique aspect of the U.S. attitude toward the poor relates to the ethical duty of charity. Doctors and hospitals in the United States acknowledge their ethical obligation to provide charity care, and many do indeed provide substantial volumes of free or discounted services. However, health care providers generally have the autonomy to determine for themselves the amount of free or discounted services they will supply, as well as the specific recipients of their charity (Priester, 1992, p. 89), although most U.S. hospitals are required to provide services in a medical emergency regardless of the patient's ability to pay. Some health care professionals who treat elderly patients under the Medicare program refuse to treat poor patients under Medicaid, in part because Medicaid pays extremely low rates for treatment of poor people.

To address these problems and promote reform, Priester and the other members of the "New Ethic" research project proposed a new framework of health care values for the United States (Priester, 1992, p. 92). Their framework contains five essential values: access, quality, efficiency, respect, and patient advocacy. It also contains several instrumental values that can promote those essential values. Most important, the project group developed a set of ordering rules for resolving potential conflicts between and among the different values. All five of the essential values should be pursued as much as possible, but any conflicts should be resolved in favor of promoting the value of fair access to care. Instrumental values may be superseded by any one of the essential values. Significantly, provider autonomy is considered an instrumental value and therefore can be superseded by the need to increase fair access to care, such as by requiring health care professionals to treat a sufficient number of underserved patients (pp. 92, 103–104). This proposed framework of values, with its ordering rules, is an important step toward health reform in the United States. In particular it could help to promote discussion and clarification of what people in the United States care about the most, and what they may be willing to give up as the unavoidable price of reform.

As Priester (1992) noted, the U.S. health system does not place a high priority on the value of social solidarity (p. 91). **Solidarity** refers to the feeling of unity that is generated by having a fair health system, one that includes everyone in the community regardless of wealth or social status and that gives people a feeling of ownership and an opportunity to participate (Priester, pp. 99–100). In contrast to the situation in the United States, solidarity is a fundamental value in the national health system of the United Kingdom (Priester, p. 99), as well as in the social health insurance systems of several industrialized countries in Western Europe (Saltman and DuBois, 2004, p. 27).

The value of solidarity is not limited to nationwide health systems or to health systems in industrialized countries. Solidarity is also an important value in systems of **community-based health insurance**, such as local systems of risk pooling in resource-poor developing countries. Community-based financing systems are local prepayment mechanisms through which villages or other small communities pool their risks of health care costs. Depending on the local circumstances, community-based insurance can be an attractive alternative for financing health care services, especially where national governments are unable to raise sufficient funds by means of taxation (Roberts and others, 2008, pp. 176–178).

Scholars from Burkina Faso and Germany have explained that community-based health insurance systems must be based on the values of solidarity and reciprocity. Moreover, in Burkina Faso and other African countries the fundamental values of solidarity and reciprocity are not imported or imposed from other countries but rather are part of the traditional culture and society (Sommerfeld and others, 2002, pp. 149, 160). The following excerpt from an article by these scholars explains the relationship between community-based health insurance and traditional, local values of reciprocity and solidarity.

EXCERPT FROM "INFORMAL RISK-SHARING ARRANGEMENTS (IRSAs) IN RURAL BURKINA FASO: LESSONS FOR THE DEVELOPMENT OF COMMUNITY-BASED INSURANCE (CBI)"

BY JOHANNES SOMMERFELD AND OTHERS

Introduction

In recent years, community-based health insurance (CBI) has been propagated as an option to extend access to health care of poor rural populations in countries lacking formal insurance markets. In contemporary Burkina Faso, a landlocked country in the West African Sahel, low access to health care is a serious impediment to the effectiveness of modern health care intervention. In Kossi Province, the site of the present study, there are only 0.3 visits per capita and per year to modern health services. The financial costs involved in seeking such care and their timing at the time of need have been identified as major factors contributing to low access.

The formal sector of the Burkinan economy comprises only 5% of the population. Social insurance for the formal sector has been limited until now to government employees, company employees and a few families living in relative economic prosperity. Some mutual health organizations, with varying success, have recently emerged without, however, providing coverage to a significant proportion of the rural population....

Fee-for-service payment is still the predominant mode of health care financing of a large majority of the population in the non-formal sectors of the economy. The Burkinian Ministry of Health has opted to follow the Bamako Initiative, with the introduction of user fees. In the study area, user fees lead to a decrease in the utilization of formal health services: the percentage of those who reported an illness episode in the preceding month and sought care at the formal health facilities dropped from 25.6% in 1993 (before the introduction of fees) to 18.7% in 1994 and 11.7% in 1995.

Burkina Faso's Ministry of Health has recently called for promoting solidarity-based modes of health care financing to increase the financial accessibility of health services in order to overcome the limitations of the existing system. The objective was to increase access to services and not to generate resources for the government, since funds would be retained and managed at the community or district levels. In June 1999, a national seminar was held to foster the creation of mutual health organizations in Burkina Faso.

Social insurance schemes, regardless of their design, reflect the history and cultural notions of solidarity and reciprocity norms of societies in which they develop. A crucial question, therefore, is whether an insurance scheme developed in one society can be applied in another. In other words the question remains whether CBI schemes are socially and culturally feasible, tapping into established notions of solidarity and reciprocity, and adapted to informal sector economies in rural Africa.

There is now an increasing awareness that CBI schemes need to be grounded in national values of solidarity and reciprocity. One of the underlying questions is whether CBI schemes can be built upon existing risk sharing arrangements and notions of solidarity. Solidarity is a common feature of 'traditional' rural communities, who have always shared the economic risks of unpredictable and cost-intensive life-events, such as deaths, accidents and weddings....

The present study was carried out in 1998–2000 in Kossi Province, in the North-Western part of Burkina Faso, as an integral part of a larger research project entitled 'The Scientific Basis of Community-Based Insurance,' conducted conjointly by the Nouna Center for Health Research (CRSN) and the Department of Tropical Hygiene and Public Health (ATHOEG) of Heidelberg University. The research intended to assess the scope and prevalence of existing IRSAs in rural Burkina Faso and to evaluate their potential role in CBI. The research was explicitly multi-disciplinary, bringing together the qualitative ethnographic interest of anthropology and the more quantifying research paradigm of economics.

Research Context

IRSAs in West Africa and Burkina Faso

Informal or 'traditional' risk sharing institutions and solidarity mechanisms in West Africa have, for a long time, attracted the curiosity of anthropologists and economists. Rural economies in West Africa have established a number of social and economic mechanisms in order to cope with the fnancial consequences of economic random shocks. A great number of traditional solidarity networks can be identified from the literature, e.g. clan relationships, burial societies, cooperative labour exchange pools, cooperative work groups, fire associations, sea rescue associations, special fund societies, Rotating Credit and Savings Associations (ROSCAs), beer societies, group borrowing schemes, credit cooperatives and regional associations . . . .

Mutual Health Institutions and Insurance in Burkina Faso

Burkina Faso's mutual health movement is still in an embryonic stage. Recently, a number of mutual health institutions have emerged . . . . A new formal law governing mutual health institutions is currently being conceived. This development has been strongly supported by the international donor community . . . .

Up until now, in Burkina Faso formal insurance institutions were limited to urban centres. In recent years, however, a number of commercial and state-owned insurance companies . . . have emerged, offering life, health and vehicle insurance and reinsurance. In addition, social security insurance is provided to salaried and state employees . . .

Results

A preliminary study of existing community-based risk sharing schemes in the project region identified a variety of community-based institutions involved in risk sharing. Forms of risk-sharing included credit saving funds, solidarity funds and rotating work assignments. Although none of these existing institutions constitutes by definition a health insurance scheme, assistance is provided to members through collective as well as individual donations, assisting hospitalized group members with loans for little or no interest . . . .

Solidarity Networks Based on Kinship, Neighbourhood, Ethnicity or Profession

Individuals and groups of people linked by kinship or place of origin, by neighbourhood, ethnic group or profession belong to widespread social networks which generate and share resources in times of need, e.g. in the case of illness.

Examples include financial solidarity within an extended family network, intra-community solidarity among families, neighbours and friends, and social funds among colleagues. For example, the catechists of the provincial parish have organized a solidarity fund which is deducted from their annual allowance and serves, among other purposes, to cover unforeseen medical expenditures . . . .

Notions of Solidarity and Reciprocity

Solidarity in non-monetarized IRSAs is characterized by friendly social relationships among families, clans, friends, peers or neighbours that are mobilized for the purpose of assistance to an individual in times of need or distress. Solidarity is based on the assumption, a loan is a given . . . thus implying a certain expectation of reciprocity. Interestingly, the Djoula term for loan is djuru or string. Credit is considered a string or link based on an obligation between two individuals. The obligation is exclusively moral and rarely legally enforced. Sometimes, it is even relegated to the divine by saying to the debtor nyi to ni allah ye (I leave you with God).

Solidarity

Solidarity in Times of Ill-Health . . .

In the case of sickness, asset sale is an important health financing strategy. Even the least privileged will own a chicken to sell. Relatives are the first resort in terms of financial arrangements. This resort is, in many cases, limited to providing immediate food support, i.e. delivering soup or fruit to the diseased patient. Giving money to buy medicines would be seen as meaning that a person does not have enough money to pay for his or her own needs.

Discussion and Conclusions

Solidarity is a crucial feature of the Burkinian social fabric in spite of a growing trend for individualism and monetarization. Without contributing to, and tapping into a varied set of solidarity mechanisms, the individual would face social and economic deprivation in the harsh economic and ecological conditions of the Sahel. Solidarity fulfills important functions. It allows people to situate themselves in extended social networks providing them with a sense of belonging and support. Deprived of social security as offered by the nation state, solidarity allows rural Burkinian farmers to participate in extended risk sharing networks that often transcend ethnic boundaries . . . .

In any society, the "mutualization" of risk is the result of associative experiences of collectivities. In Burkina Faso, the associative movement (village production groups)...[has] experienced serious organizational and financial deficits. Whereas national agrarian politics in the 1980s favoured village-wide production groups, just recently the advantages of small structures have been rediscovered.

A great variety of risk sharing institutions exist in the study area. Our ethnographic data suggest that informal, non-monetarized, so-called 'traditional' risk sharing arrangements, contrary to assumptions in the literature, are very prevalent and evidently not prone to immediate disappearance. They transport important solidarity notions inherent in the Burkinian society. Our data suggest that not all of the solidarity expressed in traditional arrangements is based on the idea of mutual reciprocity. Some arrangements are even altruistic.

Increasing monetarization of the Burkinian non-formal economy brings with it a tendency for collective group work to rise in size and in importance. Monetarization brings about egoism, even at the level of the extended family. This tendency will most likely affect future institutionalized risk sharing schemes. Proximity is a crucial and essential structural element of African institutions. As there is widespread mistrust of anonymous and bureaucratic institutions, one can, however, posit that the more institutionalized groups there are, the less effective they risk becoming. The specificity of African societies...[needs] to be taken into account when promoting institutional development in rural African areas. Before new mutual health institutions can be successful, they need to be grounded in local values of solidarity and reciprocity.

To be functional, CBI schemes need to be tailored around a number of presuppositions. There needs to be, in the community, a collective interest in financial precautions to ward off income shocks due to illness. More than that, communities need to have a positive attitude towards precautionary approaches for future ill-health. In addition, there needs to be awareness that certain health problems warrant insurance which relates to common attitudes towards, and perceptions of, health risks. Shared norms of solidarity and reciprocity can largely increase the trust in a pooling scheme. Finally, the ability to pay (ATP) and willingness-to-pay (WTP) are necessary in order to create trust in service providers....

New mutual health organizations in the rural Sahel face a number of challenges. The administrative set-up needs to fulfill popular expectations regarding leadership and transparency. New innovative ways to promote an administration based on proximity need to be conceived. Administrative skills, particularly, financial management skills, need to be strengthened. A benefit package based on issues of financial sustainability and popular expectation needs to be defined. Enrollment, modalities and the level of fee payment, membership administration and reimbursement procedures need to be developed and systematized. Potential sources for moral hazard need to be identified. The greatest challenge will be to bridge the need for proximity with the health care financing need to pool resources. One possibility to preserve the benefits of small size and proximity, yet avoiding the risks of bankruptcy inherent in small groups, would be to create a public re-insurance scheme covering high cost/low volume risks.

Finally, nation states are called upon to provide clear-cut legal frameworks for mutual health organizations. Burkina Faso needs to provide a legal framework for the rapidly emerging mutual health organizations. To be successful as stimulators of local development, CBI schemes need to enroll marginalized and disadvantaged populations into national development processes. In Burkina Faso, the law on community associations . . . provides sufficient legal framework to implement a community-based insurance scheme except that it does not provide any structure for social (i.e. public) re-insurance. The Burkinian government should assume two roles; providing a legal framework both for CBIs and reinsurance for small scale . . . [IRSAs] so that they can take on health care expenditures as additional item to share risks.

Source: Excerpted from "Informal Risk-Sharing Arrangements (IRSAs) in Rural Burkina Faso: Lessons for the Development of Community-Based Insurance (CBI)," by J. Sommerfeld and others, 2002. *International Journal of Health Planning and Management, 17*(2), 147–163 (citations, references, tables, and some text omitted). Copyright 2002 John Wiley & Sons, Ltd. Reprinted by permission.

SUMMARY

In some countries, people have accomplished the goals of universal access to care and financial security for every member of their community. In many other countries, however, people are still working toward these goals. Where these goals have been accomplished, people have identified the fundamental values of their health system and have made trade-offs that were consistent with those values. Countries that are still trying to reform their health systems also need to focus on their fundamental values and then use those values to decide on the trade-offs that they are willing to make.

This chapter analyzed the fundamental values on which different countries have based their health systems, including the value of solidarity in local African communities and in the nations of Western Europe. Finally, the chapter analyzed the meaning of fairness and evaluated the fairness of different methods of raising money for health services and designing a health insurance system.

KEY TERMS

community-based health
  insurance
financing

horizontal equity
risk pooling

solidarity
vertical equity

DISCUSSION QUESTIONS

1. Is prepayment of health costs, through taxes or insurance, fairer than payment out of pocket at the point of service? If so, why?
2. As a matter of fairness, should individuals be required to pay for health services on the basis of their actuarial risk of illness or, alternatively, on the basis of their ability to pay? Why?
3. Is an employment-based system of health insurance inherently less ethical than a system of tax-supported, national health insurance? Why or why not?
4. What are the fundamental values of each of these health systems: the system in Mexico, the system in Canada, the system in the United Kingdom, and the system in the United States?
5. How does community-based health insurance relate to traditional values in Burkina Faso and other countries?

ACTIVITY: ESTABLISHING A SYSTEM OF HEALTH COVERAGE IN A DEVELOPING COUNTRY

The developing country that we will call Yulatonga is a small island nation in the South Pacific with a population of 1 million. It is a very poor country. The average per capita income is $2,000 per year. Ten percent of the population (100,000 people) have an annual income at or below the Yulatonga government's poverty level of $1,000 per year. Some people are even poorer than that. Five percent of the population (50,000 people) have an annual income below 50 percent of the government's poverty level (that is, they have annual incomes below $500 per year).

Yulatonga does not have a national health insurance system, and 100 percent of the population is uninsured. The government does not have enough money to establish a national health insurance system, and it could not raise enough tax revenue to support that type of system. Similarly, it is not feasible to develop a social insurance system with employer and employee contributions, because only a small percentage of the population is employed in the formal sector. The health care system of Yulatonga includes several hospitals, but most residents cannot afford the services of those hospitals because they lack money and health insurance.

Recently, a nongovernmental organization (NGO) based in Switzerland agreed to give the government of Yulatonga $100 million per year for ten years for the purpose of establishing a system of health coverage. The money may not be used for any other purpose. If the government of Yulatonga does not use that money to establish a system of health coverage, the NGO will spend the money on expansion of its headquarters building in Switzerland.

If the government of Yulatonga accepts the money, the government will have flexibility to determine the details of the system. For example, the NGO will allow the government to determine which residents of Yulatonga will be eligible for coverage, the amount of that coverage, the scope of benefits, and the level of individual cost sharing.

The government of Yulatonga has decided to accept the money and has carefully considered the best way to apply $100 million per year to establish and maintain a system of health coverage. The government has no other resources for this purpose, and there is no source of additional funding. Therefore, the maximum amount that can be spent on this new system of coverage is $100 million per year. At the present time, government officials have narrowed down the possibilities to these three potential ways of using that money:

1. Provide comprehensive health coverage at no charge for the 50,000 poorest people in the country. (These are the people whose annual incomes are below $500 per year.) The government's annual cost to provide this comprehensive coverage would be $2,000 per person: 50,000 people × $2,000 per person = $100 million per year. This comprehensive (*first dollar*) coverage would not be subject to any deductibles and would not require any copayments from the individual.
2. Provide less comprehensive health coverage at no charge for all 100,000 people at or below the government's poverty level. (These are the people whose annual incomes are below $1,000 per year.) In other words, this alternative would cover more people than the first alternative, but it would provide less comprehensive coverage. The government's annual cost to provide this less comprehensive coverage would be $1,000 per person: 100,000 people × $1,000 per person = $100 million per year. Under this alternative, the coverage would be subject to an individual deductible of $300. After paying the deductible, eligible individuals would be responsible for copayments of 20 percent on their remaining health care bills.

3. Provide catastrophic health coverage at no charge for all 1 million residents of Yulatonga, regardless of their level of income. The government's annual cost to provide this catastrophic coverage would be $100 per person: 1,000,000 people × $100 per person = $100 million per year. This catastrophic coverage would have an individual deductible of $1,000 per year. This alternative would provide 100 percent coverage of all health care expenses after paying the individual deductible.

Please evaluate these three options and determine which one would be the most ethical for the government of Yulatonga to adopt. Be prepared to explain the reasons for your conclusion.

CHAPTER TEN

ETHICAL ISSUES IN THE MOVEMENT OF PATIENTS ACROSS NATIONAL BORDERS

LEARNING OBJECTIVES

- Be able to evaluate the ethical obligations to provide health care services to people who are undocumented aliens.

- Demonstrate the ability to analyze the ethical issues involved in treating patients who have limited proficiency in the language of the health care provider.

- Learn how to evaluate the ethical implications in the global phenomenon of medical tourism.

- Understand and be able to explain the additional ethical problems that arise when people from wealthy countries travel to developing countries to obtain organ transplants.

GLOBALIZATION has had profound effects on health systems and the delivery of health care services (Fried and Harris, 2007). Patients and health care workers travel across national borders. Drugs and medical equipment are regularly sold and transported between continents. Health care facilities "outsource" services to providers in other countries, such as arranging for X-rays taken in the United States to be read by radiologists in India when it is nighttime in the United States and daytime in India (Wachter, 2006). Meanwhile, the spread of communicable disease does not stop at national frontiers. As the director of the Office of Global Health Affairs in the U.S. Department of Health and Human Services put it, "From our perspective, there is no border in terms of health anymore" (Sanchez, 2007).

A useful framework for analyzing these various cross-border issues is provided by the four modes of trade in services, as set forth in the **General Agreement on Trade in Services (GATS)**. The GATS is a system through which countries may agree to make certain commitments with regard to their trade in particular types of services, including health care services (Fried and Harris, 2007, pp. 4–6). The four modes of trade in services relate to the geographical location of the provider and recipient. In Mode 1, a person or organization provides services across a national border to a recipient located in a different country: for example, a provider and a patient in separate countries might hold a medical consultation through videoconferencing (an instance of telemedicine). In Mode 2, the recipient of services physically travels to the provider's country: for example, a patient might visit another country for surgery (an instance of *medical tourism*). In Mode 3, people in one country conduct commercial activities, such as investment, in a different country. Finally, in Mode 4, service providers physically travel to the recipients' country: for example, health care professionals might move to another country to work in hospitals or clinics there.

The widespread migration of health care professionals from developing countries to developed countries is a Mode 4 activity, because it is the service providers who are traveling to different countries. The ethical issues in that movement of health care providers across borders, which is often referred to as a *brain drain*, are analyzed in Chapter Eleven. This chapter focuses on analyzing the ethical issues that arise under Mode 2, in which patients physically travel to a country that is different from their country of origin, and seek health care services in that different country.

As millions of people migrate across national borders, health care providers around the world face ethical and practical issues in providing services to these patients who come from very different countries and cultures. There are many reasons why an individual might seek health care services in a country other than his or her country of origin (Fried and Harris, 2007, p. 8). Some people travel to world-famous hospitals in other countries, if they can afford to do so, in the hope of receiving the best possible care. Other people may need medical treatment while they are traveling for reasons wholly unrelated to their health, such as education, business, tourism, or visiting family and friends. And yet other people may have moved to another country to work and live, either alone or with their families, on a long-term basis.

In some cases persons seeking care in a different country are considered to be undocumented aliens, in which case they might have fewer legal rights to medical care than the citizens and legal residents of the host country do. They might be unable to understand or communicate in the local language, and health care personnel might not be able to understand or communicate in the various languages of their patients. While in their countries of origin, patients might have suffered from types of violence and disease that are extremely uncommon in their new country (Grady, 2009). Meanwhile, some patients from wealthy countries are travelling to developing countries, in order to obtain health care services that are less expensive or more available there than in their country of residence. This medical tourism raises significant ethical issues, especially when the effect is to reduce access to care for residents of the developing country.

This chapter begins by explaining the barriers that undocumented aliens face in obtaining access to health care services. Then it explores the ways in which health care providers in various countries have attempted to balance their need to control costs with the need to provide services to undocumented aliens. The chapter evaluates the ethical obligation to provide care to individuals in need, regardless of their immigration status, in light of different ethical theories. Then it describes the global phenomenon of medical tourism and analyzes the ethical problems that arise when people from wealthy countries travel to developing countries to obtain organ transplants or other types of medical care. At the end of the chapter an activity provides an opportunity to evaluate how to balance the competing concerns in developing a hospital policy on providing care for undocumented aliens.

ETHICAL DUTIES TO PROVIDE HEALTH CARE TO UNDOCUMENTED ALIENS

Irregular migration is a global phenomenon. Millions of undocumented aliens live and work in dozens of countries across the globe. As of 2009, estimates of migrants who were staying illegally in the European Union (EU) ranged from 4.5 to 8 million people, although exact numbers are impossible to obtain (European Union, 2009). U.S. government officials have estimated that in 2000 there were approximately 7 million undocumented aliens in the United States (U.S. General Accounting Office, 2004, p. 5). In fact, many estimates of the undocumented alien population in the United States are much higher than that, with some researchers using estimates in the range of 11 to 12 million (Kaiser Commission on Medicaid and the Uninsured, 2008, p. 2). There are large numbers of undocumented aliens in other countries as well. In 2004, Solomon Benatar noted that many undocumented immigrants were seeking treatment for HIV/AIDS in postapartheid South Africa (Benatar, 2004, p. 88).

Undocumented aliens might be persons who entered a country illegally. Alternatively, they might have entered legally with visas for education, tourism, or temporary employment and then remained illegally after the expiration of their visas. In some cases they are persons who made requests for asylum but were refused (Hjern and Bouvier, 2004. p. 1538). Millions of undocumented aliens were young children when they taken to a new country by their parents. As Anders Hjern and Paul Bouvier (2004) have pointed out, a child in that situation "is obviously a suffering, unprotected, innocent third party in the conflict going on between his parents and the state" (p. 1538).

Barriers to Access, Cost Implications, and Provider Response

Because of their irregular status, undocumented aliens often lack health insurance coverage, and they often are excluded from participation in government health programs (Rosenthal, 2007, pp. 138–140). It is estimated that almost 60 percent of undocumented aliens in the United States have no health insurance (Kaiser Commission on Medicaid and the Uninsured, 2008, p. 5). Generally, these individuals are also not eligible for benefits under the Medicaid program or the State Children's Health Insurance Program, although they may be eligible for Medicaid benefits in emergency situations such as labor and delivery (Kaiser Commission on Medicaid and the Uninsured, 2008, p. 6).

In Europe, citizens of EU countries have the right to cross national borders to obtain health care services in other EU countries, and their national health plans will pay for services rendered in other EU countries under certain conditions (Bowden, 2009). However, undocumented aliens from non-EU countries are treated differently from local citizens and from citizens of EU countries in general, and they might not have complete access to health care services in the EU (Pace, 2007, p. 21). Even where care is officially permitted, undocumented aliens can be deterred from seeking care by practical barriers, such as fees, administrative requirements, and fear of deportation (Pace, 2007, pp. 21–24; Rosenthal, 2007, p. 140). A report from the International Organization for Migration described the conflict between theory and practice in many EU countries with regard to undocumented aliens, whom the report refers to as *irregular migrants*.

> In the EU, the European Commission has noted that "illegal immigrants are protected by universal human rights standards and should enjoy some basic rights i.e. emergency health care and school education for their children." . . .

> In practice, however, the irregular migrant is not granted a complete right to health care in EU Member States. For example, the Danish law on health care limits irregular migrants' access to the national health care system to urgent treatment. In Germany, in principle, irregular migrants are granted the same right to health care as asylum seekers, being entitled to emergency care, care in pain situations, or indispensable care in order to preserve health (for example avoiding long-term aggravation or complications of diseases). The implementation of these provisions conflicts, however, with the *Aufenthaltsgesetz*, under which public servants have to report the details of any irregular migrant they encounter during their job, and anyone who helps an individual without a regular residence permit can be punished if assistance is provided for financial gain, or if it is done repeatedly or for the benefit of several foreigners.

> In countries like Spain, Italy, Portugal, Belgium, the Netherlands and the UK, there are various obstacles to the implementation of national legislation guaranteeing irregular migrants' right to health care [Pace, 2007, pp. 20–22].

International conventions include lofty promises of access to care for migrant workers and their families (Hjern and Bouvier, 2004, p. 1535; Rosenthal, 2007, pp. 138, 141). However, those international conventions have not been ratified by all countries, and even where ratified, they are subject to numerous exceptions and limitations. Some countries, such as the United States, provide emergency medical care without regard to citizenship or immigration status but are more restrictive about providing nonemergency care.

One important aspect of this issue is the cost of providing care for undocumented aliens and deciding who should bear that cost. For example, hospitals in the United States complain that they are forced to pay the high costs for treating undocumented aliens who lack health insurance (Fried and Harris, 2007, pp. 8–9). The actual costs have been subject to dispute, and this is a politically-charged issue in the United States, with some people and organizations holding very strong beliefs (Blackwood, 2006).

In 2004, the U.S. General Accounting Office (GAO) was unable to determine the costs incurred by U.S. hospitals in providing uncompensated care for undocumented aliens (p. 3). Subsequently, a 2006 study by researchers at the RAND Corporation estimated that the cost in 2000 for providing care to adult undocumented aliens (aged eighteen to sixty-four) was $6.5 billion (Goldman and others, 2006). To put that in perspective, $6.5 billion represented only about 1.5 percent of U.S. health care costs at that time (Goldman and others, 2006). However, the cost of providing care to undocumented aliens is not spread evenly across the United States. In regions with large numbers of undocumented aliens, this cost has a serious financial impact on state governments and some hospitals (Fried and Harris, 2007, p. 8). For example, in Texas as of 2001, the Harris County Hospital District, which includes Houston, had spent an average of $110 million per year in caring for undocumented aliens, who represented about 23 percent of patient visits for that public hospital district (Texas House of Representatives, 2001, p. 3). In 2005, that same public hospital district spent about 14 percent of its total operating costs on providing care for undocumented aliens, primarily from Mexico (Preston, 2006).

Under these circumstances, health care professionals, facilities, and governmental agencies have struggled to develop policies that balance the need to control health care costs with the need to provide necessary services to undocumented aliens (Coyle, 2003). As a result of the severe economic recession in 2009, even community health clinics in some parts of the United States have reduced some of the nonemergency services that they previously provided to undocumented aliens (Kaiser Daily Health Report, 2009). According to one activist opposed to illegal immigration into the United States, restricting public services is appropriate because, as she put it, undocumented aliens "have absolutely no right, No. 1, to be here and, No. 2, to take the tax dollars of law-abiding American taxpayers for anything" (Gorman, 2009). However, government officials and health experts recognize that limiting primary care services could increase the much more costly visits to emergency departments (Gorman, 2009).

In the United States the general rule is that hospitals must provide services in an emergency, without regard to a patient's immigration status or ability to pay. However, there is no similar mandate for nonemergency hospital services on a national level. Thus, some hospitals choose to treat undocumented aliens on an equal basis with all other patients, but other hospitals are more restrictive about providing nonemergency care (Preston, 2006).

In fact, some U.S. hospitals have gone so far as to forcibly "repatriate" undocumented alien patients whose condition has been stabilized by the hospital but who require long-term care (Sontag, 2008). Undocumented aliens are not eligible to receive Medicaid benefits for long-term care, and they might not have private health insurance or sufficient assets to pay for extended care. Therefore, in cases involving such conditions as stroke or traumatic brain injury, hospitals may be unable to find any nursing home or rehabilitation facility to accept the patient after stabilization. Some stabilized patients in that situation have essentially become permanent residents of an acute-care hospital, even though they no longer need acute hospital care and the hospital does not receive any payment for their continued stay. Frustrated by the expense and the inefficient use of their facilities, some hospital managers in the United States have chartered private airplanes and returned the patients to their countries of origin. Although the hospital is required to make arrangements for appropriate follow-up care, the arrangements in some of these cases have been criticized as being woefully inadequate (Sontag, 2008), as in the following example.

> American immigration authorities play no role in these private repatriations, carried out by ambulance, air ambulance and commercial plane. Most hospitals say that they do not conduct cross-border transfers until patients are medically stable and that they arrange to deliver them into a physician's care in their homeland. But the hospitals are operating in a void, without governmental assistance or oversight, leaving ample room for legal and ethical transgressions on both sides of the border.

> Indeed, some advocates for immigrants see these repatriations as a kind of international patient dumping, with ambulances taking patients in the wrong direction, away from first-world hospitals to less-adequate care, if any . . . .

> Hospital administrators view these cases as costly, burdensome patient transfers that force them to shoulder responsibility for the dysfunctional immigration and health-care systems. In many cases, they say, the only alternative to repatriations is keeping patients indefinitely in acute-care hospitals (Sontag, 2008).

In contrast to these examples of restricting services, some health care providers in the United States and other countries have decided to provide care for undocumented aliens, even when that has required standing up against their own government authorities. For example, in the State of Texas, a state official determined that public hospital districts were not permitted to provide nonemergency care to undocumented aliens for free or at a discount. Nevertheless, some of those public hospital districts continued to provide nonemergency services for undocumented aliens for free or at a discount, despite the risk of criminal penalties for the hospital district or its officials (Fried and Harris, 2007, p. 9). In Sweden, pediatricians "openly defied a state policy to exclude asylum-seeking children from medical care if their asylum request was denied." The Swedish pediatricians had the support of their professional association, and their actions caused the government to provide state-funded care for undocumented children in Sweden (Hjern and Bouvier, 2004, p. 1538). Similarly, the unwillingness of health professionals in Italy to enforce a restrictive law regarding treatment of undocumented aliens caused the Italian government to change its legislation (Pace, 2007, pp. 23–24). In the United Kingdom, regulations passed in 1989 required hospitals to play a role in immigration checks, but trade unions encouraged their members to refuse to participate in such checks. This enabled many undocumented aliens to receive government health services, although subsequent actions by the government have continued to try to prevent these services (Pace, 2007, p. 24, n. 94).

Ethical Analysis of Providing Care for Undocumented Aliens

Is there an ethical obligation to provide care to individuals in need, regardless of their immigration status? Do health care providers have an ethical obligation to provide health care services to undocumented aliens? Does society as a whole have this obligation? Ethical theories and approaches can be used both to support and to oppose this proposed obligation.

The proposed obligation to provide care for undocumented aliens can be supported by ethical theories or approaches of principlism, Kantian ethics, and utilitarianism and also by the professional ethics of health care providers and health care managers. Under principlism, there is a moral duty of beneficence to provide care to people in need, regardless of their legal status. In addition, there is a moral duty of justice to provide care to undocumented aliens, because those aliens are living and working as members of society in the host country. Even assuming that resources are limited and must be rationed in some way, the moral duty of justice requires that rationing decisions be made on the basis of need and not on the basis of a person's immigration status.

The moral duty of justice also applies to the related issue of whether undocumented aliens should be allowed to receive organ transplants in the host country. This issue has arisen on a number of occasions in the United States, including the tragic case of Jesica Santillan. Jesica was an undocumented immigrant from Mexico who needed a heart-lung transplant (Williams, n.d.). At an academic medical center in the United States, Jesica was given an organ transplant. Unfortunately, the organs were not properly matched to Jesica by blood type, and her condition became critical. Subsequently, the medical center performed another transplant, despite her weakened condition, but she lost all brain function and life support was terminated. Many people have expressed ethical concerns about the medical center's decision to perform the second transplant, both because of Jesica's weakened condition at that time and because the second transplant for Jesica necessarily resulted in denying a transplant for a different potential recipient (Williams, n.d.) However, there has been less consensus about whether Jesica's status as an undocumented alien should have precluded her from receiving the first transplant. The rules of the transplant system in the United States generally allow nonresidents to receive up to 5 percent of the organ transplants at each transplant center (Vedantam, 2003). Some people argue that noncitizens, and particularly undocumented aliens, should not receive any organ transplants in the United States (Darr, 2005). However, others point out that noncitizens contribute more organs to U.S. citizens than noncitizens receive from U.S. citizens (Vedantam, 2003). Under these circumstances the ethical principle of justice supports allowing undocumented aliens to receive organ transplants in the United States or another host country, regardless of their irregular immigration status.

Kantian ethics also supports the proposed obligation to provide care for undocumented aliens. Providing care would be consistent with Kantian ethics because every person—including an undocumented alien—must be treated as an end in himself or herself. In addition, providing care to undocumented aliens in need is consistent with the categorical imperative, because we can consistently will or wish that to be a rule for all similar situations. Similarly, there is a utilitarian justification for providing medical care that would maintain the health of undocumented members of society, including those people who do the most difficult physical work in society.

Finally, the professional ethics of health care providers and health care managers support the existence of a duty to provide care to undocumented aliens. The most basic principle of professional ethics is the duty to provide care to people in need, regardless of their legal or financial circumstances. Similarly, providing care to people in need is the fundamental reason for the existence of health care facilities. Therefore, denying medical care on the basis of a person's immigration status would violate professional ethics. Some people would argue that health care professionals and managers must refuse to comply with unethical laws that limit care for undocumented aliens, as in the examples from several countries discussed previously. The American Medical Association (1994) has recognized that in "exceptional circumstances of unjust laws, ethical responsibilities should supersede legal obligations." Under some circumstances, ethical duties might even require health care professionals and managers to use—or cooperate in the use of—patient names that they know to be false, such as when an undocumented alien is entitled to employee health insurance benefits under the false name that the alien uses for purposes of employment.

Despite the foregoing analysis, some of the same ethical theories and approaches can be used to argue against the proposed obligation to provide care for undocumented aliens. Under principlism, one could argue that the duty of beneficence to undocumented aliens is outweighed by the duty of nonmaleficence, because providing care to undocumented aliens would take limited resources away from citizens and lawful residents. In every country, resources are limited and must be rationed in some way. Under this argument, health care facilities in each country should first meet the needs of people who are there lawfully, before providing services to people who are there unlawfully.

The ethical duties of nonmaleficence and justice could also be used to argue against providing scarce organ transplants to undocumented aliens. According to this argument, it would be harmful and unjust for a government to allow citizens and lawful residents to die while waiting for organ transplants, and to simultaneously allow illegal aliens to receive the scarce human organs. From a utilitarian perspective, one could argue that the greatest good for the greatest number of people would be achieved by using limited health care resources for the majority group of people in each country, those who are the citizens or lawful residents, rather than by diverting limited resources for the benefit of a minority group of people, those who are undocumented aliens.

Under Kantian ethics, the ends do not justify the means. Therefore, health care professionals and managers should not lie to health insurance companies or government health programs by signing or submitting a document that contains a patient name that they know, or have reason to know, is not the patient's legal name. Health care professionals and managers should not cooperate in misleading or defrauding insurance companies or government programs, because that is not a type of conduct that we can consistently will or wish to be a rule for all similar situations.

As discussed previously, some people argue that society in the host country has an ethical duty of justice to provide care to undocumented aliens. However, if we were to recognize or impose an ethical obligation to provide care for undocumented aliens, that could raise other potential obligations under the ethical duty of justice. It seems clear that the host country's society does not have an ethical obligation to provide medical care to every person living in every other country on the planet. Even though it would be good to help every person in every other country, the society of the host country really does not have an ethical obligation to do so, and that society would not be acting unethically by failing to do so. Therefore, this argument goes, it would not be fair or just to impose an obligation to provide care for people who have come from those other countries and are now in the host country. As a practical matter, that proposed ethical obligation would impose a duty to help only those people who had managed to "jump the fence" and get into the host country illegally. It would not impose any obligation to people who remained in their own countries, including those people too sick or disabled to travel. In addition the proposed obligation would impose a duty to help only those people who broke the law, while imposing no duty to help people who were willing to obey the law. Finally, the proposed obligation would impose a duty to help people only during those periods of time that they are physically present in the host country, but not while they are visiting their friends or relatives in their countries of origin. For all of these reasons, it could be argued that imposing the proposed ethical duty to provide care for undocumented aliens would be irrational and would raise other problems of justice and fairness. The counterargument, of course, is that society in the host country owes a greater duty to undocumented aliens in the host country than it owes to people outside the host country, because those undocumented aliens are living and working as contributing members of society in the host country.

Finally, the issue of an ethical obligation to provide care for undocumented aliens raises the related issue of whether health care providers have an ethical obligation to provide translation services for patients who are unable to communicate effectively in the language of the host country. These issues are not totally congruent, because some undocumented aliens can indeed communicate effectively in the language of the host country, whereas some aliens with proper visas have limited proficiency in the host country's language. Nevertheless, language can present an additional barrier to access for many undocumented aliens, and the need to provide translation services can impose an additional cost on the health care system of the host country.

For example, in the United States in the year 2000, more than 21 million people (more than 8 percent of the U.S. population) had **limited English proficiency** (Flores, 2006). According to a survey of U.S. hospitals conducted in 2005 and 2006, 88 percent of hospitals provided language services at all times, but only 3 percent were directly reimbursed for those services (Health Research and Educational Trust, p. 9).

Health care professionals and health care organizations have an ethical obligation to provide high-quality care. In order to provide care of high quality, health care personnel must be able to communicate with their patients. However, translation and other language services can be expensive, and health care resources are limited. Do host-country health care providers, such as hospitals and other health care facilities, have an ethical obligation to provide translation services or multilingual staff at the provider's expense? Put another way, do all patients have an ethical right to be seen by a health care professional who speaks their language or, alternatively, to have a translator provided to them by the hospital at the hospital's expense?

If you were sick or injured in a foreign country and you needed to go to a hospital, you would be very happy if someone at that hospital could speak your language. It would be a great relief to be able to explain your symptoms and your medical history in your own language, to be able to find out what is wrong with you, and to understand what you are supposed to do for your treatment. That would be a great relief, but do you really have a right to it as an ethical matter?

Using a family member or friend as translator for medical problems could be ineffective, inappropriate, and potentially dangerous. Family members and friends are probably not trained as translators, and they probably do not understand medical terminology. Moreover, using a family member or friend as translator could violate the patient's privacy or could limit the extent of communication by the patient, as he or she tries to preserve some degree of privacy. Former U.S. surgeon general Richard Carmona (2007) has written about his childhood experiences in having to translate for his grandmother, his Abuelita, during her visits to the doctor. "I felt honored to do so, but I knew it was too much responsibility to interpret words and symptoms that I did not understand. What I know now that I could not have understood then is that Abuelita's own dignity would prevent her from speaking openly about her symptoms in front of me—her young grandson. I know that my experience as a child interpreter was not unique then and is not unique now" (p. 277). Under these circumstances, some people argue that patients who have limited proficiency in the local language have an ethical right to a health care professional who speaks their language or a qualified translator at the hospital's expense. However, the ethical basis for that right needs to be considered and articulated more fully. You will have an opportunity to consider this ethical issue, together with the related ethical issue of providing care for undocumented aliens, in the activity at the end of this chapter.

ETHICAL ISSUES IN MEDICAL TOURISM

Wealthy patients have traveled to world-famous hospitals in other countries for many years in an effort to obtain the best quality of care. More recently, many patients from industrialized countries have traveled to developing countries in an effort to obtain services that are less expensive or more available than in their country of residence (Fried and Harris, 2007, p. 6). Although the term **medical tourism** has been defined in several different ways (Bookman and Bookman, 2007, p. 1; Cortez, 2008, p. 76), it is useful to distinguish the modern concept of medical tourism from more traditional forms of travel to obtain medical care. As Michael Horowitz and colleagues have explained:

> In medical tourism, citizens of highly developed nations bypass services offered in their own communities and travel to less developed areas of the world for medical care. Medical tourism is fundamentally different from the traditional

model of international medical travel where patients generally journey from less developed nations to major medical centers in highly developed countries for medical treatment that is unavailable in their own communities. The term medical tourism does not accurately reflect the reality of the patient's situation or the advanced medical care provided in these destinations. Nevertheless, this phrase has come into general usage and it provides an unambiguous way of differentiating the recent phenomenon of medical tourism from the traditional model of international medical travel [Horowitz and others, 2007].

Under the four-part framework for trade in services discussed earlier in this chapter, medical tourism fits within Mode 2, because the recipient of health care services is traveling to the country of the provider.

An estimated 50,000 people traveled from Great Britain to other countries for medical care in 2003 (Mattoo and Rathindran, 2006, p. 358). In 2005, an estimated 150,000 people traveled from various countries to India for medical care (Chinai and Goswami, 2007, p. 164). The estimated number of medical tourists traveling to Thailand ranges from 400,000 to over 1 million per year, although it is unclear whether these estimates include expatriates who were living and working in Thailand at the time they sought medical treatment (Saniotis, 2008, p. 150).

Why do people from industrialized countries travel to developing countries for medical care? The lower cost of treatment is not the only reason, but cost is certainly an important factor (Fried and Harris, 2007, p. 6). For example, knee surgery on an inpatient basis costs over $10,000 in the United States, but costs less than $2,000 at top hospitals in India or Hungary, including the cost of travel (Mattoo and Rathindran, 2006, p. 358). In the expensive U.S. health system millions of U.S. citizens are uninsured or underinsured, and this has led some U.S. citizens to seek less expensive care in other countries. In the opinion of Arnold Milstein and Mark Smith (2006), these "patients are not 'medical tourists' seeking low-cost aesthetic enhancement. They are middle-income Americans evading impoverishment by expensive, medically necessary operations, as health care services are increasingly included in international economic trade" (p. 1637).

Meanwhile, some people travel to other countries in order to obtain drugs or treatments not available in their home countries. The regulatory authorities in some countries approve new drugs more quickly than other countries' regulators do, and patients may be able to obtain those drugs only by travelling to a different country (Cortez, 2008, pp.77–78). In addition, people might travel to a country that allows more choice in reproductive decisions, such as abortion or new reproductive technologies (Cortez, p. 77). Because of the severe shortage of transplantable organs in their home countries, thousands of patients have obtained transplants in other countries, such as China and the Philippines; this is referred to as **transplant tourism** (Biggins and others, 2009, p. 831). Like other types of medical tourism, transplant tourism raises significant ethical issues, which are discussed in detail in the remainder of this section.

In analyzing the ethical issues of medical tourism, it is important to consider its effects on the host country that provides the medical services, the patient's home country, the individual patient, and those individuals in the host country who would be personally affected by the provision of services to the patient. For the host country, positive effects of medical tourism include potential increases in revenue and economic growth (Bookman and Bookman, 2007, pp. 177–178). Theoretically, medical tourism could generate revenue for countries and facilities, money that could be used to support and improve services for the local population. Medical tourism could also provide more income and opportunities for physicians and other health workers and thereby make it less likely that they will leave the country (Mattoo and Rathindran, 2006, p. 367). Although medical tourism can reduce external brain drain to other countries, it can increase internal brain drain by encouraging health workers to leave public facilities for better-paying jobs in private facilities that cater to wealthy patients. As stated by the director of WHO's Department of Human Resources for Health, "it does not augur well for the health of patients who depend largely on the public sector for their services as the end result does not contribute to the retention of well-qualified professionals in the public sector services" (Chinai and Goswami, 2007, p. 165).

In addition, medical tourism could have other negative effects on the health system of the host country. Medical tourism could perpetuate two standards of care—one for medical tourists and one for the local population. Writing in the *Indian Journal of Medical Ethics*, Thelma Narayan (2005) stated that the "policy of 'medical tourism for the classes and health missions for the masses' will only lead to a deepening of the inequities already embedded in our health care system." Other potential negative effects on the host country include increased local prices for health care services as a result of additional demand by medical tourists (Mattoo and Rathindran, 2006, p. 367), "crowding out" of domestic patients as more resources are shifted to serving the medical tourism market (Bookman and Bookman, 2007, pp. 175–177), and diverting government resources to attract international patients and subsidize the growth of medical tourism (Bookman and Bookman, p. 176; Cortez, 2008, p. 110).

For the host country the ultimate impact of medical tourism depends on whether the government of that country uses the revenues from medical tourism effectively to improve public health services for the local population (Mattoo and Rathindran, 2006, p. 367; Cortez, 2008, pp. 110–111; Bookman and Bookman,

2007, p. 179). For example, "governments could cross-subsidize care for the poor by taxing these export revenues or by requiring providers also to extend care to the poor" (Mattoo and Rathindran, p. 367). However, the experience so far in that regard has not been encouraging. Generally, it does not appear that host country governments have used revenues or taxes from medical tourism to subsidize public health services, nor have they generally required private facilities that cater to foreigners to also provide significant volumes of care for the poor (Cortez, 2008, pp. 110–111). In order to accomplish those goals, it would be necessary to implement effective systems of regulation and taxation, with explicit earmarking of funds for the use of public health facilities and their staff (Chinai and Goswami, 2007, p. 165).

The effect of medical tourism on the patient's home country is less complex but still potentially serious. Health care facilities in the patient's country could suffer financial losses from the reduction in patient volume as well as from reductions in economies of scale (Mattoo and Rathindran, 2006, p. 365). In the United States, hospitals use patient revenues to cross-subsidize their indigent care, a process that might be jeopardized to some extent by the loss of patients to hospitals in other countries (Cortez, 2008, p. 109). Medical tourism could also impose a financial burden on the home country's health system, because health care providers in that country are obligated to provide follow-up care after the patient's return, especially in cases of transplant tourism. Moreover, obtaining an organ transplant in a developing country could pose a risk to public health in the patient's home country if the patient were to become infected with a communicable disease (Budiani-Saberi and Delmonico, 2008, p. 927; Bramstedt and Xu, 2007, p. 1700). In addition, because patients pay cash to donors in other countries for their organs, transplant tourism could also have a negative effect on the system of altruistic organ donation in the patient's home country (Budiani-Saberi and Delmonico, p. 928).

For the individual patient, medical tourism can promote autonomy to choose goods and services that would not be available in the patient's home country, such as a wider choice of reproductive health services (Cortez, 2008, pp. 111–113). However, the increased autonomy for that particular patient is arguably unfair to other patients who are unable to travel to another country. Moreover, the opportunities for treatment in another country might discourage people from trying to reform their own health systems (Cortez, pp. 107–113).

Nevertheless, medical tourism can increase access to care, especially for people who lack adequate health insurance coverage (Cortez, 2008, pp. 107–108). There is some risk to the patient in traveling to another country for treatment, as there is in the performance of any medical procedure. However, individual patients should have the right to make their own decisions, after complete disclosure of the risks. In deciding whether to travel to another country for care, individuals should not be subjected to coercion or undue financial incentives from their health insurance plans or their employers (Bramstedt and Xu, 2007, p. 1700).

It is also important to consider the interests of those individuals in the host country who are personally affected by providing services to the medical tourist. In transplant tourism, some patients have received organs from executed prisoners, with serious questions about the donors' informed consent (Bramstedt and Xu, 2007, p. 1699; Biggins and others, 2009, p. 832). Other transplant tourists have purchased organs from live donors, who are referred to as **commercial living donors (CLDs)**. Budiani-Saberi and Delmonico (2008) have explained that for these transplant tourists, the "source of their allografts is mainly from the poor and vulnerable in the developing world. These vendors or commercial living donors resort to an organ sale because they have virtually no other means to provide support for themselves or their families. Selling kidneys may be a consideration of 'autonomy' in academic debate but it is not the coercive reality of experience when a kidney sale is a desperate alternative available to the poor" (p. 925). In fact, researchers have documented negative effects on CLDs after the transplant procedure, including health problems, continued financial difficulties, and regret about their organ donation (Budiani-Saberi and Delmonico, pp. 927–928).

The system of payment for organs in transplant tourism is also unfair to residents of the host country who have been waiting for organ transplants (Bramstedt and Xu, 2007, p. 1700). In transplant tourism, wealthy foreigners essentially "jump the queue" to obtain organs before local patients, who may have been waiting for many years and may die for lack of transplants.

On libertarian grounds, some people argue that individuals should be allowed to sell their organs and should be allowed to purchase organs from other people. However, others strongly disagree with the concept of an organ market, because of the unfairness to potential transplant recipients who have less money and because of the serious potential for coercion of donors, among other reasons. Merely for purposes of argument, we could assume that it might be possible to develop a lawful organ market with sufficient protections, within the limited confines of a well-regulated, industrialized country. Even with that assumption, however, it is clear that it would not be possible to provide sufficient protections in the context of a global organ market, where patients from wealthy countries would purchase organs from poor individuals in developing countries. In a global market for organ transplants, the ethical and practical problems would be insurmountable.

SUMMARY

The movement of patients across national borders is part of the globalization of health care services. This phenomenon raises important ethical issues for health care professionals and organizations. As explained in this chapter, health care providers are attempting to balance their need to limit costs with their ethical obligation to provide services to individuals in need, regardless of their immigration status. Some health care providers have adopted restrictive policies on the treatment of undocumented aliens. Other providers have decided to serve all people in need, even when that required them to stand up against their own government authorities and thereby set an inspiring example for health care professionals and organizations throughout the world.

The movement of patients across national borders also includes the modern practice of medical tourism, which raises another set of complex ethical problems. This chapter has evaluated the ethical problems of medical tourism from the perspectives of the host country, the patient's home country, the individual patient, and those individuals in the host country who would be personally affected by providing services to the medical tourist. For some types of medical tourism, the ultimate effect depends on the extent to which the government of the host country uses medical tourism revenues to promote the health of the entire population. In the case of transplant tourism, however, a global market for organ transplants raises far too many ethical and practical problems.

KEY TERMS

commercial living donors (CLDs)

General Agreement on Trade in Services (GATS)

limited English proficiency

medical tourism

transplant tourism

undocumented aliens

DISCUSSION QUESTIONS

1. Do health care professionals and health care organizations have an ethical obligation to provide services to undocumented aliens, even if the situation is not a medical emergency?
2. As an ethical matter, do you have a right to show up at a hospital in a foreign country and be helped by a person who speaks your language? Would the answer be the same if you were working or going to school in that foreign country?

3. Should the governments of developing countries promote medical tourism as a way to improve the health of their populations?

4. Should people from wealthy countries be allowed to obtain organ transplants from individuals in developing countries?

ACTIVITY: DEVELOPING A HOSPITAL POLICY ON UNDOCUMENTED ALIENS

Please assume that you are a member of the board of trustees of a general, acute-care hospital in an industrialized country. Your hospital has 400 beds and provides a wide range of inpatient and outpatient services. There is no other hospital within a fifty-mile radius.

Your hospital is a public hospital in the sense that it is owned and operated by a unit of local government. The local government appoints all members of the hospital's board of trustees, which has the authority to establish all policies for operation of the hospital. The local government also provides some financial support for the hospital from tax revenues. However, most of the hospital's operating expenses are funded by revenues from patients and their insurance plans.

During the past few years the hospital has experienced some serious financial difficulties. The economic recession has reduced the amount of tax revenue collected by the local government. Therefore the local government has reduced its level of financial support for the hospital. That reduction in government financial support has forced the hospital to rely more heavily on revenue from patients. However, patients and their insurance plans have not been willing to accept a rate increase for hospital services, and the hospital has been providing an increased volume of uncompensated care. Due to these financial difficulties, the hospital has been forced to close some of its health programs and terminate some of its employees.

A large number of undocumented aliens reside in your community. Some of those undocumented aliens have arrived recently; others have lived and worked in the community for several years. The vast majority of undocumented aliens in your community have no health insurance coverage, and they are excluded by law from participation in government health programs.

Pursuant to the applicable laws in your country, the hospital is required to provide emergency treatment without regard to the patient's citizenship or immigration status, and without regard to the patient's ability to pay for his or her care. The applicable laws are silent on the issue of providing nonemergency care for undocumented aliens. Therefore hospitals may choose to provide nonemergency care for undocumented aliens and may use their public funds to provide those services for free or at a discount. However, hospitals are not legally required to provide nonemergency care for undocumented aliens and may choose to limit their nonemergency services to those undocumented aliens who are willing and able to pay for their care.

Your hospital fully complies with legal requirements in regard to providing emergency treatment without regard to immigration status. Moreover, under its current policy, your hospital provides nonemergency care for free or at a discount to any resident of the community who cannot afford to pay for his or her care. In fact, many of the patients who have received nonemergency care from the hospital for free or at a discount have been undocumented aliens. This situation, together with the hospital's financial difficulties, has led to a discussion about possible changes in the hospital's policy about nonemergency care for undocumented aliens.

Last month, the hospital's board of trustees held a town hall meeting on this issue. The purpose of the meeting was to solicit input from the local community and to provide an opportunity for local residents and hospital personnel to express their opinions. Almost two thousand people attended the meeting, which was held in the auditorium of the local high school.

At the meeting, the head of the Local Taxpayers' Association (LTA) argued against providing any services whatsoever to undocumented aliens, other than the emergency services that the hospital is required by law to provide, and he made this statement:

> These people have no legal right to be here in our country. They are here illegally. What part of the word 'illegal' do you not understand? The hospital has a limited amount of money and cannot meet all of the needs of people who have a legal right to be here. In fact, the hospital has been closing health programs and terminating employees. The local government cannot provide any more funding, and insurance plans cannot increase the rates that they pay to the hospital. So, this is really a zero-sum game. Any resources that the hospital gives to undocumented aliens are being taken away from people who have a legal right to be here. I understand that the hospital has to provide emergency care. That's fine, but that's all. After the hospital has provided emergency treatment and stabilized the patient, he is well enough to travel. At that point, the only thing that our public hospital should give that person for free is a one-way plane ticket, economy class, back to his own country!

The representative from the Immigrant Rights Organization (IRO) strongly disagreed with the previous speaker. She made this argument:

> Health is a universal human right. Therefore, everyone has a right to health, regardless of the technicalities of their citizenship or visa status. Despite

their irregular status, many immigrants have lived and worked in this community for many years. They are your neighbors, your tenants, your customers, and your employees. Undocumented aliens contribute to the community by paying many types of taxes, and by performing difficult, low-paid work that many local residents do not want to perform. Therefore, undocumented aliens have the right to be treated like everyone else in our community.

The hospital's chief executive officer (CEO) also spoke at the meeting:

The hospital administration wants to retain the current policy of providing nonemergency care for free or at a discount to any resident of the community who cannot afford to pay for his or her care, regardless of immigration status. We don't even want to ask patients about their visa status. We run a hospital. We are not the immigration police!

Finally, the chief of the hospital's medical staff spoke at the meeting:

The fundamental concept of medical ethics is providing services to people in need. When someone needs medical care, we do not ask about things that have nothing to do with the individual's need for medical care. We provide medical care to convicts in prison, and we do not deny care on the ground that they were convicted of terrible crimes. We provide medical care to prisoners of war, and we do not deny care on the ground that they tried to kill our soldiers. We provide medical care to people who did not pay their taxes as required by law, and we do not deny care on the ground that they failed to meet their legal obligation to pay their taxes. We should not deny care to people on the ground that they don't have a proper visa.

After the meeting, the hospital's CEO prepared two policies for consideration by the hospital's board of trustees. These two policies, which set forth the alternatives discussed at the meeting, are referred to as Plan A and Plan B. Specifically, Plan A provides as follows:

1. **Emergency care**. As required by applicable laws, the hospital will provide emergency treatment without regard to the patient's citizenship or immigration status, and without regard to the patient's ability to pay for his or her care.

2. **Nonemergency care**. The hospital will continue its current policy of providing nonemergency care for free or at a discount to any resident of the community who cannot afford to pay for his or her care, regardless of the person's immigration status.

3. **Notification to police and immigration authorities**. Hospital personnel will not notify police or immigration authorities about the actual or suspected immigration status of any patient or the family member of any patient.

4. **Use of a false name by a patient**. Even if a member of the hospital staff knows or has reason to believe that a patient has provided a name that is not that patient's legal name, the staff member shall continue to use the name provided by that patient in all medical records for that patient. In addition, hospital staff shall use the name provided by that patient in billing health insurance programs and government health programs for treatment of that patient.

5. **Translation services**. If a patient requires translation services in order to communicate effectively with hospital personnel, the hospital will provide translation services at the hospital's expense, regardless of the immigration status of the patient.

In contrast, Plan B provides as follows:

1. **Emergency care**. As required by applicable laws, the hospital will provide emergency treatment without regard to the patient's citizenship or immigration status, and without regard to the patient's ability to pay for his or her care.

2. **Nonemergency care**. The hospital will provide nonemergency care to those undocumented aliens who pay the hospital's regular rates and charges, in advance. In nonemergency situations the hospital will not provide care to undocumented aliens for free or at a discount. If the undocumented alien does not require emergency care, the hospital will offer the undocumented alien, at the hospital's expense, a free, one-way plane ticket (economy class) back to the patient's country of origin.

3. **Notification to police and immigration authorities**. If any member of the hospital staff knows or has reason to believe that a patient is an undocumented alien, the staff member shall immediately notify the local police or immigration authorities about that patient.

4. **Use of a false name by a patient**. If any member of the hospital staff knows or has reason to believe that a patient has provided a name that is not that patient's legal name, the staff member shall attempt to determine the patient's legal name. To the extent possible, the staff member shall use the patient's legal name in all medical records for that patient, and shall not use the false name provided by the patient in any medical record. Under these circumstances the hospital staff shall not use the false name provided by the patient in billing any health insurance plan or government health

program for treatment of that patient, and the staff member shall not sign or submit any document that the staff member knows or has reason to believe is false.

5. **Translation services**. In an emergency situation, if a patient requires translation services in order to communicate effectively with hospital personnel, the hospital will provide translation services at the hospital's expense, regardless of the immigration status of the patient. However, in a nonemergency situation, the hospital will not provide or pay for translation services for any undocumented alien.

Please analyze the ethical issues presented by proposed plans A and B and determine which plan is more ethical. You should also evaluate whether the most ethical approach may be some modification or combination of those plans. Be prepared to explain and justify your conclusions.

CHAPTER ELEVEN

ETHICAL ISSUES IN THE MOVEMENT OF HEALTH CARE PROFESSIONALS ACROSS NATIONAL BORDERS

LEARNING OBJECTIVES

- Demonstrate the ability to explain the facts, causes, and effects of cross-border migration by health care personnel, including the movement of workers from resource-poor to resource-rich countries.

- Acquire proficiency in analyzing the ethical issues involved in the large-scale recruitment of health care workers from developing countries.

- Be prepared to debate alternative solutions to this problem from an ethical perspective, and to compare and evaluate proposals for codes of ethical recruiting practices.

- Understand and be able to explain the ethical issues involved in the fair treatment of health care workers from other countries.

BECAUSE of technological changes in transportation and communications, it is now easier than ever to travel to other countries and continents, including travel for the purpose of living and working in another part of the world. Other factors that contribute to large-scale human migration include changes in political, economic, and social systems. In our globalized world, many patients and health professionals travel across national borders in order to obtain health care services or to provide those services.

Chapter Ten of this book analyzed the ethical implications in the movement of patients across national borders. The issues in that chapter included obligations to provide care for undocumented aliens, problems of medical tourism and transplant tourism, and ethical issues in treating patients with limited proficiency in the language of the host country. In contrast, this chapter analyzes the ethical issues in the movement of health care professionals across national boundaries. The migration to wealthier countries by highly educated workers, including health care professionals, is commonly referred to as **brain drain** (Mullan, 2005, p. 1811; Wright and others, 2008). Those countries to which professionals migrate are described as **destination countries** or **recipient countries**, whereas countries from which they migrate are described as **source countries** (Dwyer, 2007, p. 42; Mullan, 2005, p. 1813).

This chapter explains the global migration of health care workers, including the causes of migration and the consequences for those people who are left behind in the worker's home country. It also analyzes the ethical issues that arise in recruiting and employing health care workers from countries that have severe shortages of health personnel and high burdens of disease. Then this chapter evaluates proposed solutions to the problem and analyzes the ethical issues in those proposed solutions. An activity at the end of this chapter provides an opportunity to evaluate the ethical implications in developing a code of practice for recruiting health care personnel. Finally, this chapter analyzes the ethical issues involved in the fair treatment of health care workers while they are working in a country other than their country of origin.

ETHICAL ISSUES IN THE MIGRATION OF HEALTH PROFESSIONALS

Many of the physicians and nurses who care for patients in wealthy countries were born and educated in resource-poor developing countries. In the United States, about 25 percent of the physicians are **international medical graduates (IMGs)**, which means that they received their medical education outside the United States (Mullan, 2005, p. 1811). Only 3 percent of U.S. physicians are U.S. citizens who attended medical school in other countries, whereas 22 percent of U.S. physicians migrated to the United States from other countries (Mullan, pp. 1812–1814). Similar patterns exist in other wealthy, English-speaking countries, such as the United Kingdom, where over 28 percent of physicians are IMGs, and Australia and Canada, where IMGs represent more than 26 percent and 23 percent of physicians, respectively (Mullan, pp. 1811). With regard to nursing, foreign-educated nurses constitute approximately 10 percent of the U.K.'s nursing workforce, and more nurses who were trained outside that country registered to practice there in 2001 than did nurses who were trained in the United Kingdom (Dwyer, 2007, p. 37). Data are extremely limited or unavailable about the migration of other categories of health workers, such as pharmacists and allied health professionals (World Health Organization, 2006, p. 98).

Many of the source countries from which health professionals migrate are suffering as a result of severe shortages of health workers, low life expectancy, and high burdens of disease (Dwyer, 2007, pp. 36–37, 40). In both the United States and the United Kingdom, the largest number of IMGs is from India, and many more IMGs come from Pakistan. Another major source for IMGs in the United States is the Philippines. When these numbers are calculated as percentages, they reveal that countries in sub-Saharan Africa provide particularly large percentages of their limited number of physicians to the wealthy destination countries (Mullan, 2005, 1812–1816). For example, out of the 500 physicians who were trained in Zambia since that nation became an independent country, only 60 are still practicing medicine in Zambia (Johnson, 2005, p. 3). Out of a total of 3,240 physicians in Ghana, 926, or about 29 percent, were working in eight wealthy countries (World Health Organization, 2006, p. 100). Moreover, Ghana reached a dreadful equilibrium in 1999 by losing as many nurses to migration as it certified, and then it lost twice that number in 2000 (Chaguturu and Vallabhaneni, 2005, p. 1762). South Africa loses health care professionals to more industrialized countries, but it is a destination country for physicians from less developed countries in Africa (Dwyer, 2007, p. 37; Wright and others, 2008).

The causes of medical migration include both **pull factors**, which draw health care professionals to more developed countries, and **push factors**, which cause professionals to leave their home countries. According to the World Health Organization (2006), "Workers' concerns about lack of promotion prospects, poor management, heavy workload, lack of facilities, a declining health service, inadequate living conditions and high levels of violence and crime are among the push factors for migration . . . Prospects for better remuneration, upgrading qualifications, gaining experience, a safer environment and family-related matters are among the pull factors . . . In Zimbabwe, for example, a startling 77% of final university students were being encouraged to migrate by their families" (pp. 99–101).

In some cases, patterns of medical migration reflect former colonial relationships, such as migration of physicians from the Philippines to the United States and from India and Pakistan to the United Kingdom (Mullan, 2005, pp. 1812, 1816). As stated earlier, the United States receives the largest number of its IMGs from India, which was never a colony of the United States, but that migration is facilitated by the use of the English language in both India and the United States, both of which are former colonies of England (Mullen, 2005). The use of English in the Commonwealth countries of Africa makes health workers from those former British colonies more desirable in wealthy, English-speaking countries (Johnson, 2005, p. 2). Interestingly, some former colonial powers do not rely extensively on IMGs from their former colonies. Despite France's historical and linguistic relationships in Africa and Asia, only 3 percent of France's physicians are IMGs (Mullen, 2005, p. 1816).

For source countries the consequences of brain drain are severe. According to the World Health Organization's World Health Report 2006, fifty-seven countries have a critical shortage of health workers (p. 12). Many of the source countries also experience an internal brain drain of health professionals from the countryside to the cities and from public health care facilities to private facilities (Dwyer, 2007, p. 38; Organisation for Economic Co-operation and Development, 2008, p. 68). For countries that suffer from HIV/AIDS and lack sufficient health workers to meet the United Nation's Millennium Development Goals, the further losses of health professionals have been described as "fatal flows" (Chen and Boufford, 2005, p. 1851). As James Johnson (2005) has pointed out, "Although the developed countries of the North are giving aid with one hand, they are robbing African countries with the other by siphoning off their most precious resource—trained doctors and nurses" (p. 2). Similarly, Sreekanth Chaguturu and Snigdha Vallabhaneni (2005) have noted that international assistance has increased the availability of drugs for AIDS in developing countries, but wealthy countries are draining off the nurses needed to deliver those drugs: "It seems like a cruel joke to play: providing funds for AIDS care but simultaneously taking away the nurses who can give that care" (p. 1762). In addition, medical migration deprives poor countries of the money that they invested in educating their health professionals (Chen and Boufford, 2005, p.1851; Dwyer, 2007, p. 37), and distorts medical education in source countries by preparing prospective migrants to treat diseases that are more relevant to wealthy countries than to local populations (Mullan, 2005, p. 1816).

However, as Francesca Colombo and others noted in an Organisation for Economic Co-operation and Development (OECD) report (2008), migration of health professionals, while making an existing problem worse, is not the primary cause of the human resource crisis in developing countries (p. 63). As explained in that report, "The World Health Organization's estimates of regional health professional shortages largely outstrip the number of foreign-born health professionals who have emigrated to OECD countries. This means that even considering an unrealistic hypothetical scenario where migration from developing countries were to stop, these countries would still face up to considerable health human resource gaps" (p. 63). Moreover, some of the source countries that have severe shortages of nurses also have high rates of unemployment among nurses. Qualified nurses in those countries are unable to find jobs because their health systems have insufficient funds or are subject to hiring restrictions in programs of reform or because the jobs appear to be filled by "ghost workers," people who are paid but do not actually work (Kingma, 2007, p. 1287). Thus, in some of the impoverished source countries, stopping the migration of nurses would not necessarily increase the number of nurses available to treat patients.

Migration of health care personnel to wealthier countries could provide some benefits to source countries, but the extent of those potential benefits is questionable. In theory, migrants could acquire skills that would help their home country when they return, but many migrants do not return to their country of origin, and those who do return will find that some of the skills they acquire in wealthy countries are not relevant to the needs of the local population (Organisation for Economic Co-operation and Development, 2008, p. 67). Some migrants assist their home countries on a temporary basis by teaching or providing medical services (Organisation for Economic Co-operation and Development, p. 67), but it is difficult to quantify the extent or effects of those activities.

Migrants often send money home to their families, and those **remittances** can represent an important share of the source country's gross domestic product (Kingma, 2007, pp. 1291–1292). The Philippines has adopted a policy of promoting temporary migration of health care workers and using remittances to promote development of the country (World Health Organization, 2006, p. 101). However, the 2008 Organisation for Economic Co-operation and Development report concludes that remittances probably do not compensate a source country for the loss of health care professionals and do not promote development of the local health system. Moreover, these well-educated health workers probably come from families that are relatively wealthy, and therefore their remittances are benefitting those people in the source country that need this help the least (p. 64). For that reason, James Dwyer (2007) rejected the approach of trying to weigh the advantages and disadvantages of medical migration for source countries and instead advocated an approach of social justice and international justice, saying: "This concern with the least advantaged is missing from accounting models of international justice that simply tally up the average gains and losses in the respective countries. Balance sheets that try to calculate what a source country loses and what it gains in remittances and partnerships tend to ignore the distribution. The least advantaged in the source countries are often left behind because the remittances rarely benefit them, and the out-migrations undermine the public sector on which they depend. The private gains do not compensate fairly for the public losses" (p. 41).

Moreover, the destination countries are not mere passive recipients of individual health workers who choose to exercise their right to emigrate. First, the right of an individual health professional to emigrate does not necessarily require any particular destination country to admit that individual. Destination countries choose to grant entry visas to potential immigrants who are considered desirable, including health care professionals, while denying visas to many prospective immigrants who lack professional skills (Dwyer, 2007, pp. 38–39). In considering individual applications for visas, destination countries could consider the effect of immigration on the applicant's home country but ordinarily do not consider that factor. Moreover, some destination countries permit the operation of for-profit recruiting firms, with little or no effective regulation of their recruiting practices. From an ethical perspective, governments of destination countries cannot disclaim all responsibility for unethical recruiting practices by insisting that the recruiting is conducted by private firms that those governments do not regulate.

In addition, some destination countries have intentionally created their own need for migrant health professionals by failing to produce sufficient numbers of domestic professionals. Those countries have relied instead on less expensive migrant workers, who can be sent home when they are no longer needed. As Lisa Eckenwiler (2009) has written, "the growing reliance by some affluent countries on migrant health workers is not merely the result of poor planning, but increasingly, an integral part of health and labour policy" (p. iii). The 2008 Organisation for Economic Co-operation and Development report describes this as a "free rider" situation: "Countries have inadequate incentives to train sufficient health workers so long as they can rely on immigration to fill any gaps between supply and demand. Also, training more health professionals than necessary may be costly in terms of public expenditure. The resulting temptation is to risk shortages and to export them, if they arise" (pp. 35–36). The United States, for example, relies heavily on IMGs to provide indigent care, as medical residents in urban hospitals, and as practitioners in rural areas (Dow and Harris, 2002, pp. 68–69; Dwyer, 2007, p. 39).

Wealthy destination countries also have substantial influence over the policies of international lenders. Therefore, those wealthy countries bear some responsibility for the structural adjustment programs and other policies that limit public sector spending in developing countries, thereby contributing to shortages of health workers and increasing the incentive for remaining workers to emigrate (Kingma, 2007, p. 1286; Dovlo, 2007, p. 1375; Eckenwiler, 2009, p. iii). For all of these reasons, wealthy destination countries cannot claim to be mere passive recipients of individual migrants but rather bear substantial responsibility for the migration of health professionals and for the effects of that migration on developing countries.

The following excerpt from an article by David Wright and colleagues describes the history of medical brain drain, as well as the ways in which perceptions of the phenomenon and its ethical implications have changed over time. As Wright and colleagues explain here, those changes in perception are consistent with the recent trend in bioethics, described in Chapter One of this book, to consider important issues of social justice and population health.

EXCERPT FROM "THE 'BRAIN DRAIN' OF PHYSICIANS: HISTORICAL ANTECEDENTS TO AN ETHICAL DEBATE, C. 1960–79"

BY DAVID WRIGHT AND OTHERS

Background

The recruitment of health care practitioners from developing to developed countries is now an important topic in global health ethics. The intense public policy interest in foreign-trained doctors and nurses, however, is not new. During the mid-1960s, most western countries revised their immigration policies to focus on highly-trained professionals. These immigration changes facilitated the migration of hundreds of thousands of health care personnel from poorer jurisdictions to western countries to solve what were then deemed to be national physician and nursing shortages. Although we are now beginning to understand the broad socio-geographical impact of this massive international migration of health care workers, little has been written about the historical origins of this important era of post-war medical migration.

This paper will examine the emergence of the debate over what is now popularly called the "Brain Drain"—the migration of physicians from developing to developed countries and between industrialized nations. It will demonstrate how the early scholarship on the brain drain arose not from a concern over the impact on developing countries, but from a recognition in Britain of the loss of post-war NHS physicians to North America. Occasionally, early research acknowledged that the migration of health human resources from developing to developed countries (which was also occurring apace) raised concerns. However, writings in immigrant receiving countries—such as Canada, the United States, Britain or Australia—did not conceptualize physician immigration as ethically problematic. The responsibility for such a transfer of what was then commonly referred to as "highly skilled manpower" was understood as the accumulation of thousands of defensible individual decisions made by the doctors themselves. Indeed, much of the literature emphasized the value of advanced medical training being provided by industrialized countries. Moreover, since so much of the medical migration in this period occurred between developed countries the ripple effect on third and fourth countries was seldom fully appreciated or commented upon.

By contrast, the literature over the last decade has witnessed a dramatically different conceptual framework, informed by globalization, the rise in South Africa as a leading "donor" country, and the ongoing catastrophe of the AIDS epidemic. Unlike the literature a generation ago, new scholarship has focussed on the responsibility (financially or otherwise) of receiving countries to donor countries. Such ideas reflect in part, the rise (and partial acceptance) of international treaties (such as the Kyoto Accord) whereby countries have obligations to the global community for policy decisions they make domestically. This paper explores the historical antecedents to this important ethical debate in global health care.

The Transnational Migration of Physicians, c.1960–79

By the early 1960s, governments in western industrialized nations recognized with alarm that the domestic production of professionals—university professors, engineers, scientists—was insufficient to provide the same level, let alone a surging demand, for professional services within their respective societies. Nowhere was this more acutely felt than in the domain of health care where rising affluence and technological advances in the treatment of diseases led to a growing need for medical personnel. In English-speaking Commonwealth countries, this demand for health care services was accelerated by the advent and extension of universal state-run health insurance systems which unleashed a seemingly insatiable appetite for state-funded procedures. Western, industrialized English-speaking countries were thus to experience in the 1960s and

1970s an acute problem of access to physicians which would be characterized, by the press, as national doctor "shortages"....

The "Brain Drain" of Physicians from Britain to North America

The term "brain drain" appears to have become popularized in the context of a substantial body of work about the impact of physician migration on countries in the *developed* rather than developing world. Mainly written by American and British scholars, this literature was the first to address the impact of medical migration on the health systems of the "first world". In *Geographical Mobility and the Brain Drain*, McKay characterised the term "brain drain" as a "peculiarly British invention" that was coined in the mid-1950s (by the Royal Society) to capture the social and professional impact of British medical graduates leaving the country to seek opportunities in North America. McKay's study traced large numbers of Scottish medical graduates who flocked south to England, across the Atlantic to the United States and Canada, and down under to Australia and New Zealand....

Western Bioethics Meets Global Social Justice

There appear to be several reasons why the migration of physicians from developing to developed countries did not coalesce in the 1960s and early 1970s into a major ethical debate. The first concerns the unpredictable movement of the physicians themselves. While plenty of statistical information was available regarding the inflow of migrating physicians to wealthy countries, the outflow (emigration) records of developing countries were fragmented, if they existed at all. Social scientists had to, in effect, piece together the larger puzzle by working backwards from data in recipient nations. In addition, this poorly understood drain of resources was supposed by most scholars to be only temporary. It was frequently assumed that many foreign-born or trained physicians who had migrated would eventually return home following a period of additional or "advanced training" in the developed country. The reality that most of these physicians settled abroad permanently or migrated to yet other developed countries was not widely recognized. The degree and nature of permanent international migration of physicians from poorer to richer countries had to be determined before it could be assessed or judged to be explicitly unethical.

Complicating matters...was the phenomenon of certain developed countries—like Britain and Canada—being in the then top nations as both donor and recipient countries, owing to their status as countries used as "stepping stones" to elsewhere. In these cases, nations simultaneously received physicians from abroad while they themselves were losing health human resources to medical migration elsewhere. Further, there were a small number of countries who began *supporting* the migration of physicians either for geo-political, historical or financial reasons. Castro embarked on a self-conscious policy of training physicians for export, in order to support the ideal of socialized medicine and socialist politics. Ireland, a country that had a long history of out-migration, reconciled itself to the fact that many physicians would leave for elsewhere by generating a capacity to graduate more doctors than the country could absorb. Finally, in a manner analogous to its support of nurse and caregiver migration, the Philippines appears to have encouraged the out-migration of physicians in order to facilitate the flow of millions of dollars of remittances.

Cultural attitudes and racial prejudices also played an important role. Most scholars of the 1960s and 1970s viewed foreign-born and -trained physicians—especially those from underdeveloped nations—as inferior to the medical graduates from developed countries. In other words, most early sources that investigate doctor migration demonstrate a prejudice towards the quality of care provided by foreign medical graduates, even though many countries were relying heavily on these foreign workers to fill the gaps in their health service systems. It took a good decade for international medical graduates to prove themselves worthy of being considered and discussed as equals with physicians trained in industrialized countries. Only then could the ethical problems begin to be articulated with respect to the drain of medical personnel from developing countries to developed ones. Foreign physicians had to be appreciated as being valuable resources before ethical, transnational concerns could be conceived of, and applied to, their situation.

Finally, there seems to have been an implicit understanding that it was ultimately the physician's choice to leave his or her home country—which removed culpability from developed countries for "stealing" medical personnel. As health economist Alfonso Mejia put it rather elegantly, "Learned men (and women) have always travelled abroad seeking a more congenial intellectual milieu to realise their full potential". The physician's decision to migrate was understood to be a very personal calculation based upon a unique set of factors for each individual, the prevention of which would itself be both impossible and unethical. How could the post-war Western World embrace refugees and economic migrants but deny the right of educated individuals to better their personal situations? . . .

Thus even those who were coming to understand the magnitude of the problem recoiled from suggesting interventionist measures to stop it. There appeared to be a conceptual chasm: how could thousands of defensible . . . [individual] moral decisions constitute one large collective ethical problem?

The conceptual leap—from an individualistic bioethics attitude which framed ethical issues within the doctor-patient-relationship to one that began to conceptualize collective rights and identify problems of global social justice—was a long time in formation. Bioethics was, for the longest time, rooted in moral dilemmas arising from the increasing use of medical technologies particularly within North American and Western settings. Bioethics was thus preoccupied with micro-ethical issues and has only recently begun to focus on what are increasingly called global health ethics. This intellectual shift is reflected in the growing use of the term "global health" in medical literature, one which took off in the 1990s as a term to replace international health. As Brown et al. explain, global health in contradistinction to "international health . . . recognizes the growing importance of actors beyond governmental or intergovernmental organizations and agencies". The transnational migration of health workers clearly falls within this "global" realm and outside the traditional discourses of Western bioethics.

Out of Africa

During the 1980s and early 1990s, the interest in the international migration of foreign-trained doctors subsided in concert with the dramatic decline in the licensing of IMGs in most western countries. By the late 1990s, however, the issue of national doctor and nursing shortages had emerged as a major topic of concern and public interest. By this time, rural regions of industrialized countries were finding themselves denuded of primary care and looked abroad to foreign-trained doctors as a solution. For the last decade then, western countries have ramped up their licensing of foreign-trained doctors. But, unlike a generation ago an ethical and public policy debate has emerged around this phenomenon. In this current era of globalization, politicians and policy makers could no longer claim ignorance about the impact of medical migration on donor countries.

Within the new ethical debate, South Africa has played a totemic role. Devastated by the AIDS pandemic and struggling with rebuilding a post-apartheid civil society, the dramatic exodus of (mainly) white doctors, aided and abetted by western countries, has touched raw nerves. The exact number of doctors who are practising abroad is unknown, but the South African Medical Association estimated in 2002 that over 3,500 (approximately 50%) of its domestically-trained doctors were living abroad. Ironically, South Africa itself backfills, by recruiting African doctors from poorer states, such as Uganda and Tanzania. The *South African Medical Journal* describes a "medical carousel", in which doctors seem to be continually moving to countries with a perceived higher standard of living.

The ethical debate currently revolves around several related issues. Critics point to the purposeful underproduction of health human resources in the West to be supplemented, as a matter of policy, by foreign medical graduates. This results, they argue, in the depletion of health human resources in countries that are not only poorer but often plagued by serious public health challenges. On the opposite side, commentators suggest that it would be unethical to restrict the free movement of skilled labour in an era of globalization. Physicians, they argue, have as much a right to safe working conditions, or decent pay, as anyone else does. Some have even argued that the poor public health conditions in Africa are "a result of factors unrelated to international movement of health professionals". Others lament that, even if a restriction on the emigration of health professionals may be desirable, it would be largely impossible to enforce. Nevertheless, the embarrassing optics of rich countries exploiting the health human resources of African countries devastated by the AIDS epidemic—one that has unfortunate trappings of neo-colonialism—has led to some intermittent policy initiatives. Britain, for example, recently pledged to tighten the loopholes in its three-year old commitment to stop recruiting from the "developing world"....

At the 2005 World Health Assembly, the WHO resolved that World Health Day in 2006 should focus on the crisis of international migration of health personnel. Additionally, the assembly determined that their General Programme of Work, 2006–2015 should focus on the complexity of issues involved in international health human resource migration. Yet, despite recognition at the highest public policy levels, the question of physician migration and recruitment has failed to gain much traction from the lay public. Perhaps there is little popular appeal in industrialized countries to solutions that may, in many unpredictable ways, make the complex problem of doctor shortages worse. And so the brain drain continues and threatens to worsen over the next decade. As this article has demonstrated, the current wave of international physician migration, accelerated in part by health policy and immigration decisions made in industrialized countries, has a longer history to it than many current scholarly articles acknowledge. An historical perspective assists us in understanding the broader social and economic forces at work, as well as the changing ethical framework within which we understand this complex issue facing the world today....

PROPOSED SOLUTIONS AND THEIR ETHICAL IMPLICATIONS

In addressing the problem of brain drain, some of the potential solutions require separate actions by source countries or by destination countries. Other potential solutions require the source countries and destination countries to work together toward cooperative solutions, in either a bilateral or multilateral context. The potential solutions also have important ethical implications.

For example, is it ethical for source countries to prohibit health care professionals from leaving their home country? In the source country, health care professionals are an extremely valuable resource. Other residents of the source country depend on those professionals for their lives and health. Moreover, those health professionals obtained their skills, at least in part, at the expense of the public and the taxpayers in the source country. Would it be ethical to prevent them from leaving their home country, in order to seek more lucrative work in a wealthy country, one that did not pay for their education?

The United Nation's Universal Declaration of Human Rights recognizes that "[e]veryone has the right to leave any country, including his own" (1948, art. 13). As Dwyer (2007) explained, the right of emigration protects other human rights by making it possible for people to leave a country when those other rights are violated or threatened (p. 38). However, Dwyer also recognized that the right to emigrate must be balanced against the duty of health workers to the society that trained them. Under these circumstances, most commentators conclude that it would be unethical for a country to prevent its health professionals from ever leaving the country (Chen and Boufford, 2005, p. 1851; Chaguturu and Vallabhaneni, 2005, p. 1763; Johnson, 2005, p. 3). Dwyer (2007) argued, however, that it would be ethical for source countries to require their health professionals to meet an obligation of public service prior to emigration or graduation, or to require health professionals to pay their source country if they leave without completing their obligation of service (p. 38). As a practical matter, however, public service requirements and bonding requirements may be ineffective or difficult to enforce (Organisation for Economic Co-operation and Development, 2008, p. 69). Meanwhile, source countries could take other actions to help build capacity and retain health personnel. These actions include training cost-effective community health workers, who would not have internationally recognized credentials that would enable them to migrate, and improving living and working conditions for highly trained health professionals (Organisation for Economic Co-operation and Development, 2008, p. 68; Chen and Boufford, 2005, p. 1851; Dwyer, 2007, p. 42; World Health Organization, 2006, p. 102).

It will cost money to improve working and living conditions for health professionals in developing countries, and wealthy destination countries should provide financial assistance and training to help developing countries in that effort (Chen and Boufford, 2005, p. 1851). Some people have gone even further, and argued that destination countries should enter into compensation schemes with source countries, which currently subsidize the training of health professionals for wealthy destination countries (Organisation for Economic Co-operation and Development, 2008, p. 71; Wright and others, 2008). This type of compensation arrangement could be set forth in a bilateral agreement between a source country and a destination country. Governments of wealthy countries can also regulate private recruiting companies, which facilitate medical migration and profit from it (Organisation for Economic Co-operation and Development, 2008, pp. 70–71). In addition, destination countries should increase their own programs to educate and train domestic health professionals (Chen and Boufford, 2005, p. 1851), and should take steps to reduce attrition among nurses by improving their working conditions and professional status (Chaguturu and Vallabhaneni, 2005, p. 1763).

Another widely discussed alternative is for governments, employers, and recruiting agencies to adopt a code of ethical recruiting practices (Organisation for Economic Co-operation and Development, 2008, pp. 69–71). In 2001, the U.K. Department of Health issued the Code of Practice for NHS Employers Involved in the International Recruitment of Healthcare Professionals. That 2001 code was superseded in 2004 by the Code of Practice for the International Recruitment of Healthcare Professionals (U.K. Department of Health, 2004). Meanwhile, the Commonwealth Code of Practice for the International Recruitment of Health Workers was issued in 2003, together with the Companion Document to the Commonwealth Code, a source of additional information and explanation (Commonwealth Secretariat, 2003a, 2003b). In 2008, a coalition of health care organizations in the United States issued the Voluntary Code of Ethical Conduct for the Recruitment of Foreign-Educated Nurses to the United States

(Alinsao and others, 2008). Finally, the World Health Organization (2009) has been developing the Global Code of Practice on the International Recruitment of Health Personnel, and a revised draft of that code was issued in December of 2009.

The first issue to consider in developing a code is whether it will be mandatory or voluntary. If the code will be mandatory, how will it be enforced? The Commonwealth Code of Practice and the Companion to the Commonwealth Code are purely voluntary and are not binding on the governments of Commonwealth countries (paras. 10 and 4, respectively). The 2004 U.K. Code of Practice offers benchmarks of best practices and provides that "healthcare organisations utilizing the services of recruitment agencies for international recruitment are commended to use those agencies that are included on the list of agencies whose business is carried out in accordance with this Code of Practice" (p. 15). This Code of Practice also provides that organizations in the private sector can agree to comply and that recruiting agencies must comply with the code if they want to provide staff for the National Health Service (pp. 5–6). The Global Code of Practice from WHO is also to be voluntary, although "Member States and other stakeholders are strongly encouraged to comply with the code" (art. 2.1). Some commentators have criticized the voluntary nature of these codes (Eckenwiler, 2009, p. ii), but others have argued that even a voluntary code can help to establish a mechanism for cooperation on this important issue (Dayrit and others, 2008).

Like most of the codes, the Commonwealth Code of Practice explicitly recognizes the right of individual health professionals to migrate to another country (paras. 4, 18). The draft of the WHO's Global Code of Practice encourages member states to balance the health professional's individual right to migrate against the right of people who live in the source country "to the highest attainable standard of health" (art. 3.4). However, it also explicitly provides that "nothing in this code should be interpreted as limiting the freedom of health personnel, in accordance with international law, to migrate to countries that wish to admit and employ them" (art. 3.4).

Another important variable in these codes is whether they prohibit the recruiting of health care professionals from countries that have been identified as having a severe shortage of health personnel. The 2004 U.K. Code of Practice generally prohibits targeting developing countries for recruitment, but employers may accept unsolicited applications from individuals who live in developing countries, provided those individuals are not using the services of a recruiting agency (pp. 7, 10). Moreover, this code permits recruiting from developing countries when the U.K. government has entered into a bilateral agreement on recruitment with the government of the source country (pp. 7, 10).

A bilateral agreement between governments may include a commitment by a destination country to provide financial support for training in the source country, or may limit the period of time that health professionals may remain in the destination country before returning home (Organisation for Economic Co-operation and Development, 2008, p. 70). In that regard the draft of the WHO's Global Code of Practice provides that "Member States should abstain from active recruitment of health personnel from developing countries unless there exist equitable bilateral, regional or multilateral agreement(s) to support recruitment activities" (art. 5.3). The U.K. government has entered into bilateral agreements with several countries on the subject of recruiting health personnel (Organisation for Economic Co-operation and Development, 2008, p. 70; U.K. Department of Health, 2004, p. 14).

The Voluntary Code of Ethical Conduct for the Recruitment of Foreign-Educated Nurses to the United States includes an aspirational goal of discouraging active recruitment of nurses from countries that have severe shortages of health personnel. When that code was issued, an official of the U.S. Department of State objected to what he perceived as the code's implication that migrants from developing countries were acting unethically by coming to the United States.

> The . . . article . . . on the new code of ethics for hiring nurses from overseas, noted the laudable focus on protecting foreign nurses from exploitation in the United States. Unfortunately, the code also discourages U.S. companies from hiring nurses from countries with severe shortages of health workers, implying that a qualified nurse from a developing country has less right to apply for migration than a counterpart in a developed country.
>
> The U.S. government is uncomfortable with the notion that nurses from poor countries are behaving in an unethical manner when they seek better opportunities overseas. Many factors drive health workers to migrate, including poor working conditions, unpromising economic prospects, lack of professional development opportunities and the desire for a better life for their families.
>
> The code contains many positive suggestions for responsible recruitment, but the provision regarding recruiting nurses in developing countries is not one of them [Witten, 2008, p. B06].

In fact the Voluntary Code of Ethical Conduct includes a footnote (n. 3) clarifying that this particular provision refers to active recruitment in developing countries, and recognizing that employers in the United States may not discriminate against any applicant for employment on the basis of that applicant's country of origin.

Some codes discourage recruiting any individual health professional who still has an obligation of service to his or her home country. According to the

Commonwealth Code of Practice, "Recruiters should not seek to recruit health care workers who have an outstanding obligation to their own country, for example, contract of service agreed to as a condition of training" (para. 14). The Commonwealth Code of Practice provides, however, that it is the obligation of the individual to promptly disclose that information to the recruiter (para. 14). Similarly the draft of the WHO's Global Code of Practice discourages recruiting "health care personnel who have an outstanding legal responsibility to the health system of their own country such as a fair and reasonable contract of service" (art. 4.2). However, the WHO code does not specify the terms that would be considered fair and reasonable in a contract of service, and does not indicate when contract terms would be sufficiently unfair and unreasonable that the individual's outstanding obligation could be ignored by recruiters and destination countries.

Finally, these codes vary in describing the obligation of destination countries to provide compensation or assistance to the source countries from which they recruit health personnel. The Commonwealth Code of Practice is extremely vague about listing ways in which "[g]overnments recruiting from other Commonwealth countries should/[may wish to] consider how to reciprocate for the advantages gained by doing so" (para. 21). The draft WHO Global Code of Practice is similarly vague about the assistance that destination countries should provide "to the extent possible," and it provides that "[v]oluntary financial mechanisms...should be explored" (arts. 3.3, 11.4). However, this code also urges countries to develop bilateral or multilateral agreements, which could include provisions for financial and technical support to developing and transitional countries (art. 5.2).

In summary, codes of ethical recruiting can be categorized and evaluated on the basis of several variables. These variables are (1) whether the code is mandatory or voluntary; (2) whether it attempts to limit the freedom of individuals to migrate; (3) whether it prohibits recruiting from countries with a severe shortage of health personnel; (4) whether and to what extent it tries to discourage or prevent the recruiting of individuals who still have obligations to the health system or government of their home country; and (5) whether and how it describes the obligations of destination countries to provide compensation to source countries. The impact of a code is also likely to depend on several factors. According to the 2008 Organisation for Economic Co-operation and Development report, the "effectiveness of ethical codes and intergovernmental agreements will depend on: the content (principles envisaged, practical details), the coverage (countries and employers involved), and the compliance (mechanisms utilised, effectiveness) of these arrangements" (p. 70). The activity at the end of this chapter provides an opportunity to consider the variables and alternatives in developing a code of international recruiting practices that is likely to be effective and ethical.

FAIR TREATMENT OF HEALTH CARE WORKERS FROM OTHER COUNTRIES

As discussed previously, health care workers often travel to wealthier countries in order to improve their living conditions and professional opportunities. When they arrive in the destination country, these foreign workers should receive the same treatment accorded to locally recruited employees. Indeed, one of the guiding principles of the 2004 U.K. Code of Practice is this: "All staff, regardless of country of origin, have the same legal protections within the workplace" (p. 8). Similarly, the Commonwealth Code of Practice emphasizes that employees who have been recruited from other countries are entitled to the same level of compensation and the same professional opportunities as employees of equal grade who have been recruited locally (para. 17). As a practical matter, however, many health workers from other countries have been subjected to misrepresentation by recruiters, exploitation by employers, or discrimination by patients or fellow employees.

In some cases, recruiters have seriously misrepresented the nature of the job, the level of compensation, or the living arrangements for recruited workers in the destination country. Foreign nurses working in the United Kingdom have complained that recruiting agencies charged them additional fees, and even withheld their passports (Commonwealth Secretariat, 2003b, p. 11). In addition, nurses can be paid lower wages for several months during their probationary period before registration, and some recruiting agencies or employers have delayed this registration so that they can continue to pay these lower wages (Maybud and Wiskow, 2006, p. 234). Meanwhile, foreign nurses can find themselves going deeper and deeper into debt to the recruiting agencies or employers, who make regular deductions from the nurses' salaries to pay various expenses or to repay loans that the agencies or employers were only too willing to extend. Foreign health workers are afraid to complain, because they depend on the recommendation of their employer for the work permits and registration needed to remain in the destination country, and therefore they remain subject to exploitation (Maybud and Wiskow, 2006, pp. 233–236). It is seriously unethical for a recruiting agency or employer to use its control over a foreign worker's visa or passport as a way to force consent to unreasonable demands, demands that could not be made of a citizen of the destination country.

Aside from exploitation by employers and recruiting agencies, foreign health workers have been subjected to discrimination by fellow employees and by patients. Mireille Kingma (2007) has described some of the problems of racism and discrimination for nurses who migrate for work in other countries: "Migrant nurses are frequent victims of poorly enforced equal opportunity policies and pervasive double standards. To determine how frequently this occurs is difficult as incidents are often hidden by a blanket of silence and rarely openly acknowledged. Some migrant nurses have, however, reported dramatic situations on the job where colleagues purposefully misunderstand, undermine their professional skills, refuse to help, and sometimes bully them, thus increasing their sense of isolation" (pp. 1289–1290, citations omitted). Health care facilities and their managers have an obligation to ensure that all their employees are treated with equality, dignity, and respect. Moreover, health care facilities should not allow patients to demand to be treated by a caregiver of a particular race or national origin. Thus the World Health Organization (2006) stressed the importance of establishing policies to address racist attitudes among patients as well as employees (p. 103).

In one particularly egregious case (*Matter of Vinluan* v. *Doyle*, 2009), a number of nurses from the Philippines who were working at a nursing home in the United States resigned from their jobs in a dispute over their working conditions and terms of employment. An official of the nursing home then filed a complaint against the nurses with the state occupational licensing agency, on the ground of alleged abandonment of patients, including ventilator-dependent children. However, the licensing agency found that the nurses had not abandoned their patients, because they had not resigned during their shifts and the nursing home had obtained other coverage for those patients. Subsequently, the nurses were charged with having committed criminal offenses by resigning from their jobs. However, a state appellate court ruled in favor of the nurses, finding that prosecution of the nurses under these circumstances violated the constitutional prohibition in the United States against slavery and involuntary servitude. As the appellate court explained:

> the indictment handed down . . . explicitly makes the nurses' conduct in resign-ing their positions a component of each of the crimes charged. Thus, the indict-ment places the nurses in the position of being required to remain in [the com-pany's] service after submitting their resignations, even if only for a relatively brief period of notice, or being subject to criminal sanction. Accordingly, the prosecution has the practical effect of exposing the nurses to criminal penalty for exercising their right to leave their employment at will. The imposition of such a limitation upon the nurses' ability to freely exercise their right to resign from the service of an employer who allegedly failed to fulfill the promises and commitments made to them is the antithesis of the free and voluntary system of labor envisioned by the framers of the Thirteenth Amendment. While we are, of

course, mindful that protecting vulnerable children from harm is of enormous importance, the fact that the prosecution may serve a legitimate societal aim does not suspend the nurses' constitutional right to be free from involuntary service [*Matter of Vinluan* v. *Doyle*, 2009, pp. 80–81].

For those reasons, the appellate court prohibited the prosecutor from continuing the criminal case against the nurses.

SUMMARY

Although brain drain is not a new phenomenon, the consequences for source countries have become much more severe in recent years. This chapter explained the facts about global migration of health professionals, including its causes and effects. It also evaluated the ethical implications of recruiting health professionals from developing countries that have severe shortages of human resources for health care and very high burdens of disease. The chapter analyzed the ethical issues in alternative solutions to the problem of brain drain, and analyzed the ethical issues of treating health workers fairly while they are working in a country that is not their country of origin.

Chen and Boufford (2005) have explained that in taking decisive action to solve the problem of brain drain, the motivation of a wealthy country should be "based not simply on humanitarianism but also enlightened self-interest" (p. 1851). As these authors noted, a wealthy country has an interest in preventing the transmission of diseases and pandemics across national borders, but such prevention is hindered when less wealthy countries are being drained of necessary health personnel. Similarly, the 2008 Organisation for Economic Co-operation and Development report recognized the global "interdependence" that arises when the health systems in individual nations are affected by the circumstances and actions of systems in other nations. As the authors of that report wrote, "structural shortage of health personnel in low-income countries, no matter what their causes, could weaken health systems, and thus, in the long run, jeopardise global public health" (p. 58).

KEY TERMS

brain drain

destination countries

international medical
   graduates (IMGs)

pull factors

push factors

recipient countries

remittances

source countries

DISCUSSION QUESTIONS

1. As an ethical matter, do wealthy destination countries bear responsibility for the migration of health professionals and for the effects of that migration on developing countries?
2. Is it ethical for source countries to prohibit health professionals from ever leaving their home country?
3. Is it ethical for source countries to require health professionals to complete obligations of service or to repay the cost of their education and training before being allowed to leave the source country?
4. Do governments of source countries have an ethical obligation to improve the living and working conditions of health professionals in their countries?
5. Do governments of destination countries have an ethical obligation to provide financial assistance to source countries from which they receive health care personnel?

ACTIVITY: DEVELOPING A CODE OF ETHICAL PRACTICES FOR INTERNATIONAL RECRUITING OF HEALTH CARE PERSONNEL

This exercise provides an opportunity to evaluate the variables and alternatives in developing a code of international recruiting practices that is likely to be effective and ethical. As explained in the text of this chapter, codes of ethical recruiting can be distinguished on the basis of several variables: (1) whether the code is mandatory or voluntary; (2) whether it attempts to limit the freedom of individuals to migrate; (3) whether it prohibits recruiting from countries with a severe shortage of health personnel; (4) whether and to what extent it tries to discourage or prevent the recruiting of individuals who still have obligations to the health system or government of their home country; and (5) whether and how it describes the obligations of destination countries to provide compensation to source countries.

The following proposal for a code of ethical recruiting lists these five variables and for each variable it offers three alternative provisions. Please evaluate the alternative provisions for each variable and then select the alternative that you think is most likely to be effective and ethical, or propose your own provision for that variable. Be prepared to justify your decision and to explain how your chosen alternative is the most effective and ethical.

1. Is the Code Voluntary or Mandatory?

A. This code is voluntary, but all governments, health care organizations, recruiting firms, and employers are strongly urged to comply with all provisions of this code.

B. This code is voluntary, but all governments, health care organizations, recruiting firms, and employers are strongly urged to comply with all provisions of this code. Moreover, governments, health care organizations, and employers that agree to comply with this code may not use the services of any recruiting firm that does not comply with this code. In addition, governments that agree to comply with this code may not permit any health care organization that does not comply with this code to participate in any government-funded health program.

C. This code is mandatory and is binding on all governments, health care organizations, recruiting firms, and employers that agree to be bound by the code.

D. Other [*please describe*].

2. What Does It Say About Freedom to Emigrate?

A. This code does not impose any limitation on the right of individuals to migrate.

B. This code does not impose any limitation on the right of individuals to migrate, but the right to migrate must be balanced against the rights of the populations in source countries.

C. This code does not impose any limitation on the right of individuals to migrate, provided, however, that source countries retain the right to limit emigration by any health worker who has not yet satisfied his or her obligation under a contact for funding of that worker's education or training.

D. Other [*please describe*].

3. What Does It Say About Recruiting from Countries with Shortages of Health Workers?

A. Governments, health care organizations, employers, and recruiting firms that agree to comply with this code may not target countries for recruitment of health workers when those countries have been identified by WHO as having a severe shortage of human resources for health care.

B. Governments, health care organizations, employers, and recruiting firms that agree to comply with this code may not target countries for recruitment of health workers when those countries have been identified by WHO as having a severe shortage of human resources for health care. However, they may accept unsolicited applications from individuals who live in one of those countries, provided those individuals are not using the services of a recruiting agency.

C. Governments, health care organizations, employers, and recruiting firms that agree to comply with this code may not discriminate, in recruiting or employment, on the basis of the country of residence of any health worker.

D. Other [*please describe*].

4. What Does It Say About Individuals' Obligations to Their Home Country?

A. Governments, health care organizations, employers, and recruiting firms that agree to comply with this code may not recruit, employ, or grant a work visa to any individual who has not yet satisfied his or her obligation under a contact for funding of that worker's education or training.

B. Governments, health care organizations, employers, and recruiting firms that agree to comply with this code may not recruit, employ, or grant a work visa to any individual who has not yet satisfied his or her reasonable obligation under a contract for funding of that worker's education or training. For purposes of this provision, a reasonable obligation is an obligation of service that does not exceed [*specify a period from one to ten years*].

C. Governments, health care organizations, employers, and recruiting firms that agree to comply with this code may not recruit, employ, or grant a work visa to any individual who has not yet satisfied his or her reasonable obligation under a contract for funding of that worker's education or training. For purposes of this provision, a reasonable obligation is an obligation of service that does not impose a significant hardship on the individual or the family of that individual.

D. Other [*please describe*].

5. What Does It Say About Providing Compensation to Source Countries?

A. Governments of destination countries are strongly encouraged to evaluate ways in which they may be able to provide compensation to source countries for the costs of education and training of health professionals.

B. Governments of destination countries and governments of source countries are strongly encouraged to communicate and to negotiate bilateral agreements that make provisions to compensate source countries for the costs of education and training of health professionals.

C. For every health professional who is granted a visa to work in a destination country, the government of that destination country shall provide financial compensation to the government of the source country, in an amount sufficient to compensate the source country for the costs of education and training of that individual.

D. Other [*please describe*].

CHAPTER TWELVE

CORRUPTION AND INFORMAL PAYMENTS IN HEALTH SYSTEMS

LEARNING OBJECTIVES

- Develop an appreciation for the relationship between corruption and the health of a population.

- Demonstrate the ability to describe the practice of paying unofficial fees to health care professionals, which is common in developing and transitional countries.

- Understand and be able to explain the consequences and ethical implications of collecting unofficial fees from patients and their families.

- Learn how to evaluate potential methods of reducing the level of corruption in health systems, including the collection of informal fees.

IMAGINE that you go to a doctor's office and pay the fee for the doctor's consultation. Then you are told that if you want to see the doctor, you really need to pay an additional fee in cash "under the table." The additional, unofficial fee might be even higher than the official fee for that particular service.

Alternatively, imagine that you go to a hospital and find that the hospital workers routinely collect extra fees from patients or their families, in addition to the official fees established by governmental agencies or insurance programs. These additional fees might include payments to doctors for examination and treatment, payments to nurses for bedding, medications, and food, and even a payment to the guard in order to get in the door and obtain an appointment. As explained in this chapter, these types of fees are very common in developing and transitional countries. They create barriers to access for health services and cause financial hardship to millions of people.

The common practice of collecting unofficial fees from patients or their families is just one part of the broader topic of corruption in health systems. **Corruption** is often defined as "using public office for private gain" (Lewis, 2007, p. 985). In addition to the collection of unofficial fees, health system corruption includes conduct such as the theft or "siphoning off" of public resources, bribery of government health officials, and taking kickbacks from pharmaceutical companies or other potential vendors (Ensor and Duran-Moreno, 2002, pp. 107–112). Where health care facilities are public entities and health care workers are public employees, unethical conduct by professionals and managers could also constitute corruption. For example, many physicians who are employed in the public sector also engage in private practice, during the time they are paid to serve public patients. Those physicians might use public facilities and resources to treat patients on a private basis or might regularly abandon their public responsibilities in order to practice at private clinics (Ensor and Duran-Moreno, 2002, pp. 109–110).

This chapter analyzes both the specific issue of unofficial fees and the broader issue of health system corruption, in all of its various forms. From an ethical perspective the problem of unofficial fees requires separate consideration, because some people have questioned whether collecting unofficial fees is corrupt and unethical. Unofficial fees are unique in this regard. No one could seriously dispute that it is corrupt and unethical to steal resources from public health programs or to steal drugs that are needed by seriously ill patients. In contrast, some people argue that collecting unofficial fees is a cultural practice, which might not be corrupt or might be only "petty corruption." The first part of this chapter, therefore, analyzes the specific issue of collecting unofficial or informal fees from patients and their families, including the various types of fees, the reasons they are paid, the effects on patients and families, the ethical implications, and the potential solutions to this problem.

The second part of this chapter analyzes the broader issue of health system corruption in general as well as the effect of corruption on health. Specifically, it analyzes the relationship between the level of corruption in a country and the health status of its population, using a country's level of HIV prevalence as one way to measure population health. (This is not meant to suggest that HIV prevalence is the only effect of corruption or the only measure of population health, merely that HIV prevalence is a useful metric for analyzing the relationship between corruption and the health of a population.) The ethical issue in this second part is not evaluating whether the corrupt conduct is unethical, which is obvious, but rather determining the most ethical solution to the problem of corrupt conduct in health systems. For example, as an ethical matter, should international organizations and lenders refuse to provide money to corrupt officials and their governments? Is it ethical for international public health programs to work toward changing social systems and cultural practices in developing and transitional countries when they consider those social systems and cultural practices to be corrupt? For both the specific issue of unofficial payments and the broader issue of corruption in general, this chapter analyzes the effects of the conduct, the relevant ethical issues, and the potential solutions to these problems. At the end of this chapter, an activity provides an opportunity to evaluate the ways in which collection of unofficial fees could be reduced or eliminated.

PAYMENT OF INFORMAL FEES BY PATIENTS AND THEIR FAMILIES

Informal payments are defined as payments "to individual and institutional providers, in kind or in cash, that are made outside official payment channels or are purchases meant to be covered by the health system" (Lewis, 2007, p. 985). This definition includes payments made to doctors or hospitals under the table and the cost of drugs, supplies, or amenities that are bought by patients or families but that should have been provided by the public facility or program (Lewis, 2007, p. 985; Tatar and others, 2007).

In 2008, Anne Cockcroft and others published a study of informal payments in the Baltic States of Estonia, Latvia, and Lithuania, which had formerly been parts of the Soviet Union. Almost half of the participants in this household survey believed that informal fees are not really corruption. However, the authors concluded that the "lack of consensus on whether informal payment is corruption is a subject for concern. Some believe that the very lack of consensus encourages corruption" (Cockcroft and others, 2008).

How should we react to the payment of informal fees for health services in developing and transitional countries? It seems that people who study the issue tend to go through several stages in their reaction to the use of informal fees for health services. These stages are similar in some ways to the well-known stages of grief. As discussed in the following section, these stages are outrage, multicultural acceptance, research, rationalization, and developing practical solutions.

The Stage of Outrage.   The first stage is to be outraged and acrimonious at the unethical behavior of health workers who take advantage of poor patients in developing and transitional countries. These informal fees create barriers to access for essential health care services, cause financial hardship or even ruination for patients and their families, and reduce equity in the health system (Lewis, 2007, p. 990). Because developing countries typically lack systems of health insurance to prepay expenses and pool the risks, a large share of health spending comes from out-of-pocket payment by patients and their families. As Maureen Lewis (2007) has pointed out, compared to populations generally, people in poor countries pay the highest percentage of their income out of pocket for health services, in part because their governments lack the capacity to raise revenues by taxation to finance health services (p. 984). Under these circumstances, requiring payment of additional fees under the table is particularly burdensome. Experts have also noted that informal fees can result in distortion of priorities and misallocation of resources (Ensor, 2004, pp. 241, 244), lead to understatement of actual levels of health spending (Tatar and others, 2007, p. 1037), and interfere with efforts toward health reform (Ensor, 2004, p. 244; Tatar and others, 2007, p. 1038).

The Stage of Multicultural Acceptance.   Who are we to judge or criticize the deeply ingrained cultural practice of expressing gratitude to those members of a community who provide necessary services to fellow community members? According to some researchers, making a "donation" to a physician is a cultural or social practice (Tatar and others, 2007, p. 1036). The study by Cockcroft and others (2008) in the Baltic States found that many people consider gifts for health professionals to be an appropriate statement of gratitude. Moreover, the practice of collecting informal fees is arguably analogous to some of the ways in which health care providers in industrialized countries distinguish among their patients on the basis of wealth, insurance status, and source of payment.

The Stage of Research.   When all else fails, let's look at the actual data. The data indicate that informal fees are usually paid before receiving the health service and therefore are not post hoc expressions of gratitude (Tatar and others, 2007, pp. 1035–1037). Rather, informal fees may be paid to obtain services to which patients were already entitled, get more attention, reduce waiting times, increase hospital length of stay, have a choice of physician, or even for mothers in maternity homes to be allowed to see their babies (Tatar and others, 2007, pp. 1035–1037; Lewis, 2007, pp. 989–990; Ensor and Duran-Moreno, 2002, p. 118). Informal fees might also be paid as a type of implicit health insurance for future medical services (Lewis, 2007, pp. 984–985). Finally, data indicate that many patients and their families do not like having to pay informal fees, which undercuts the argument that informal fees are an accepted cultural practice (Tatar and others, 2007, p. 1037).

The Stage of Rationalization.   After all, informal fees are small potatoes. The focus on informal fees may distract our attention from the much more important issue of large-scale corruption in health systems of developing and transitional countries (Ensor and Duran-Moreno, 2002, p. 118). Some government officials might even want us to focus on informal fees, in order to distract attention from their own large-scale bribery and diversion of resources. Moreover, informal fees are necessary to support the health system, in light of inadequate government funding and ridiculously low salaries for health workers. "Where earnings are low, individuals have second and third jobs, but they also perceive that low wages entitle them to demand contributions from patients" (Lewis, 2007, p. 993). Under these circumstances, Tim Ensor and Antonio Duran-Moreno (2002) attempted to distinguish informal fees that constitute the extraction of "rents" from other informal fees that are merely a "coping strategy" or "survival strategy." They reasoned that physicians in industrialized countries (members of the Organisation for Economic Co-operation and Development) usually earn between 2.5 and 4 times the average wage in their countries. Therefore, if physicians in other countries collect informal fees from their patients, it is arguably not corruption or is merely "petty corruption" so long as the physicians are not taking in more than twice the average income in their respective countries (pp. 114–117). From an ethical perspective, however, that approach is problematic. In fact, Ensor (2004) subsequently wrote that "unofficial payments might be given to ensure that staff employed in the facility reach their reservation wage—the wage which ensures retention of staff and provision of a good quality service . . . . Yet giving tacit acceptance to the practice of 'reasonable bribes' to medical practitioners to perform procedures that they are officially required to provide without charge is hard to accept from an ethical point of view, even if it is understandable from the point of view of personal survival" (p. 239).

The Stage of Developing Practical Solutions.   Although it is crucial to address high-level corruption in health systems, it is also important to reduce the burden of informal payments, especially as they affect access to care and financial hardship for the poorest segment of the population. Writing about informal payments in Turkey, Mehtap Tatar and others (2007) explained that when "extended to the whole country, the impact of these payments could exceed that of large-scale corruption, and their consequences could be more serious and direct, both on the health system and on patients" (p. 1039). Similarly, Cockcroft and others (2008) have argued that on a cumulative basis, so-called petty corruption, including informal fees, can have a serious effect on the health system and the delivery of health services. Having decided that we want to eliminate—or at least reduce—the collection of informal fees, how can we best accomplish that goal? If we simply outlaw the collection of informal fees, that could have the adverse results of (1) being unenforceable; (2) reducing the actual income of health workers; or (3) causing health workers to leave public health care facilities for work in the private sector (Ensor and Duran-Moreno, 2002, p. 117) or leave the country altogether. Most experts conclude that it is necessary to raise the official income of health workers (Ensor and Duran-Moreno, pp. 117–118), but governments may be unable or unwilling to provide the additional funding. Moreover, pay increases alone will not solve the problem, unless they are accompanied by other reforms to provide more appropriate incentives for health workers, greater accountability, and elimination of informal fees (Lewis, 2007, pp. 993–994). It is also necessary to consider how to enforce the prohibition against informal fees, so that patients are not required to pay both an increased official fee and an informal fee. It is particularly important that local managers have the ability to discipline and even fire health workers who violate the rules against collection of informal fees or fail to provide appropriate care (Lewis, 2007, p. 994). Under these circumstances, most proposals for reform involve increasing the official fees to be paid by patients, as part of a comprehensive plan to reduce informal fees. This strategy, which is described as **formalization of fees**, has been implemented with promising results in a few locations such as Cambodia and the Kyrgyz Republic (Ensor and Duran-Moreno, 2002, p. 118; Lewis, 2007, pp. 992–999; Barber and others, 2004). Even after formalization, however, patients might still be forced to pay informal fees, and some patients might even prefer to pay informal fees as a way to have their choice of physician (Ensor, 2004, p. 242; Ensor and Duran-Moreno, 2002, pp. 118, 121). Fundamentally, informal fees in the health system are part of the broader problems of corruption, lack of accountability, and inadequate governance, and the ultimate solution to informal fees will require reform of incentives and regulation on a much broader level (Lewis, 2007, pp. 992, 995; Ensor, 2004, p. 244).

The activity at the end of this chapter presents an opportunity to consider the practical aspects of developing a hospital plan to stop collection of informal fees from patients in a developing country. As described in the activity, the goal is to effectively prevent collection of informal fees from patients, without reducing the income of health workers and without increasing expenditures by the government.

IS CORRUPTION BAD FOR YOUR (AND OTHER PEOPLE'S) HEALTH?

We often hear about things that are bad for our health. What about corruption, including informal fees and other types of corrupt conduct in health systems? Is it possible that corruption could be bad for our health and also bad for other people's health?

The first part of this chapter analyzed one specific type of corruption, the collection of informal fees, and described some of its adverse effects, such as creating barriers to access and causing financial hardship. The next part of this chapter applies a broader approach, by analyzing the effects of corruption, in all of its various forms, on the health status of a population.

The relationship between good governance and good health is complex (Lewis, 2006, pp. 8–13). One possibility is that poor governance, including a high level of corruption, can cause or contribute to poor health status in a population or even to a large-scale crisis in public health. Another possibility is that a health crisis, or some other type of crisis such as war or natural disaster, can cause or contribute to an increase in corruption. In a time of crisis, extreme shortages exist, and many people struggle to save themselves and their families. Meanwhile, large sums of money may be allocated in a relatively short period of time, with an urgent mandate to spend that money as soon as possible to alleviate the widespread suffering. Under those circumstances, opportunities can arise to take advantage of the needs of other people, by means of theft, bribery, or other forms of corruption. This may involve small-scale theft or bribery, engaged in as a means of survival, as well as large-scale corruption by public officials at the highest levels.

Another possibility is that some other factor can cause or contribute to both corruption and low health status. Among other factors, illiteracy or poverty could lead to both corruption and problems in health. In fact, this might be the familiar phenomenon of the chicken and the egg, in which each factor contributes to the other in a cyclical fashion. By analogy, it has been well documented that poverty leads to illness, which in turn leads to more poverty. Perhaps the relationship between corruption and health is similar, with corruption leading to low health status or a large-scale crisis in health, which in turn leads to even more corruption.

In the article excerpt that follows, Anatole Menon-Johansson explores the relationship between health and poor governance, including a high level of corruption. Menon-Johansson used the level of HIV prevalence in each country as one way to measure the health of a population, and relied on data from the World Bank and UNAIDS. (Readers who are interested in more information about the underlying data should refer to the full text of the article as originally published.)

EXCERPT FROM "GOOD GOVERNANCE AND GOOD HEALTH: THE ROLE OF SOCIETAL STRUCTURES IN THE HUMAN IMMUNODEFICIENCY VIRUS PANDEMIC"

BY ANATOLE MENON-JOHANSSON

Some of the shared societal structures underpinning economic growth and health are the absence of violence, government effectiveness, the rule of law, lack of corruption and the ability to select a government. Even though all of these are clearly desirable the relative weight of each societal structure necessary for a strong nation state is debatable. The risk of infectious disease is determined not only by pathogens and the response of the patient but also by powerful societal forces that override individual knowledge and choice. Paul Farmer has coined the phrase "structural violence" that reflects the limit of life choices, particularly of women, by racism, sexism, political violence, and grinding poverty.

The 2004 World Health Report discusses the challenges of tackling the HIV pandemic. In the African continent, HIV is implicated in poor economic performance and falling gross domestic product (GDP). Within this document it describes the wide range of international support garnered to meet this challenge. However, even though the requirement of local and national government co-operation is stressed within this document, it does not elaborate on the massive heterogeneity inherent within this mandatory component.

In order to investigate the strength of the relationship between the quality of societal structures and the HIV pandemic, World Bank and UNAIDS sources were used to test the null hypothesis: "HIV prevalence is not associated with governance".

Methods

A recent World Bank paper entitled Governance Matters III collated governance indicators for 199 countries/regions. Governance in this document has been broken down into six dimensions...Using these definitions, this research collected data for each country from 18 sources...Governance data were then aggregated for each country and plotted along a continuum. Only the 2002 governance data has been used in this paper....

The 2002 HIV prevalence estimates were obtained for each country. HIV prevalence is the percentage of adults aged between 15 and 49 years of age infected with HIV. One hundred and forty nine of the 199 countries/regions cited by the World Bank paper had published UNAIDS 2002 HIV prevalence estimates....

In addition to separate analysis of each governance dimension, an average governance figure was obtained based on the assumption that each governance dimension was of equal importance. The null hypothesis was tested by measuring association between ranked governance and HIV prevalence data across the whole spectrum of countries...

Results

There were fifty distinct HIV prevalence rankings from the 149 countries with UNAIDS HIV prevalence estimates in 2002. Botswana had the highest HIV prevalence estimates (38.8%) in the world that year whilst the majority of countries were placed within the lowest ranking, where HIV prevalence estimates were reported by UNAIDS to be < 0.1% (written as 0.05%)....

The negative correlations indicate that HIV prevalence falls as the governance improves for each governance dimension and mean governance. The three most influential dimensions of governance were government effectiveness, the rule of law and corruption. All correlations were significant thus rejecting the null hypothesis.

Discussion

It is possible to divide those nations affected by HIV/AIDS into three groups that approximate to governance ranking. The higher governance group is characterized by significant wealth and effective healthcare systems. The main challenges for these countries...[consist] of the provision of sexual health services, health care access to marginalized groups, continuation of education and research into new and improved prevention and treatment strategies.

The HIV prevalence is generally low in higher governance group however this figure conceals differences found within specific population groups. For example in the USA, HIV prevalence amongst African American women is almost twenty three times that in whites. Whilst in the UK, the prevalence of HIV amongst men who have sex with men (MSM) within London in 2001 was 100 times the national average. The disparity in HIV prevalence amongst "at risk" groups in the UK and US highlight the general difficulty of using the UNAIDS country HIV prevalence estimates. The quality of surveillance methods has been discussed and graded by UNAIDS surveillance teams, and it is clear that some HIV prevalence estimates are inaccurate . . . .

The null hypothesis 'HIV prevalence is not associated with governance' is rejected for each dimension of governance with variations in the relative importance of different governance dimensions. Previously, Fareed Zakaria has argued that democracy is less important in the development of a strong nation than the rule of law, corruption and political stability. The correlation coefficient of the voice and accountability dimension of governance with HIV prevalence was the lowest in this analysis somewhat supporting this contention.

Those countries in the lowest governance ranking group of governance are defined by poverty, ineffective health care systems, elevated HIV prevalence and significant international debt. The elevated HIV prevalence in many of these vulnerable countries was predicted more than a decade ago following the analysis of health, economic and human rights data. Historically, international support has focused on short-term "vertical" disease control strategies to tackle healthcare problems. Long-term, "horizontal" capacity building strategies are vital if HIV/AIDS is going to be . . . [effectively] managed in nations with limited healthcare infrastructure. It has been shown in a number of resource poor settings that the provision of voluntary counselling and testing (VCT) for HIV is facilitated by the provision of free primary care services and ART [antiretroviral therapy]. The provision of effective primary care support to pregnant women is the most effective way to provide VCT services for HIV and thereby identify HIV positive mothers, prevent mother to child transmission and facilitate VCT of their partner(s). Like surveillance, this strategy though relatively effective fails to test and treat vulnerable "high risk" groups within the population.

The poor are those most at risk of infectious disease. The role of poverty as a risk factor for disease has been clear for over 300 years. Health and wealth are inextricably linked. All who become chronically ill enter a negative cycle of limited horizons. Indeed, what is true for the individual is equally true for the nation state. The effect of HIV on economic under performance and negative growth is testament to this. It is vital that essential healthcare is free, so that those that catch treatable infectious diseases are allowed to live. Encouragingly there are a few positive examples in resource poor countries, such as Uganda, Senegal and Cuba, where leadership, good communication and support of civil society have made a difference in their respective HIV epidemics. There are however many countries within this group of vulnerable nations that need the bulk of international healthcare and financial institution commitment in order to address their devastating health-care challenges.

Cuba and Haiti are islands with a similar population size and GDP-PPP [gross domestic product—purchasing power parity] per capita yet the HIV prevalence estimates are 0.05% and 6.1% respectively. HIV is thought to have entered Haiti from the USA via the sex trade in the early 1980s. The main exposure risk for Cuban nationals was from military and healthcare worker interaction with sub-Saharan Africa. Cuba was one of the first countries in the Americas to launch a nationwide HIV policy to contain transmission and care for those people living with HIV/AIDS. Healthcare in Cuba is provided free to its citizens by the state and there is strong political commitment supporting health as well as national and international HIV/AIDS action. In contrast, there have been 33 coups in Haiti in the last two centuries of independence. Political instability in addition to other governance factors...[has] been attributed to the lack of development of a responsive healthcare system.

As governance improves fewer women die in childbirth, more physicians exist per population, there is better access to improved water and life expectancy is longer. In addition with improvements in governance there is more GDP-PPP per capita, more equitable distribution of income and greater investment in health and education compared to the military....Russia has over 3 million intravenous drug users and relatively expensive ART that help to fuel the HIV epidemic. The collapse of the USSR produced significant strain on the health of the people. Life expectancy in Russia fell 9 years following its transition to a market economy and there has been a significant rise in 'social diseases' of Tuberculosis (TB), HIV and Hepatitis. Intravenous drug use accounts for approximately 80% of those infected with HIV however recently a new phase of the epidemic has developed that is driven by sexual transmission. It is only since 2003 that there has been an increase in leadership and commitment at higher political levels to combat HIV and AIDS.

UNAIDS reported in 2002 that the number of overall infections in China increased 30% since 1998, with over 1 million people infected with HIV. It is feared that China may soon experience an explosive and widespread HIV epidemic. Intravenous drug use and the sharing of contaminated needles in the south and north-west of China was one mechanism of initial transmission. The other was unsafe practices among paid blood donors. Unsafe blood collections in the 1990s led to the appearance of HIV and subsequent AIDS deaths in China's central provinces. In response to this the Chinese authorities have recently announced that they are providing free ART in central provinces.

The first main focus of HIV in India was Mumbai where there is a large commercial sex work industry and the HIV prevalence reported amongst these workers is 50%. It is expected that HIV will become the largest cause of adult mortality in India in the coming decade. Despite the government making HIV its national topmost priority, any attempt to address the problem is hampered by its fractured health care infrastructure, poor literacy figures and widespread poverty. At the end of 2003 the Indian government began providing free ART in eight government hospitals with the plan to expand it to a total of 25 centres.

The aim of this paper was to attempt to dissect out the role of governance in the HIV pandemic. It is not possible yet to determine if the relationship seen represents correlation or causation. Even though this first analysis alludes to causation, for those 149 countries with UNAIDS HIV prevalence data, the relationship will become clearer over time when it is possible to compare nations that appear similar today. Currently Brazil and India have equivalent overall governance and HIV prevalence estimates at 0.8% and 0.7% respectively. However when other health and economic indices are examined it is clear that India . . . [invests] less than Brazil in health and education, has one quarter the number of physicians and double the MMR [maternal mortality rate]. The GDP-PPP per capita is three times greater in Brazil but it is more equitably distributed in India which is likely to contribute to equivalent life expectancy seen in both countries. India and Brazil are the main producers of generic ART. However Brazil, unlike India, has consistently provided strong political support for HIV/AIDS patients after the end of the military dictatorship in 1990. In 1996, the Brazilian government guaranteed by national law the permanent allocation of financial resources and universal access to care, including ART. The current disparities between India and Brazil's HIV treatment policy predicts that the Indian epidemic will progress more rapidly and is likely to impact on its development. . . .

HIV/AIDS control in Russia, China and India will only be possible if they follow the example set by Brazil. International institutions need to support national civil society groups within these nations to focus the attention and resources of their respective governments for progressive healthcare changes. The global plan to stop TB outlines the possibilities and challenges that will be faced treating chronic illness, such as HIV. It is pertinent that international health and financial institutions work together to influence change so that robust healthcare networks and responsive government are developed in order to apply best healthcare and economic practice.

The WHO goal of three million HIV positive persons being on ART by 2005 would be readily met if civil society in resource rich countries was able to precipitate progressive societal changes. Health is a fundamental human right, consequently each global institution, organization and citizen needs to work towards stable and progressive societal structures that can facilitate the provision of healthcare "access for all". The current HIV pandemic represents collective inaction and indifference towards global health. The promotion of good governance is a necessary step to enable national civil society to engineer long-term healthcare changes to deal with HIV/AIDS and future healthcare challenges.

Conclusion

Using World Bank governance data and UNAIDS HIV prevalence estimates for 2002 this paper tests the hypothesis "HIV prevalence is not associated with governance". Additional health and economic indices are used to highlight the development needs for each country. The accuracy of both governance and HIV prevalence estimates are discussed and some country comparisons are made. HIV prevalence is significantly associated with poor governance. International public health programs need to address societal structures in order to create strong foundations upon which effective healthcare interventions can be implemented.

In the article excerpted here, Menon-Johansson (2005) found that the prevalence of HIV is associated with poor governance in a significant manner and that corruption is one of the most influential aspects of governance. He recognized that the association might indicate merely correlation rather than causation, but stated that "this first analysis alludes to causation." Let's assume that Menon-Johansson's first analysis is correct. As a practical matter, how could corruption cause poor health status, such as a high rate of HIV prevalence?

One way in which corruption could reduce the health status of the population is by diverting resources from health programs and facilities. As discussed in the introduction to this chapter, many physicians in the public sector divert resources and time to treat patients on a private basis. Other types of diversion include the siphoning off of money by government officials or by the managers of health programs and facilities, as well as the theft of drugs and supplies. Theft of drugs is particularly harmful, because people in need of treatment often refrain from seeking care at public facilities that routinely have insufficient supplies of drugs (Lewis, 2006, p. 21). In cases of high-level corruption, some of the money designated for health programs may be sent out of the country to secret bank accounts owned by government officials or members of their families. Some government officials may require the payment of unofficial license fees, consulting fees, taxes, or customs duties, as conditions of developing or operating health programs in their country. In other situations, charges for construction of health facilities may be artificially inflated. These types of corruption harm the health of the population by making it more costly to develop, build, and operate health facilities and by leaving less money available to provide desperately needed health programs and services.

Another type of corruption involves increasing the costs that must be paid by patients, and thereby reducing access to care. One example of this type of corruption is the collection of informal fees, as discussed in detail in the first part of this chapter. Another example in this category is the payment of kickbacks from pharmaceutical companies to doctors for prescribing a company's drugs. At a superficial level, it might appear that these payments would not increase the costs to be paid by patients, because the payments are made by pharmaceutical companies rather than patients. However, these kickbacks often lead to supplier-induced demand, including the purchase of unnecessary and potentially harmful drugs. In addition, kickbacks might raise the cost of marketing drugs, and those cost increases might be passed on to the ultimate consumer. Similarly, when a vendor of equipment or supplies pays a bribe to the purchasing officer of a health care facility, as an inducement to make a purchase from that particular vendor, the bribe might ultimately result in higher prices to the health care facility and its patients. Bribes and kickbacks can also distort the competitive market and lead to the purchase of lower quality goods and services. In some countries, health workers need to pay bribes to obtain jobs or promotions in public health care facilities. As Lewis (2006) has pointed out, these practices lead to a "corruption spiral," because health workers who pay bribes need to obtain the money for their bribes from other people (p. 20).

Another way in which corruption can reduce the health status of the population is by increasing the level of instability in the country. Instability can lead to violence, with direct physical and emotional harm to individuals and their families. In addition, instability can displace large portions of the population, causing people to become refugees or internally displaced persons. Corruption and instability also encourage health workers to emigrate, thereby increasing the problem of brain drain, as discussed in Chapter Eleven. Finally, corruption can have an adverse effect on health status by reducing economic development in a country, which could in turn reduce the living standards of the population.

For all of these reasons, a strong case can be made that corruption reduces the health status of individuals and populations. What we should do about it is much less clear. Should international organizations and lenders, such as the World Bank, stop giving money or lending money to corrupt dictators and their governments? On a superficial level that approach might seem appropriate, but it would be tantamount to punishing the victims, the people who are already suffering from poverty as well as corruption. Perhaps the answer is to use some type of staged process with clear incentives, such as providing grants or loans in installments, with additional funds dependent on making progress in reducing corruption.

Menon-Johansson's article is a good first step toward understanding the problem of corruption and HIV prevalence. However, the article does not provide any specific methods to reduce the level of corruption and thereby reduce the prevalence of HIV and possibly other health problems.

How can nations and international organizations reduce the level of corruption, especially in developing and transitional countries? Although there is no simple solution, experts have identified several approaches that, taken together, could have a significant impact in reducing the level of corruption. These approaches include improving systems of management and accountability, creating incentives to encourage good performance and discourage corruption, and improving systems of regulation (Lewis, 2006, pp. 35–45; Ensor and Duran-Moreno, 2002, pp. 117–122). Improvements in the management and accountability of health systems include giving local managers the authority to hire, discipline, and fire workers in public health facilities, as well as implementing effective mechanisms of community oversight (Lewis, 2006, pp. 35–38). Although it may be costly to increase the salaries and benefits of health workers, such increases may help to limit the amount of corruption in the health system (Ensor and Duran-Moreno, 2002, pp. 117–118). Increasing the compensation of workers may reduce their need to spend time on other employment and may also reduce the perception of unfair treatment that leads workers to rationalize their corrupt behavior (Lewis, 2006, p. 36). Regulation and the rule of law are other important tools in the fight against corruption. As explained by Ensor and Duran-Moreno (2002), a "country that does not have a clear system of property rights, an independent legal system and an accountable public sector may produce more corruption opportunities than countries that do have these institutions" (p. 119). Regulation requires more than mere adoption of written laws and rules. Effective implementation requires the development of agencies with the authority, resources, and motivation to enforce the regulatory regime, as well as continuous training to build regulatory capacity.

Ensor and Duran-Moreno (2002) also recognized that efforts to eliminate corruption from a health system may require broader, cross-sector reforms, if the root cause is endemic corruption in the society as a whole (p. 117). In those circumstances, reducing corruption in the health system, as a way to improve health status, would necessarily be a long-term strategy. In the meantime it may be more useful to focus on other ways to reduce HIV prevalence and improve overall health status in countries that are extremely corrupt and likely to remain so for the foreseeable future.

Menon-Johansson (2005) arrives at this conclusion: "International public health programs need to address societal structures in order to create strong foundations upon which effective healthcare interventions can be implemented." That sounds inspirational and seems appropriate, but it raises a potentially controversial issue. On one hand it makes very good sense to say that reducing corruption, promoting the rule of law, and increasing regulatory capacity are necessary components of international public health programs. Those legal and regulatory issues are integral parts of the societal structures that public health programs need to address, and they should be recognized as important components of the public health agenda.

On the other hand we need to consider whether it is appropriate for international programs, which are run primarily by organizations outside developing countries, to work toward changing the societal structures in developing and transitional countries. Is that an appropriate role for international organizations such as the World Bank? Would addressing the societal structures in recipient countries amount to improper interference by foreign public health and development programs?

The alternative of working in cooperation with a local nongovernmental organization (NGO) would not necessarily resolve the ethical dilemma. Even if an international organization were working with a local NGO in trying to change the societal structures in a country, that international organization would nevertheless be assisting a relatively small minority in trying to change the society and the practices of the majority. If it is problematic from an ethical perspective for international organizations to change a local society, it may be just as problematic for international organizations to assist a local minority, such as a group of Western-educated professionals, in attempting to change that society and the practices of the majority.

This dilemma could be resolved by reconsidering what it means to address societal structures. Rather than reading the phrase *address societal structures* as meaning "attempt to change the local practices," we could interpret that phrase as meaning "be aware of and design around the practices and conditions of the local society." For example, assume that two methods exist to support improvements in the public health of a developing country. One method would pose a risk that a large share of the financial and material resources would be stolen or siphoned off, whereas the other method would make it much more likely that the resources would be used to benefit the health of the population. Under those circumstances, international public health programs could address the local society by being cognizant of local conditions and practices and by designing their support in ways that would maximize the benefit to the public.

Finally, Menon-Johansson's conclusion brings us back to an issue raised in the first chapter of this book with regard to the issue of universal values. Are there any universal values that transcend the cultural values and practices of particular societies? If good governance and the rule of law are indeed universal values, it would be ethical and appropriate for international organizations to assist in making changes to local societies, in order to reduce the level of corruption and improve the public health.

SUMMARY

Corruption can divert resources from health programs and facilities, increase the costs for patients, and reduce access to care. As explained in this chapter, a persuasive case can be made that corruption reduces the health of individuals and the public. This chapter described the widespread practice of paying informal fees to health care professionals, and analyzed the ethical implications of collecting those fees from patients and their families. This chapter also evaluated methods to reduce the level of health system corruption in general and the collection of informal fees in particular. These methods include improving systems of management and accountability, creating positive and negative incentives, and giving authority to local managers to remove health workers who continue to collect informal fees or violate other rules. It is also important to develop effective systems of regulation, including implementing rules and building capacity for regulation. Ultimately, the search for the best way to fight corruption raises another important question, which was addressed in Chapter One of this book: how can we best encourage individuals and organizations in the health system to *do the right thing*?

KEY TERMS

corruption

formalization of fees

informal payments

DISCUSSION QUESTIONS

1. Is it ethical for physicians to collect informal fees from their patients, if the total of official and unofficial fees collected by each physician is less than two times the average wage in the particular country?
2. What are the best ways to eliminate or reduce the collection of informal fees from patients and their families?
3. How could corruption reduce the health status of the population, such as causing or contributing to a high rate of HIV prevalence?
4. What are the most effective ways to reduce the level of corruption in a health system, especially in developing and transitional countries?

ACTIVITY: DEVELOPING A HOSPITAL PLAN TO STOP COLLECTION OF INFORMAL FEES FROM PATIENTS IN A DEVELOPING COUNTRY

The hospital we will call Peaceful Valley Hospital (PVH) is a 200-bed, acute-care general hospital in a developing country. PVH is the only hospital within a 150-mile radius, and it is the only source of hospital care for the people who reside in that area.

PVH is owned by the national Ministry of Health (MOH). All of the physicians, nurses, and other workers at the hospital are employees of PVH. There are five doctors at PVH, six nurses, and one guard. There are no other employees at PVH. Therefore, the one guard and six nurses are responsible for the cleaning and maintenance of the facility in addition to all of their other duties. The employees receive monthly salaries from PVH, but those salaries are extremely low. For example, the monthly salaries of doctors are less than the monthly income of taxi drivers in that country.

Under these circumstances, the doctors, nurses, and guard at the hospital routinely collect informal fees from patients or their families. Patients are not happy about paying those additional fees, but they understand that they must pay those fees to obtain hospital care.

The expenses and revenues for PVH are described in the following paragraphs. All monetary figures are in the local currency (the main unit is the "dollar"), and all the figures are stated on a monthly basis.

The salary for each of the five doctors is $1,000 per month, for a total of $5,000 per month for the doctors. The salary for each of the six nurses is $500 per month, for a total of $3,000 per month for the nurses. The one guard is paid $200 per month. Thus, the total salary expense at PVH is $8,200 per month.

Aside from the salary expense, supplies and utilities at PVH cost $1,800 per month. Finally, the national MOH provides $5,000 per month in administrative services for PVH. Carried out for PVH by personnel who work at MOH's central office in the capital city, these services include management, budgeting, accounting, human resources, purchasing, planning, and oversight. PVH is required to pay $5,000 per month to the national MOH for those central office services. Thus, the total expense to operate PVH is $15,000 per month ($8,200 for salaries, $1,800 for supplies and utilities, and $5,000 for central office services).

Each patient pays a fee to PVH. This fee was set by the government at a relatively low level in order to avoid creating a financial barrier to access. The patient fee is $10 per visit, regardless of the diagnosis, treatment, or length of stay. The fee is the same whether the patient is treated as an inpatient or outpatient. On average, 1,500 new patients are treated each month at PVH (approximately 50 new patients each day). So at $10 per patient, the formal patient fee yields $15,000 per month in revenue for PVH.

Each month, PVH uses the $15,000 in formal patient fees to pay its expense for salaries of $8,200, its expense for supplies and utilities of $1,800, and its expense for central office services by MOH of $5,000. The national MOH is not willing to reduce the cost of those central office services and is not willing to allow PVH to use any of that money for employee salaries. Moreover, PVH is required to use those central office services provided by MOH; it cannot decline those services. MOH cannot afford to provide any additional funds to PVH.

As stated previously, the doctors, nurses, and guard at the hospital routinely collect additional, informal fees from patients or their families. In order to get in the door and obtain an appointment, patients pay a fee of $1 to the guard at the entrance to the hospital. Patients pay an additional fee of $10 to a doctor for examination or treatment. Finally, they pay an additional fee of $4 to a nurse for items such as bedding, medications, and food. This amounts to a total of $15 per patient for informal fees, aside from the formal fee of $10 per patient.

At 1,500 new patients per month, the revenue from informal fees of $15 per patient equals $22,500 per month (1,500 patients × $15 = $22,500). The guard's share of this income from informal fees is $1,500 per month (1,500 patients × $1 = $1,500). The six nurses' share is $6,000 per month, which equals $1,000 for each nurse (1,500 patients × $4 = $6,000 ÷ 6 nurses = $1,000 per nurse).

The five doctors receive a total of $15,000 per month from these informal fees (1,500 patients × $10 = $15,000). However, this income is not divided equally among the five doctors. Some doctors treat more patients per day than other doctors, because they are willing to work harder or because patients think these doctors provide care of a higher quality. Therefore, some doctors receive more and some receive fewer informal fees. Unlike the nurses, the doctors do not pool their informal fees; rather each doctor keeps the informal fees that he or she receives from the patients.

In its latest plan for national health reform, MOH has decided that hospitals should stop the practice of collecting informal fees from patients or their families. MOH has directed each hospital to develop a written plan that will prohibit hospital employees from requesting or receiving any informal fees. However, MOH cannot afford to provide any additional funds to hospitals. Even after the reforms, MOH will continue to provide central office services for every hospital at the current monthly rate, and hospitals may not refuse to use those services. MOH is not willing to reduce the cost of those central office services, and will not allow hospitals to use any of that money for salaries of hospital employees.

As part of this reform, MOH is willing to allow each hospital to increase the formal fee that is charged to each patient. However, there is a risk that increasing the formal fees could create a financial barrier to access. Advocacy organizations have expressed their serious concerns about permitting hospitals to increase their formal patient fees. Meanwhile, doctors, nurses, and other hospital employees are very worried that their income will be reduced as a result of these changes.

Please develop a plan to stop the collection of informal fees from patients at PVH, without reducing the income of hospital employees and without increasing expenditures by the government. Indicate how you will divide the revenue from formal patient fees among the various doctors and other hospital employees. In addition, please be sure to include a way to enforce the prohibition against informal fees, so that patients will not be required to pay more under the new system than they now pay under the current system for the combination of formal and informal fees.

REFERENCES

Chapter One

Beauchamp, T., and Childress, J. *Principles of Biomedical Ethics.* (4th ed.) New York: Oxford University Press, 1994.

Beauchamp, T., and others (eds.). *Contemporary Issues in Bioethics.* (7th ed.) Belmont, Calif.: Thomson/Wadsworth, 2008.

Blackhall, L., and others. "Bioethics in a Different Tongue: The Case of Truth-Telling." *Journal of Urban Health*, 2001, *78*(1), 59–71.

Blocker, H. (ed.). *Ethics: An Introduction.* New York: Haven, 1986.

Brock, D. "Broadening the Bioethics Agenda." *Kennedy Institute of Ethics Journal*, 2000, *10*(1), 21–38.

Chen, J. *Chinese Law: Towards an Understanding of Chinese Law, Its Nature and Development.* The Hague, Netherlands: Kluwer Law International, 1999.

Illingworth, P., and Parmet, W. "The Ethical Implications of the Social Determinants of Health: A Global Renaissance for Bioethics." *Bioethics*, 2009, *23*(2), ii–v. Editorial.

Kilner, J. "Who Shall Be Saved? An African Answer." *The Hastings Center Report*, 1984, *14*(3), 18–22.

King, M. "Letter from Birmingham Jail" [originally titled "The Negro Is Your Brother"]. *The Atlantic*, 1963, *212*(2), 78–88. [http://www.theatlantic.com/ideastour/civil-rights/king-excerpt.mhtml]. (Accessed Jan. 31, 2010.)

Marshall, P., and Koenig, B. "Accounting for Culture in a Globalized Bioethics." *Journal of Law, Medicine & Ethics*, 2004, *32*(2), 252–266.

Shaw, W., and Barry, V. *Moral Issues in Business.* (5th ed.) Belmont, Calif.: Thomson/Wadsworth, 1992.

Steinbock, B., and others. *Ethical Issues in Modern Medicine.* (6th ed.) New York: McGraw Hill, 2003.

Chapter Two

Akabayashi, A., and Slingsby, B. "Informed Consent Revisited: Japan and the U.S." *American Journal of Bioethics*, 2006, *6*(1), 9–14.

Akabayashi, A., and others. "Family Consent, Communication, and Advance Directives for Cancer Disclosure: A Japanese Case and Discussion." *Journal of Medical Ethics*, 1999, *25*, 296–301.

American Medical Association. "Opinion 10.01: Fundamental Elements of the Patient-Physician Relationship." *Code of Medical Ethics*. June 1992. [http://www.ama-assn.org/ama/pub/ physician-resources/medical-ethics/code-medical-ethics/opinion1001.shtml]. (Accessed Jan. 30, 2010.)

Blackhall, L., and others. "Bioethics in a Different Tongue: The Case of Truth-Telling." *Journal of Urban Health*, 2001, *78*(1), 59–71.

Humayun, A., and others. "Patients' Perception and Actual Practice of Informed Consent, Privacy and Confidentiality in General Medical Outpatient Departments of Two Tertiary Care Hospitals of Lahore." *BMC Medical Ethics*, 2008, *9*(14). [http://www.biomedcentral.com/1472-6939/ 9/14]. (Accessed Jan. 30, 2010.)

Katz J. "Informed Consent—Must It Remain a Fairy Tale?" *Journal of Contemporary Health Law and Policy*, 1994, *10*, 69–91.

Marshall, P., and Koenig, B. "Accounting for Culture in a Globalized Bioethics." *Journal of Law, Medicine & Ethics*, 2004, *32*(2), 252–266.

Moazam, F., and Jafarey, A. "Pakistan and Biomedical Ethics: Report from a Muslim Country." *Cambridge Quarterly of Healthcare Ethics*, 2005, *14*, 249–255.

Pakistan Medical and Dental Council. *Code of Ethics for Medical and Dental Practitioners*. 2001. [http://www.pmdc.org.pk/Ethics/tabid/101/Default.aspx]. (Accessed Sept. 14, 2010.)

People's Republic of China. *Law of the People's Republic of China on Medical Practitioners*. June 26, 1999. [http://www.fdi.gov.cn/pub/FDI_EN/Laws/law_en_info.jsp?docid=50965]. (Accessed June 26, 2010.)

Rodriguez del Pozo, P., and Fins, J. "Islam and Informed Consent: Notes from Doha." *Cambridge Quarterly of Healthcare Ethics*, 2008, *17*, 273–279.

Sastry, J., and others. "Optimizing the HIV/AIDS Informed Consent Process in India." *BMC Medicine*, 2004, *2*(28). [http://www.biomedcentral.com/1741-7015/2/28]. (Accessed Jan. 30, 2010.)

Schloendorff v. *Society of New York Hospital*, 105 N.E. 92 (N.Y. 1914).

World Health Organization. *Health Systems: Improving Performance*. The World Health Report 2000. 2000. [http://www.who.int/whr/2000/en/whr00_en.pdf]. (Accessed Jan. 24, 2010.)

World Medical Association. *WMA International Code of Medical Ethics*. Oct. 2006. [http://www .wma.net/en/30publications/10policies/c8/index.html]. (Accessed Jan. 30, 2010.)

Wu, A., and others. "To Tell the Truth: Ethical and Practical Issues in Disclosing Medical Mistakes to Patients." *Journal of General Internal Medicine*, 1997, *12*(12), 770–775.

Yousuf, R. M., and others. "Awareness, Knowledge and Attitude Towards Informed Consent Among Doctors in Two Different Cultures in Asia: A Cross-Sectional Comparative Study in Malaysia and Kashmir, India." *Singapore Medical Journal*, 2007, *48*(6), 559–565.

Chapter Three

Albar, M. "Seeking Remedy, Abstaining from Therapy and Resuscitation: An Islamic Perspective." *Saudi Journal of Kidney Diseases and Transplantation*, 2007, *18*(4), 629–637.

American Medical Association. "Opinion 2.211—Physician-Assisted Suicide." *Code of Medical Ethics*. June 1994a. [http://www.ama-assn.org/ama/pub/physician-resources/medical-ethics/code-medical-ethics/opinion2211.shtml]. (Accessed Mar. 14, 2010.)

American Medical Association. "Opinion 2.215—Treatment Decisions for Seriously Ill Newborns." *Code of Medical Ethics*. June 1994b. [http://www.ama-assn.org/ama/pub/physician-resources/medical-ethics/code-medical-ethics/opinion2215.shtml]. (Accessed Mar. 14, 2010.)

American Medical Association. "Opinion 2.20—Withholding or Withdrawing Life-Sustaining Medical Treatment." *Code of Medical Ethics*. June 1996. [http://www.ama-assn.org/ama/pub/physician-resources/medical-ethics/code-medical-ethics/opinion220.shtml]. (Accessed Mar. 14, 2010.)

American Medical Association. "Opinion 2.037—Medical Futility in End-of-Life Care." *Code of Medical Ethics*. June 1997. [http://www.ama-assn.org/ama/pub/physician-resources/medical-ethics/code-medical-ethics/opinion2037.shtml]. (Accessed Mar. 14, 2010.)

American Medical Association. "Opinion 2.201—Sedation to Unconsciousness in End-of-Life Care." *Code of Medical Ethics*. June 2008. [http://www.ama-assn.org/ama/pub/physician-resources/medical-ethics/code-medical-ethics/opinion2201.shtml]. (Accessed Mar. 14, 2010.)

Arras, J. "Physician-Assisted Suicide: A Tragic View." *Journal of Contemporary Health Law and Policy*, 1997, *13*, 361–389.

Ball, D., and Mengewein, J. "Assisted-Suicide Pioneer Stirs a Legal Backlash." *Wall Street Journal*, Feb. 6, 2010, pp. A1, A10. [http://online.wsj.com/article/SB100014240527487 03414504575001363599545120.html]. (Accessed Mar. 14, 2010.)

Battin, M. "The Least Worst Death." *Hastings Center Report*, 1983, *13*(2), 13–16.

Beauchamp, T., and others (eds.). *Contemporary Issues in Bioethics*. (7th ed.) Belmont, Calif.: Thomson/Wadsworth, 2008.

Blackhall, L., and others. "Bioethics in a Different Tongue: The Case of Truth-Telling." *Journal of Urban Health*, 2001, *78*(1), 59–71.

Brasor, P. "No Brains When it Comes Down to Transplants." *Japan Times*, Aug. 2, 2009. [http://search.japantimes.co.jp/print/fd20090802pb.html]. (Accessed Mar. 14, 2010.)

Brody, H. "Withdrawing Versus Withholding Therapy: Still a Pernicious Distinction." *Journal of the American Geriatrics Society*, 1995, *43*(6), 716–717.

Callahan, D. "The Goals of Medicine: Setting New Priorities." *Hastings Center Report*, 1996, *26*(6), S1–S27.

Cortez, N. "Patients Without Borders: The Emerging Global Market for Patients and the Evolution of Modern Health Care." *Indiana Law Journal*, 2008, *83*, 71–132.

Dworkin, R. "Introduction." In R. Dworkin and others, "Assisted Suicide: The Philosophers' Brief." *New York Review of Books*, 1997, *44*(5), 41–47. [http://www.nybooks.com/articles/1237]. (Accessed Mar. 14, 2010.)

Fagerlin, A., and Schneider, C. "Enough: The Failure of the Living Will." *Hastings Center Report*, 2004, *34*(2), 30–42.

Graham, J. "Bishops Change Feeding Tube Guidelines." *Chicago Tribune*, Feb. 8, 2010. [http://www.chicagotribune.com/health/ct-met-catholic-hospitals-20100208,0,3456275.story]. (Accessed Mar. 14, 2010.)

Johnson, K. "Montana Ruling Bolsters Doctor-Assisted Suicide." *New York Times*, Dec. 31, 2009. [http://www.nytimes.com/2010/01/01/us/01suicide.html]. (Accessed Mar. 14, 2010.)

Lanre-Abass, B. "Recommending Euthanasia for a Developing Country." *Eubios Journal of Asian and International Bioethics*, 2008, *18*(5), 152–157.

Löfmark, R., and others. "Physicians' Experiences with End-of-Life Decision-Making: Survey in 6 European Countries and Australia." *BMC Medicine*, 2008, *6*(4). [http://www.biomedcentral .com/1741-7015/6/4]. (Accessed Mar. 14, 2010.)

Miljeteig, I., and Norheim, O. "My Job Is to Keep Him Alive, But What About His Brother and Sister? How Indian Doctors Experience Ethical Dilemmas in Neonatal Medicine." *Developing World Bioethics*, 2006, *6*(1), 23–32.

Pickett, J. "Can Legalization Improve End-of-Life Care? An Empirical Analysis of the Results of the Legalization of Euthanasia and Physician-Assisted Suicide in the Netherlands and Oregon." *The Elder Law Journal*, 2009, *16*(2), 333–373.

Quill, T., and Brody, R. "You Promised Me I Wouldn't Die Like This: A Bad Death as a Medical Emergency." *Archives of Internal Medicine*, 1995, *155*, 1250–1254.

Rebagliato, M., and others. "Neonatal End-of-Life Decision Making: Physicians' Attitudes and Relationship with Self-Reported Practices in 10 European Countries." *JAMA*, 2000, *284*(19), 2451–2459.

"Recognition of Brain Death." Editorial. *Japan Times*, June 20, 2009. [http://search.japantimes .co.jp/cgi-bin/ed20090620a1.html]. (Accessed Mar. 14, 2010.)

Searight, H., and Gafford, J. "Cultural Diversity at the End of Life: Issues and Guidelines for Family Physicians." *American Family Physician*, 2005, *71*(3), 515–522.

Stevens, L., and others. "Palliative Care." *JAMA*, 2006, *296*(11), 1428.

Sulmasy, D., and Sugarman, J. "Are Withholding and Withdrawing Therapy Always Morally Equivalent?" *Journal of Medical Ethics*, 1994, *20*, 218–224.

Teno, J. "Advance Directives: Time to Move On." *Annals of Internal Medicine*, 2004, *141*(2), 159–160.

Truog, R. "Brain Death: Too Flawed to Endure, Too Ingrained to Abandon." *Journal of Law, Medicine & Ethics*, 2007, *35*(2), 273–281.

Tucker, K., and Steele, F. "Patient Choice at the End of Life: Getting the Language Right." *Journal of Legal Medicine*, 2007, *28*, >305–325.

United States Conference of Catholic Bishops. *Ethical and Religious Directives for Catholic Health Care Services*. (5th ed.) Nov. 2009. [http://www.usccb.org/meetings/2009Fall/docs/ERDs_5th_ed_ 091118_FINAL.pdf]. (Accessed Mar. 14, 2010.)

World Medical Association. *WMA Statement on Physician-Assisted Suicide*. May 2005. [http://www .wma.net/en/30publications/10policies/p13/index.html]. (Accessed Mar. 14, 2010.)

Yardley, W. "First Death for Washington Assisted-Suicide Law." *New York Times*, May 22, 2009. [http://www.nytimes.com/2009/05/23/us/23suicide.html]. (Accessed Mar. 14, 2010.)

Chapter Four

American College of Obstetricians and Gynecologists Committee on Ethics. *The Limits of Conscientious Refusal in Reproductive Medicine: ACOG Committee Opinion No. 385*. Nov. 2007. [http://www.acog.org/from_home/publications/ethics/co385.pdf]. (Accessed Jan. 10, 2010.)

Cantor, J. "Conscientious Objection Gone Awry—Restoring Selfless Professionalism in Medicine." *New England Journal of Medicine*, 2009, *360*(15), 1484–1485.

Catholics Bishops Conference of the Philippines. *Standing Up for the Gospel of Life: CBCP Pastoral Statement on Reproductive Health Bill*. Nov. 2008. [http://www.cbcponline.net/documents/2000s/html/2008-STANDING%20UP%20FOR%20THE%20GOSPEL%20OF%20LIFE.html]. (Accessed Jan. 10, 2010.)

Centers for Disease Control and Prevention. *Assisted Reproductive Technology (ART)*. Feb. 18, 2010. [http://www.cdc.gov/ART/]. (Accessed Sept. 14, 2010.)

Diniz, D., and others. "Reproductive Health Ethics: Latin American Perspectives." *Developing World Bioethics*, 2007, *7*(2), ii–iv.

Ethics Committee of the American Society for Reproductive Medicine. "Donating Spare Embryos for Stem Cell Research." *Fertility and Sterility*, 2009, *91*(3), 667–670.

John Paul II. *Evangelium Vitae: On the Value and Inviolability of Human Life*. 1995. [http://www.vatican.va/edocs/ENG0141/_PQ.HTM]. (Accessed Jan. 10, 2010.)

Kluge, E. "Female Circumcision: When Medical Ethics Confronts Cultural Values." *Canadian Medical Association Journal*, 1993, *148*(2), 288–289.

LaFleur, W. "Contestation and Consensus: The Morality of Abortion in Japan." *Philosophy East & West*, 1990, *40*(4), 529–542.

LaFleur, W. "Silences and Censures: Abortion, History, and Buddhism in Japan: A Rejoinder to George Tanabe." *Japanese Journal of Religious Studies*, 1995, *22*(1–2), 185–196.

Larijani, B., and Zahedi, F. "Changing Parameters for Abortion in Iran." *Indian Journal of Medical Ethics*, 2006, *3*(4), 130–131.

"Minnesota's Muslim Cab Drivers Face Crackdown." *Thomson Reuters/Reuters.Com*, Apr. 17, 2007. [http://www.reuters.com/article/idusn1633289220070417]. (Accessed Jan. 10, 2010.)

Mohr, J. *Abortion in America: The Origins and Evolution of National Policy, 1800–1900*. New York: Oxford University Press, 1979.

Phillips, K. "As a Matter of Faith, Biden Says Life Begins at Conception." *New York Times*, Sept. 7, 2008. [http://www.nytimes.com/2008/09/08/us/politics/08campaign.html]. (Accessed Jan. 10, 2010.)

President. Memorandum of January 23, 2009. "Mexico City Policy and Assistance for Voluntary Population Planning." *Federal Register* 74, no. 17 (Jan. 28, 2009), 4903–4904.

Roe v. *Wade*, 410 U.S. 113 (1973).

Sandel, M. "The Case Against Perfection: What's Wrong with Designer Children, Bionic Athletes, and Genetic Engineering." *The Atlantic Monthly*, Apr. 2004, 51–62.

Sherwin, S. *No Longer Patient: Feminist Ethics and Health Care*. Philadelphia: Temple University Press, 1992.

Syahlul, D., and Amir, L. "Do Indonesian Medical Practitioners Approve the Availability of Emergency Contraception over-the-Counter? A Survey of General Practitioners and Obstetricians in Jakarta." *BMC Women's Health*, 2005, *5*(3). [http://www.biomedcentral.com/1472-6874/5/3]. (Accessed Jan. 10, 2010.)

Tanabe, G. "Review: William R. LaFleur, *Liquid Life: Abortion and Buddhism in Japan*." *Japanese Journal of Religious Studies*, 1994, *21*(4), 437–440.

Tanabe, G. "Sounds and Silences: A Counterresponse." *Japanese Journal of Religious Studies*, 1995, *22*(1–2), 197–200.

Thomson, J. "A Defense of Abortion." *Philosophy and Public Affairs*, 1971, *1*(1), 47–66.

U.K. National Health Service. "NHS Choices: Emergency Contraception." 2009. [http://www.nhs.uk/Conditions/Emergency-contraception/Pages/Introduction.aspx]. (Accessed Jan. 10, 2010.)

United States Conference of Catholic Bishops. *Reproductive Technology (Evaluation & Treatment of Infertility) Guidelines for Catholic Couples.* 2009. [http://www.usccb.org/LifeGivingLove/Reproductive-Technology-Guidelines.pdf]. (Accessed Jan. 10, 2010.)

U.S. Department of Health and Human Services. "Ensuring That Department of Health and Human Services Funds Do Not Support Coercive or Discriminatory Policies or Practices in Violation of Federal Law." Proposed Rule. *Federal Register 73*, no. 166 (Aug. 26, 2008), 50274–50285.

U.S. Food and Drug Administration. *Highlights of Prescribing Information.* 2009. [http://www.accessdata.fda.gov/drugsatfda_docs/label/2009/021998lbl.pdf]. (Accessed Jan. 10, 2010.)

Verlinsky, Y., and others. "Preimplantation Diagnosis for Fanconi Anemia Combined with HLA Matching." *JAMA*, 2001, *285*(24), 3130–3133.

World Medical Association. *Declaration on Therapeutic Abortion.* 2006. [http://www.wma.net/en/30publications/10policies/a1/index.html]. (Accessed Jan. 10, 2010.)

Chapter Five

Althaus, F. "Female Circumcision: Rite of Passage or Violation of Rights?" *International Family Planning Perspectives*, 1997, *23*(3), 130–134. [http://www.guttmacher.org/pubs/journals/2313097.html]. (Accessed Jan. 25, 2010.)

Center for Reproductive Rights. "Legislation on Female Genital Mutilation in the United States." Briefing Paper. Nov. 2004. [http://reproductiverights.org/sites/crr.civicactions.net/files/documents/pub_bp_fgmlawsusa.pdf]. (Accessed Jan. 26, 2010.)

Center for Reproductive Rights. "Female Genital Mutilation (FGM): Legal Prohibitions Worldwide." Fact Sheet. 2009. [http://reproductiverights.org/en/document/female-genital-mutilation-fgm-legal-prohibitions-worldwide]. (Accessed Sept. 14, 2010.)

Criminalization of Female Genital Mutilation Act of 1996. U.S. Code 18 (2006), § 116.

Egyptian National Council for Childhood and Motherhood. "Cairo Declaration for the Elimination of FGM." Paper presented at the Afro-Arab Expert Consultation "Legal Tools for the Prevention of Female Genital Mutilation," Cairo, Egypt, June 2003. [http://www.childinfo.org/files/fgmc_Cairodeclaration.pdf]. (Accessed Jan. 26, 2010.)

Egyptian National Council for Childhood and Motherhood. *Cairo Declaration on FGM +5: High Level Meeting.* 2008. [http://www.npwj.org/No+Peace+Without+Justice/Female+Genital+Mutilation/History/Cairo+2008/Background]. (Accessed Jan. 26, 2010.)

El Guindi, F. "Had *This* Been Your Face, Would You Leave It as It Is? Female Circumcision Among the Nubians of Egypt." In R. Abusharaf (ed.), *Female Circumcision: Multicultural Perspectives.* Philadelphia: University of Pennsylvania Press, 2006. [http://books.google.com/books?id=t2vMxOzujlQC&pg=PA1&lpg=PA1&dq=Female+Circumcision+by+Abusharaf,+Rogaia+Mustafa&source=bl&ots=BrfIwhnKkg&sig=SnJ4QT8fHPkhctQl9kVbpVMiCgs&hl=en&ei=5pBkSt-BGtORtgfH3OX7Dw&sa=X&oi=book_result&ct=result&resnum=2]. (Accessed Jan. 26, 2010.)

Fam, M. "How a Muslim Cleric Rattles Cairo." *Wall Street Journal*, Oct. 19, 2007, p. A8.

Female Genital Mutilation Act. London: Her Majesty's Stationary Office, 2003.

Gibeau, A. "Female Genital Mutilation: When a Cultural Practice Generates Clinical and Ethical Dilemmas." *Journal of Obstetric, Gynecologic & Neonatal Nursing*, 1998, *27*(1), 85–91.

Hellsten, S. "From Human Wrongs to Universal Rights: Communication and Feminist Challenges for the Promotion of Women's Health in the Third World." *Developing World Bioethics*, 2001, *1*(2), 98–115.

Kaplan-Marcusan, A., and others. "Perception of Primary Health Professionals About Female Genital Mutilation: From Healthcare to Intercultural Competence." *BMC Health Services Research*, 2009. [http://www.biomedcentral.com/1472-6963/9/11]. (Accessed Sept. 14, 2010.)

Kluge, E. "Female Circumcision: When Medical Ethics Confronts Cultural Values." *Canadian Medical Association Journal*, 1993, *148*(2), 288–289.

Schroeder, P. "Female Genital Mutilation—A Form of Child Abuse." Editorial. *New England Journal of Medicine*, 1994, *331*(11), 739–740.

Schwartz, R. "Multiculturalism, Medicine, and the Limits of Autonomy: The Practice of Female Circumcision." *Cambridge Quarterly of Healthcare Ethics*, 1994, *3*(3), 431–441.

Toubia, N. "Female Circumcision as a Public Health Issue." *New England Journal of Medicine*, 1994, *331*(11), 712–716 (with correction).

Toubia, N. "Female Circumcision." Correspondence. *New England Journal of Medicine*, 1995, *332*(3), 188–190.

Turillazzi, E., and Fineschi, V. "Female Genital Mutilation: The Ethical Impact of the New Italian Law." *Journal of Medical Ethics*, 2007, *33*(2), 98–101.

World Health Organization. *Islamic Ruling on Male and Female Circumcision*. Alexandria, Egypt: World Health Organization Regional Office for the Eastern Mediterranean, 1996.

World Health Organization. *Eliminating Female Genital Mutilation: An Interagency Statement*. 2008. [http://www.unfpa.org/upload/lib_pub_file/756_filename_fgm.pdf]. (Accessed Jan. 26, 2010.)

World Medical Association, *The World Medical Association Statement on Female Genital Mutilation*. 2005. [http://www.wma.net/en/30publications/10policies/c10/index.html]. (Accessed Jan. 26, 2010.)

Chapter Six

Abdullahi v. *Pfizer, Inc.* 562 F.3d 163 (2d Cir. 2009).

Ballantyne, A. "Benefits to Research Subjects in International Trials: Do They Reduce Exploitation or Increase Undue Inducement?" *Developing World Bioethics*, 2008, *8*(3), 178–191.

Benatar, S. "Commentary: Justice and Medical Research: A Global Perspective." *Bioethics*, 2001, *15*(4), 333–340.

Brandt, A. "Racism and Research: The Case of the Tuskegee Syphilis Study." *Hastings Center Report*, 1978, *8*(6), 21–29. [http://www.jstor.org/pss/3561468]. (Accessed Jan. 30, 2010.)

Cha, A. "AIDS Drug Trial Turned Away: Protests by Prostitutes in Cambodia Ended Tenofovir Testing." *Washington Post*, May 23, 2006. [http://www.washingtonpost.com/wp-dyn/content/article/2006/05/22/AR2006052201190_pf.html]. (Accessed Jan. 30, 2010.)

Childress, J., and others (eds.). *Belmont Revisited: Ethical Principles for Research with Human Subjects*. Washington, D.C.: Georgetown University Press, 2005.

Christakis, N. "The Ethical Design of an AIDS Vaccine Trial in Africa." *Hastings Center Report*, 1988, *18*(3), 31–37.

Council for International Organizations of Medical Sciences. "International Ethical Guidelines for Biomedical Research Involving Human Subjects." 2002. [http://www.cioms.ch/frame_guidelines_nov_2002.htm]. (Accessed Jan. 30, 2010.)

Dalton, R. "Trauma Trials Leave Ethicists Uneasy." *Nature*, 2006, *440*(7083), 390–392.

Epstein, R. "The Erosion of Individual Autonomy in Medical Decisionmaking: Of the FDA and IRBs." *Georgetown Law Journal*, 2008, *96*, 559–582.

Frimpong-Mansoh, A. "Culture and Voluntary Informed Consent in African Health Care Systems." *Developing World Bioethics*, 2008, *8*(2), 104–114.

Hawkins, J. "Justice and Placebo Controls." *Social Theory and Practice*, 2006, *32*(3), 467–496.

Hyder, A., and Wali, S. "Informed Consent and Collaborative Research: Perspectives from the Developing World." *Developing World Bioethics*, 2006, *6*(1), 33–40.

Hyman, D. "Institutional Review Boards: Is This the Least Worst We Can Do?" *Northwestern University Law Review*, 2007, *101*(2), 749–774.

Kao Tha and others. "The Tenofovir Trial Controversy in Cambodia: Can a Trial Be Considered Ethical If There Is No Long-Term Post-Trial Care?" *Research for Sex Work*, 2004, *7*, 10–11.

Lie, R., and others. "The Standard of Care Debate: The Declaration of Helsinki Versus the International Consensus Opinion." *Journal of Medical Ethics*, 2004, *30*(2), 190–193.

Lurie, P., and Wolfe, S. "Unethical Trials of Interventions to Reduce Perinatal Transmission of the Human Immunodeficiency Virus in Developing Countries." *New England Journal of Medicine*, 1997, *337*(12), 853–856.

Oduro, A., and others. "Understanding and Retention of the Informed Consent Process Among Parents in Rural Northern Ghana." *BMC Medical Ethics*, 2008, *9*(12). [http://www.biomedcentral.com/1472-6939/9/12]. (Accessed Jan. 30, 2010.)

Pfizer, Inc. "Pfizer Responds to Divided Ruling by U.S. Court of Appeals for 2nd Circuit in Cases Related to Trovan Study in Nigeria." *Pfizer News*, Jan. 30, 2009.

Schüklenk, U. "The Standard of Care Debate: Against the Myth of an 'International Consensus Opinion.'" *Journal of Medical Ethics*, 2004, *30*(2), 194–197.

Shapiro, H., and Meslin, E. "Ethical Issues in the Design and Conduct of Clinical Trials in Developing Countries." *New England Journal of Medicine*, 2001, *345*(2), 139–142.

Stephens, J. "Panel Faults Pfizer in '96 Clinical Trial in Nigeria: Unapproved Drug Tested on Children." *Washington Post*, May 7, 2006, p. A01. [http://www.washingtonpost.com/wp-dyn/content/article/2006/05/06/AR2006050601338.html]. (Accessed Jan. 30, 2010.)

U.S. Food and Drug Administration. *Code of Federal Regulations* 21, § 312.120 and 314.106 (2009).

U.S. Government Accountability Office. *Human Subjects Research: Undercover Tests Show the Institutional Review Board System Is Vulnerable to Unethical Manipulation.* Testimony before the Subcommittee on Oversight and Investigations, Committee on Energy and Commerce, House of Representatives. Washington, D.C.: U.S. Government Printing Office, 2009.

U.S. National Commission for the Protection of Human Subjects of Biomedical and Behavioral Research. *The Belmont Report: Ethical Principles and Guidelines for the Protection of Human Subjects of Research.* Apr. 18, 1979. [http://www.hhs.gov/ohrp/humansubjects/guidance/belmont.htm]. (Accessed Jan. 30, 2010.)

Weijer, C., and LeBlanc, G. "The Balm of Gilead: Is the Provision of Treatment to Those Who Seroconvert in HIV Prevention Trials a Matter of Moral Obligation or Moral Negotiation?" *Journal of Law, Medicine & Ethics*, 2006, *34*(3), 793–808.

World Medical Association. *Declaration of Helsinki: Ethical Principles for Medical Research Involving Human Subjects.* Ferney-Voltaire, France: World Medical Association, Oct. 2000.

World Medical Association. *Declaration of Helsinki: Ethical Principles for Medical Research Involving Human Subjects.* Ferney-Voltaire, France: World Medical Association, Oct. 2001.

World Medical Association. *Declaration of Helsinki: Ethical Principles for Medical Research Involving Human Subjects.* Ferney-Voltaire, France: World Medical Association, Oct. 2004.

World Medical Association. *Declaration of Helsinki: Ethical Principles for Medical Research Involving Human Subjects.* Oct. 2008. [http://www.wma.net/en/30publications/10policies/b3/index.html]. (Accessed Jan. 30, 2010.)

Zywicki, T., "Institutional Review Boards as Academic Bureaucracies: An Economic and Experiential Analysis." *Northwestern University Law Review*, 2007, *101*(2), 861–896.

Chapter Seven

Abbott, F., and Van Puymbroeck, R. *Compulsory Licensing for Public Health: A Guide and Model Documents for Implementation of the Doha Declaration Paragraph 6 Decision.* Washington, D.C.: World Bank, 2005.

Alexander, C., and Wynia, M. "Ready and Willing? Physicians' Sense of Preparedness for Bioterrorism." *Health Affairs*, 2003, *22*(5), 189–197.

American Medical Association. "Opinion 10.01—Fundamental Elements of the Patient-Physician Relationship." *Code of Medical Ethics.* 1993. [http://www.ama-assn.org/ama/pub/physician-resources/medical-ethics/code-medical-ethics/opinion1001.shtml]. (Accessed Jan. 24, 2010.)

American Medical Association. "Opinion 9.065—Caring for the Poor." *Code of Medical Ethics.* June 1994. [http://www.ama-assn.org/ama/pub/physician-resources/medical-ethics/code-medical-ethics/opinion9065.shtml]. (Accessed Jan. 24, 2010.)

American Medical Association. *Principles of Medical Ethics.* June 2001. [http://www.ama-assn.org/ama/pub/physician-resources/medical-ethics/code-medical-ethics/principles-medical-ethics.shtml]. (Accessed Jan. 24, 2010.)

American Medical Association. "Opinion 10.05—Potential Patients." *Code of Medical Ethics.* Dec. 2003. [http://www.ama-assn.org/ama/pub/physician-resources/medical-ethics/code-medical-ethics/opinion1005.shtml]. (Accessed Jan. 24, 2010.)

American Medical Association. "Opinion 9.067—Physician Obligation in Disaster Preparedness and Response." *Code of Medical Ethics.* Dec. 2004. [http://www.ama-assn.org/ama/pub/physician-resources/medical-ethics/code-medical-ethics/opinion9067.shtml]. (Accessed Jan. 24, 2010.)

Arras, J., and Fenton, E. "Bioethics & Human Rights: Access to Health-Related Goods." *Hastings Center Report*, 2009, *39*(5), 27–38.

Balicer, R., and others. "Local Public Health Workers' Perceptions Toward Responding to an Influenza Pandemic." *BMC Public Health*, 2006, *6*(99). [http://www.biomedcentral.com/content/pdf/1471-2458-6-99.pdf]. (Accessed Jan. 23, 2010.)

Barr, H., and others. "Ethical Planning for an Influenza Pandemic." *Clinical Medicine*, 2008, *8*(1), 49–52.

Brody, B. "Why the Right to Health Care Is Not a Useful Concept for Policy Debates." In T. Bole III and W. Bondeson (eds.), *Rights to Health Care*. Philosophy and Medicine, vol. 38. Dordrecht: Springer Netherlands, 1991.

Cohen, J. "AIDS Drugs: Brazil, Thailand Override Big Pharma Patents." *Science*, 2007, *316*, 816.

Daniels, N. "Is There a Right to Health Care, and, If So, What Does It Encompass?" In H. Kuhse and P. Singer (eds.), *A Companion to Bioethics*. Oxford, U.K.: Blackwell, 1998.

Emanuel, E. "The Lessons of SARS." *Annals of Internal Medicine*, 2003, *139*(7), 589–591.

Ensor, T., and Duran-Moreno, A. "Corruption as a Challenge to Effective Regulation in the Health Sector." In R. Saltman and others (eds.), *Regulating Entrepreneurial Behavior in European Health Care Systems*. 2002. [http://www.euro.who.int/document/e74487.pdf]. (Accessed Jan. 23, 2010.)

Epstein, R. *Mortal Peril: Our Inalienable Right to Health Care?* Reading, Mass.: Addison-Wesley, 1997.

Fox, E. "Thou Shall Not Stand Idly By: Health Care Is a Human Right." *Bridges: A Jewish Feminist Journal*, 2006, *11*(1), 7–17.

Giesen, D. "A Right to Health Care: A Comparative Perspective." In A. Grubb and M. Mehlmann (eds.), *Justice and Health Care: Comparative Perspectives*. New York: Wiley, 1995.

Heins, V. "Human Rights, Intellectual Property, and Struggles for Recognition." *Human Rights Review*, 2008, *9*(2), 213–232.

Norheim, O. "Rights to Specialized Health Care in Norway: A Normative Perspective." *Journal of Law, Medicine & Ethics*, 2005, *33*(4), 641–649.

O'Neill, O. "The Dark Side of Human Rights." *International Affairs*, 2005, *81*(2), 427–439.

President's Commission for the Study of Ethical Problems in Medicine and Biomedical and Behavioral Research. *Securing Access to Health Care: The Ethical Implications of Differences in the Availability of Health Services*: Vol. 1. *Report*. 1983. [http://bioethics.georgetown.edu/pcbe/reports/past_commissions/securing_access.pdf]. (Accessed Aug. 19, 2010.)

Priester, R. "A Values Framework for Health System Reform." *Health Affairs*, 1992, *11*(1), 84–107.

Ruderman, C., and others. "On Pandemics and the Duty to Care: Whose Duty? Who Cares?" *BMC Medical Ethics*, 2006, *7*(5). [http://www.biomedcentral.com/1472-6939/7/5]. (Accessed Jan. 24, 2010.)

Sade, R. "Medical Care as a Right: A Refutation." In R. Veatch (ed.), *Cross-Cultural Perspectives in Medical Ethics*. (2nd ed.) Sudbury, Mass.: Jones and Bartlett, 2000.

Sade, R. "Ethical Foundations of Health Care System Reform." *Annals of Thoracic Surgery*, 2007, *84*, 1429–1431. [http://ats.ctsnetjournals.org/cgi/content/full/84/5/1429]. (Accessed Jan. 24, 2010.)

Schüklenk, U. "The Standard of Care Debate: Against the Myth of an 'International Consensus Opinion.'" *Journal of Medical Ethics*, 2004, *30*(2), 194–197.

Sherwin, S. *No Longer Patient*. Philadelphia: Temple University Press, 1992.

Steinbrook, R. "Controlling Conflict of Interest—Proposals from the Institute of Medicine." *New England Journal of Medicine*, 2009, *360*(21), 2160–2163.

Thompson, A., and others. "Pandemic Influenza Preparedness: An Ethical Framework to Guide Decision-Making." *BMC Medical Ethics*, 2006, *7*(12). [http://www.biomedcentral.com/content/pdf/1472-6939-7-12.pdf]. (Accessed Jan. 24, 2010.)

Toebes, B. "Towards an Improved Understanding of the International Human Right to Health." *Human Rights Quarterly*, 1999, *21*(3), 661–679.

Torda, A. "Ethical Issues in Pandemic Planning." *Medical Journal of Australia*, 2006, *185*(10), S73–S76.

United Nations. *Universal Declaration of Human Rights*. 1948. [http://www.un.org/en/documents/udhr/index.shtml#a25]. (Accessed Jan. 24, 2010.)

World Health Organization. *Constitution of the World Health Organization.* 1946. [http://www.searo.who .int/LinkFiles/About_SEARO_const.pdf]. (Accessed Jan. 23, 2010.)

World Health Organization. *Health Systems: Improving Performance.* The World Health Report 2000. 2000. [http://www.who.int/whr/2000/en/whr00_en.pdf]. (Accessed Jan. 24, 2010.)

World Health Organization. *Ethical Considerations in Developing a Public Health Response to Pandemic Influenza.* Epidemic and Pandemic Alert and Response Report. 2007. [http://www.who.int/ csr/resources/publications/WHO_CDS_EPR_GIP_2007_2c.pdf]. (Accessed Jan. 24, 2010.)

Zuger, A., and Miles, S. "Physicians, AIDS, and Occupational Risk: Historic Traditions and Ethical Obligations." *JAMA*, 1987, *258*(14), 1924–1928.

Zywicki, T. "Institutional Review Boards as Academic Bureaucracies: An Economic and Experiential Analysis." *Northwestern University Law Review*, 2007, *101*(2), 861–896.

Chapter Eight

Aaron, H., and others. *Can We Say No? The Challenge of Rationing Health Care.* Washington, D.C.: Brookings Institution Press, 2005.

Avorn, J. "Debate About Funding Comparative-Effectiveness Research." *New England Journal of Medicine*, 2009, *360*(19), 1927–1929.

Brock, D. "Ethical Issues in the Use of Cost Effectiveness Analysis for the Prioritisation of Health Care Resources." In S. Anand and others (eds.), *Public Health, Ethics, and Equity.* New York: Oxford University Press, 2004.

Chalkidou, K., and others. "Comparative Effectiveness Research and Evidence-Based Health Policy: Experience from Four Countries." *Milbank Quarterly*, 2009, *87*(2), 339–367.

Cheng, M. "British Agency Makes Tough Choices on Costly Drugs." *Washington Post*, May 26, 2009. [http://www.washingtonpost.com/wp-dyn/content/article/2009/05/22/AR20090522023- 70.html]. (Accessed Jan. 24, 2010.)

Connolly, C. "Comparison Shopping for Medicine." *Washington Post*, Mar. 17, 2009, p. A02. [http:// www.washingtonpost.com/wp-dyn/content/article/2009/03/16/AR2009031602913.html]. (Accessed Jan. 24, 2010.)

Cutler, D. "The Lifetime Costs and Benefits of Medical Technology." *Journal of Health Economics*, 2007, *26*, 1081–1100.

Drummond, M. "Challenges in the Economic Evaluation of Orphan Drugs." *Eurohealth*, 2008, *14*(2), 16–17.

Freeman, V., and others. "Lying for Patients: Physician Deception of Third-Party Payers." *Archives of Internal Medicine*, 1999, *159*(19), 2263–2270.

Garber, A., and Tunis, S. "Does Comparative Effectiveness Research Threaten Personalized Medicine?" *New England Journal of Medicine*, 2009, *360*(19), 1925–1927.

Jamison, D., and others (eds.). *Priorities in Health.* Washington, D.C.: World Bank, 2006.

Kilner, J. "Who Shall Be Saved? An African Answer." *The Hastings Center Report*, 1984, *14*(3), 18–22.

Maynard, A. "Rationing Health Care: An Exploration." *Health Policy*, 1999, *49*, 5–11.

McGuire, A., and others. "Pricing Pharmaceuticals: Value Based Pricing in What Sense?" *Eurohealth*, 2008, *14*(2), 3–6.

Morreim, E. "Fiscal Scarcity and the Inevitability of Bedside Budget Balancing." *Archives of Internal Medicine*, 1989, *149*, 1012–1015.

National Institute for Health and Clinical Excellence. *NICE Draft Recommendation on the Use of Drugs for Renal Cancer*. Press Release 2009/009. 2009. [http://www.nice.org.uk/media/420/AD/2009009DraftNICEGuidanceDrugsRenalCancerv2.pdf].(Accessed Jan. 24, 2010.)

Newdick, C. "Accountability for Rationing—Theory into Practice." *Journal of Law, Medicine & Ethics*, 2005, *33*(4), 660–669.

Owen-Smith, A., and others. " 'I Can See Where They're Coming from, But When You're on the End of It . . . You Just Want to Get the Money and the Drug': Explaining Reactions to Explicit Healthcare Rationing." *Social Science & Medicine*, 2009, *68*, 1935–1942.

Persad, G., and others. "Ethical Criteria for Allocating Health-Care Resources—Authors' Reply." *Lancet*, 2009a, *373*(9673), 1425–1426.

Persad, G., and others. "Principles for Allocation of Scarce Medical Interventions." *Lancet*, 2009b, *373*(9661), 423–431.

President's Commission for the Study of Ethical Problems in Medicine and Biomedical and Behavioral Research. *Securing Access to Health Care: The Ethical Implications of Differences in the Availability of Health Services*: Vol. 1. *Report*. 1983. [http://bioethics.georgetown.edu/pcbe/reports/past_commissions/securing_access.pdf]. (Accessed Aug. 19, 2010.)

Rawlins, M., and Culyer, A. "National Institute for Clinical Excellence and Its Value Judgments." *BMJ*, 2004, *329*(7459), 224–227.

Rosen, S., and others. "Rationing Antiretroviral Therapy for HIV/AIDS in Africa: Choices and Consequences." *PLoS Medicine*, 2005, *2*(11), 1098–1104 (e303).

Sage Crossroads. "Should Age Count in Allocating Health Care Resources? Debate Between Daniel Callahan and Christine Cassell." July 10, 2003. [http://www.sagecrossroads.net/webcast06]. (Accessed Jan. 24, 2010.)

Sanders, D., and Dukeminier, J. "Medical Advance and Legal Lag: Hemodialysis and Kidney Transplantation." *UCLA Law Review*, 1968, *15*, 357–413.

Starfield, B., and others. "Contribution of Primary Care to Health Systems and Health." *Milbank Quarterly*, 2005, *83*(3), 457–502.

U.S. Congressional Budget Office. *CBO Testimony: Options for Controlling the Cost and Increasing the Efficiency of Health Care*. Statement of Douglas W. Elmendorf, Director, Before the Subcommittee on Health, Committee on Energy and Commerce, U.S. House of Representatives. Mar. 10, 2009. [http://www.cbo.gov/ftpdocs/100xx/doc10016/Testimony.1.1.shtml]. (Accessed Jan. 24, 2010.)

World Health Organization. *Health Systems: Improving Performance*. The World Health Report 2000. 2000. [http://www.who.int/whr/2000/en/whr00_en.pdf]. (Accessed Jan. 24, 2010.)

Chapter Nine

Carey, D., and others. *Health Care Reform in the United States*. Economics Department Working Paper no. 665. Paris: Organisation for Economic Co-operation and Development, 2009.

Davis, K. "Slowing the Growth of Health Care Costs—Learning from International Experience." *New England Journal of Medicine*, 2008, *359*(17), 1751–1755.

Emanuel, E., and Fuchs, V. "Health Care Vouchers—A Proposal for Universal Coverage." *New England Journal of Medicine*, 2005, *352*(12), 1255–1260.

European Observatory on Health Systems and Policies. *Health Systems in Transition: HiT Summary: Germany.* 2004. [http://www.euro.who.int/Document/E85472sum.pdf]. (Accessed Jan. 24, 2010.)

European Observatory on Health Systems and Policies. *Health Systems in Transition: HiT Summary: Canada.* 2005. [http://www.euro.who.int/Document/E87954sum.pdf]. (Accessed Jan. 24, 2010.)

Frenk, J., and Gómez-Dantés, O. "Ideas and Ideals: Ethical Basis of Health Reform in Mexico." *Lancet*, 2009, *373*(9673), 1406–1408.

Fuchs, V. "Three 'Inconvenient Truths' About Health Care." *New England Journal of Medicine*, 2008, *359*(17), 1749–1751.

Galvin, R. "Still in the Game—Harnessing Employer Inventiveness in U.S. Health Care Reform." *New England Journal of Medicine*, 2008, *359*(14), 1421–1423.

Gottret, P., and Schieber, G. *Health Financing: A Practitioner's Guide.* Washington, D.C.: World Bank, 2006.

Jecker, N. "Can an Employer-Based Health Insurance System Be Just?" *Journal of Health Politics, Policy and Law*, 1993, *18*(3), 657–673.

Jecker, N., and Meslin, E. "United States and Canadian Approaches to Justice in Health Care: A Comparative Analysis of Health Care Systems and Values." *Theoretical Medicine*, 1994, *15*, 181–200.

Light, D. "The Practice and Ethics of Risk-Rated Health Insurance." *JAMA*, 1992, *267*(18), 2503–2508.

Murray, C., and Frenk, J. "A Framework for Assessing the Performance of Health Systems." *Bulletin of the World Health Organization*, 2000, *78*(6), 717–731.

Priester, R. "A Values Framework for Health System Reform." *Health Affairs*, 1992, *11*(1), 84–107.

Roberts, M., and others. *Getting Health Reform Right: A Guide to Improving Performance and Equity.* New York: Oxford University Press, 2008.

Saltman, R., and Dubois, H. "The Historical and Social Base of Social Health Insurance Systems." In R. Saltman and others (eds.), *Social Health Insurance Systems in Western Europe.* New York: Open University Press, 2004.

Sommerfeld, J., and others. "Informal Risk-Sharing Arrangements (IRSAs) in Rural Burkina Faso: Lessons for the Development of Community-Based Insurance (CBI)." *International Journal of Health Planning and Management*, 2002, *17*(2), 147–163.

U.K. Department of Health. *The NHS Constitution for England.* 2009. [http://www.dh.gov.uk/en/Publicationsandstatistics/Publications/PublicationsPolicyAndGuidance/DH_093419]. (Accessed Jan. 24, 2010.)

World Health Organization. *Health Systems: Improving Performance.* The World Health Report 2000. 2000. [http://www.who.int/whr/2000/en/whr00_en.pdf]. (Accessed Jan. 24, 2010.)

Chapter Ten

American Medical Association. "Opinion 1.02: The Relation of Law and Ethics." *Code of Medical Ethics.* 1994. [http://www.ama-assn.org/ama/pub/physician-resources/medical-ethics/code-medical-ethics/opinion102.shtml]. (Accessed Jan. 16, 2010.)

Benatar, S. "Health Care Reform and the Crisis of HIV and AIDS in South Africa." *New England Journal of Medicine*, 2004, *351*(1), 81–92.

Biggins, S., and others. "Transplant Tourism to China: The Impact on Domestic Patient-Care Decisions." *Clinical Transplantation*, 2009, *23*(6), 831–838.

Blackwood, H. "Immigration Testimony Displeases Norwood." *Gainesville Times*, Aug. 16, 2006. [http://archive.gainesvilletimes.com/news/stories/20060816/localnews/117599.shtml]. (Accessed Jan. 16, 2010.)

Bookman, M., and Bookman, K. *Medical Tourism in Developing Countries.* New York: Palgrave Macmillan, 2007.

Bowden, H. "EU Cross-Border Health Care Proposals: Implications for the NHS." *Eurohealth*, 2009, *15*(1), 18–20.

Bramstedt, K., and Xu, J. "Checklist: Passport, Plane Ticket, Organ Transplant." *American Journal of Transplantation*, 2007, *7*, 1698–1701.

Budiani-Saberi, D., and Delmonico, F. "Organ Trafficking and Transplant Tourism: A Commentary on the Global Realities." *American Journal of Transplantation*, 2008, *8*, 925–929.

Carmona, R. "Improving Language Access: A Personal and National Agenda." *Journal of General Internal Medicine*, 2007, *22*(Suppl. 2), 277–278.

Chinai, R., and Goswami, R. "Medical Visas Mark Growth of Indian Medical Tourism." *Bulletin of the World Health Organization*, 2007, *85*(3), 164–165.

Cortez, N. "Patients Without Borders: The Emerging Global Market for Patients and the Evolution of Modern Health Care." *Indiana Law Journal*, 2008, *83*, 71–132.

Coyle, S. "Ethics Case Study: Providing Care to Undocumented Immigrants." *The Hospitalist*, July–Aug. 2003, 24–27.

Darr, K. *Ethics in Health Services Management.* (4th ed.) Baltimore, Md.: Health Professions Press, 2005.

European Union. "Cracking Down on Illegal Employment." Press Release. IP/09/298. Feb. 19, 2009. [http://europa.eu/rapid/pressReleasesAction.do?reference=IP/09/298&format=HTML& aged=0&language=EN&guiLanguage=en]. (Accessed Jan. 16, 2010.)

Flores, G. "Language Barriers to Health Care in the United States." *New England Journal of Medicine*, 2006, *355*(3), 229–231.

Fried, B., and Harris, D. "Managing Healthcare Services in the Global Marketplace." *Frontiers of Health Services Management*, 2007, *24*(2), 3–18.

Goldman, D., and others. "Immigrants and the Cost of Medical Care." *Health Affairs*, 2006, *25*(6), 1700–1711.

Gorman, A. "California Counties Cut Healthcare to Illegal Immigrants." *Los Angeles Times*, Apr. 27, 2009. [http://articles.latimes.com/2009/apr/27/local/me-immighealth27]. (Accessed Jan. 16, 2010.)

Grady, D. "Foreign Ways and War Scars Test Hospital." *New York Times*, Mar. 28, 2009. [http://www.nytimes.com/2009/03/29/health/29immig.html?_r=1&scp=1&sq=Foreign%20Ways %20and%20War%20Scars%20Test%20Hospital&st=cse]. (Accessed Jan. 16, 2010.)

Health Research and Educational Trust. *Hospital Language Services for Patients with Limited English Proficiency: Results from a National Survey.* 2006. [http://www.aone.org/hret/languageservices/ content/languageservicesfr.pdf]. (Accessed Jan. 17, 2010.)

Hjern, A., and Bouvier, P. "Migrant Children—A Challenge for European Paediatricians." *Acta Paediatrica*, 2004, *93*, 1535–1539.

Horowitz, M., and others. "Medical Tourism: Globalization of the Healthcare Marketplace." *Medscape General Medicine*, 2007, *9*(4), 33. [http://www.pubmedcentral.nih.gov/articlerender.fcgi?artid= 2234298&tool=pmcentrez]. (Accessed Jan. 15, 2010.)

Kaiser Commission on Medicaid and the Uninsured. *Five Basic Facts on Immigrants and Their Health Care.* Mar. 2008. [http://www.kff.org/medicaid/upload/7761.pdf]. (Accessed Jan. 15, 2010.)

Kaiser Daily Health Report. "Economic Recession Forcing Local Health Departments to Reduce Services to Undocumented Immigrants." Mar. 2009. [http://www.kaisernetwork.org/ Daily_reports/print_report.cfm?DR_ID=57497&dr_cat=3]. (Accessed Jan. 15, 2010.)

Mattoo, A., and Rathindran, R. "How Health Insurance Inhibits Trade in Health Care." *Health Affairs*, 2006, *25*(2), 358–368.

Milstein, A., and Smith, M. "America's New Refugees—Seeking Affordable Surgery Offshore." *New England Journal of Medicine*, 2006, *355*(16), 1637–1640.

Narayan, T. "Challenges of the National Rural Health Mission." Editorial. *Indian Journal of Medical Ethics*, Apr.–June 2005, *2*(2). [http://www.issuesinmedicalethics.org/132ed042.html]. (Accessed Jan. 15, 2010.)

Pace, P. *Migration and the Right to Health: A Review of European Community Law and Council of Europe Instruments.* Geneva: International Organization for Migration, 2007.

Preston, J. "Texas Hospitals Reflect Debate on Immigration." *New York Times*, July 18, 2006. [http://www.nytimes.com/2006/07/18/us/18immig.html?_r=1]. (Accessed Jan. 15, 2010.)

Rosenthal, A. "Battling for Survival, Battling for Moral Clarity: 'Illegality' and Illness in the Everyday Struggles of Undocumented HIV+ Women Migrant Workers in Tel Aviv." *International Migration*, 2007, *45*(3), 134–156.

Sanchez, M. "Health Care Lost in Translation." *Washington Post*, Nov. 19, 2007, p. B3.

Saniotis, A. "Medical Bioethics and Medical Tourism in Thailand." *Eubios Journal of Asian and International Bioethics*, 2008, *18*, 150–151.

Sontag, D. "Immigrants Facing Deportation by U.S. Hospitals." *New York Times*. Aug. 3, 2008. [http://www.nytimes.com/2008/08/03/us/03deport.html?bl]. (Accessed Jan. 15, 2010.)

Texas House of Representatives, House Research Organization. *Health Care for Undocumented Immigrants: Who Pays?*. Focus Report no. 77-13, Oct. 29, 2001.

U.S. General Accounting Office. "Undocumented Aliens: Questions Persist About Their Impact on Hospitals' Uncompensated Care Costs." GAO Highlights. Washington, D.C.: U.S. General Accounting Office, 2004.

Vedantam, S. "U.S. Citizens Get More Organs Than They Give." *Washington Post*, Mar. 3, 2003, p. A03.

Wachter, R. "The 'Dis-location' of U.S. Medicine—The Implications of Medical Outsourcing." *New England Journal of Medicine*, 2006, *354*(7), 661–665.

Williams, H. "Allocating a Future: Ethics and Organ Transplantation." n.d. [http://scu.edu/ ethics/publications/submitted/allocating_organs.html]. (Accessed Jan. 15, 2010.)

Chapter Eleven

Alinsao, V., and others. "Voluntary Code of Ethical Conduct for the Recruitment of Foreign-Educated Nurses to the United States." 2008. [http://www.fairinternationalrecruitment.org/ TheCode.pdf]. (Accessed Feb. 28, 2010.)

Chaguturu, S., and, Vallabhaneni, S. "Aiding and Abetting—Nursing Crises at Home and Abroad." *New England Journal of Medicine*, 2005, *353*(17), 1761–1763.

Chen, L., and Boufford, J. "Fatal Flows—Doctors on the Move." *New England Journal of Medicine*, 2005, *353*(17), 1850–1852.

Commonwealth Secretariat. *The Commonwealth Code of Practice for the International Recruitment of Health Workers.* 2003a. [http://www.thecommonwealth.org/Internal/190698/172879/documents/]. (Accessed Feb. 28, 2010.)

Commonwealth Secretariat. *Companion Document to the Commonwealth Code of Practice for the International Recruitment of Health Workers.* 2003b. [http://www.thecommonwealth.org/Internal/190698/172879/documents/]. (Accessed Feb. 28, 2010.)

Dayrit, M., and others. "WHO Code of Practice on the International Recruitment of Health Personnel." *Bulletin of the World Health Organization*, 2008, *86*(10), 739.

Dow, W., and Harris, D. "Exclusion of International Medical Graduates from Federal Health-Care Programs." *Medical Care*, 2002, *40*(1), 68–72.

Dovlo, D. "Migration of Nurses from Sub-Saharan Africa: A Review of Issues and Challenges." *Health Services Research*, 2007, *42*(3, Part II), 1373–1388.

Dwyer, J. "What's Wrong with the Global Migration of Health Care Professionals? Individual Rights and International Justice." *Hastings Center Report*, 2007, *37*(5), 36–43.

Eckenwiler, L. "The WHO Code of Practice on the International Recruitment of Health Personnel: We Have Only Just Begun." *Developing World Bioethics*, 2009, *9*(1), ii–v.

Johnson, J. "Stopping Africa's Medical Brain Drain." *British Medical Journal*, 2005, *331*, 2–3.

Kingma, M. "Nurses on the Move: A Global Overview." *Health Services Research*, 2007, *42*(3, Part II), 1281–1298.

Matter of Vinluan v. *Doyle*, 873 N.Y.S.2d 72 (App. Div., 2nd Dept., 2009).

Maybud, S., and Wiskow, C. "Care Trade: The International Brokering of Health Care Professionals." In C. Kuptsch (ed.), *Merchants of Labour*. 2006. [http://www.ilo.org/public/english/bureau/inst/download/merchants.pdf]. (Accessed Feb. 28, 2010.)

Mullan, F. "The Metrics of the Physician Brain Drain." *New England Journal of Medicine*, 2005, *353*(17), 1810–1818.

Organisation for Economic Co-operation and Development. *The Looming Crisis in the Health Workforce—How Can OECD Countries Respond?* 2008. [http://lysander.sourceoecd.org/vl=17208080/cl=16/nw=1/rpsv/ij/oecdthemes/99980142/v2008n11/s1/p1l]. (Accessed Feb. 28, 2010.)

U.K. Department of Health. *Code of Practice for NHS Employers Involved in the International Recruitment of Healthcare Professionals.* 2001. (Superseded). [http://www.dh.gov.uk/dr_consum_dh/groups/dh_digitalassets/@dh/@en/documents/digitalasset/dh_4034651.pdf]. (Accessed Feb. 28, 2010.)

U.K. Department of Health. *Code of Practice for the International Recruitment of Healthcare Professionals.* 2004. [http://www.dh.gov.uk/prod_consum_dh/groups/dh_digitalassets/@dh/@en/documents/digitalasset/dh_4097734.pdf]. (Accessed Feb. 28, 2010.)

United Nations. *Universal Declaration of Human Rights.* 1948. [http://www.un.org/en/documents/udhr/index.shtml#a25]. (Accessed Feb. 28, 2010.)

Witten, S. "A Fair Way to Find Nurses." *Washington Post*, Sept. 28, 2008, p. B06.

World Health Organization. *Working Together for Health.* The World Health Report 2006. 2006. [http://www.who.int/whr/2006/whr06_en.pdf]. (Accessed Feb. 28, 2010.)

World Health Organization. *International Recruitment of Health Personnel: Draft Global Code of Practice.* Report by the Secretariat. EB 126/8. Dec. 3, 2009. [http://apps.who.int/gb/ebwha/pdf_files/EB126/B126_8-en.pdf]. (Accessed Feb. 28, 2010.)

Wright, D., and others. "The 'Brain Drain' of Physicians: Historical Antecedents to an Ethical Debate, c. 1960–79." *Philosophy, Ethics, and Humanities in Medicine*, 2008, *3*, 24. [http://www.peh-med.com/content/3/1/24]. (Accessed Feb. 28, 2010.)

Chapter Twelve

Barber, S., and others. "Formalizing Under-the-Table Payments to Control out-of-Pocket Hospital Expenditures in Cambodia." *Health Policy and Planning*, 2004, *19*(4), 199–208.

Cockcroft, A., and others. "An Inter-Country Comparison of Unofficial Payments: Results of a Health Sector Social Audit in the Baltic States." *BMC Health Services Research*, 2008, *8*, 15. [http://www.biomedcentral.com/1472–6963/8/15]. (Accessed Jan. 16, 2010.)

Ensor, T. "Informal Payments for Health Care in Transition Economies." *Social Science & Medicine*, 2004, *58*, 237–246.

Ensor, T., and Duran-Moreno, A. "Corruption as a Challenge to Effective Regulation in the Health Sector." In R. Saltman and others (eds.), *Regulating Entrepreneurial Behavior in European Health Care Systems*. 2002. [http://www.euro.who.int/document/e74487.pdf]. (Accessed Jan. 16, 2010.)

Lewis, M. *Governance and Corruption in Public Health Care Systems*. CGD Working Paper 78. Washington, D.C.: Center for Global Development, 2006.

Lewis, M. "Informal Payments and the Financing of Health Care in Developing and Transition Countries." *Health Affairs*, 2007, *26*(4), 984–997.

Menon-Johansson, A. "Good Governance and Good Health: The Role of Societal Structures in the Human Immunodeficiency Virus Pandemic." *BMC International Health and Human Rights*, 2005, *5*(4). [http://www.biomedcentral.com/1472–698X/5/4]. (Accessed Jan. 16, 2010.)

Tatar, M., and others. "Informal Payments in the Health Sector: A Case Study from Turkey." *Health Affairs*, 2007, *26*(4), 1029–1039.

INDEX

Page references followed by *fig* indicate an illustrated figure.